Follow Nature's Path to

The Chinese natural health care system is a set of principles and practices based on the Taoist view of life and nature. Within this system, the bond between human beings and nature is seen as organic and inseparable. In order to attain physical well-being and spiritual satisfaction, we must live in harmony with nature.

Chinese Health Care Secrets presents the Tao secrets of increased energy, youthfulness, and vigor. You'll discover nature's abundance of age-old healing therapies and exercises that you can easily incorporate into your daily activities: diet, sleep and rest, massage and light movement, sexual activity, and breathing.

Let the time-proven and holistic healing wisdom of China start you on nature's path to health and well-being.

About the Author

Henry B. Lin has been a health/life/feng shui consultant for many years. Profoundly studied in traditional Chinese culture, he has been providing quality services to people from all over the world in natural health care and self-healing consultation, instruction of Chinese fitness exercises and martial arts, feng shui design, and astrological readings for life and business planning. For almost thirty years, he has been a close student of Dr. Wan Laisheng, the great modern Chinese martial artist and medico-athlete, a famous medical doctor and philosopher in China. Mr. Lin has published articles in local periodicals such as *The New Times* and *Seattle Journal* and is the author of the book *What Your Face Reveals*.

To Write to the Author

If you wish to contact the author or would like more information about this book, please write to the author in care of Llewellyn Worldwide, and we will forward your request. Both the author and publisher appreciate hearing from you. Llewellyn Worldwide cannot guarantee that every letter written to the author can be answered, but all will be forwarded. Please write to:

Henry Lin
c/o Llewellyn Worldwide
P.O. Box 64383, Dept. K434-0
St. Paul, MN 55164-0383, U.S.A.

Please enclose a self-addressed, stamped envelope for reply, or $1.00 to cover costs.
If outside the U.S.A., enclose international postal reply coupon.

CHINESE HEALTH CARE SECRETS

A **NATURAL** LIFESTYLE APPROACH

Henry Lin

2000
Llewellyn Publications
St. Paul, Minnesota, 55164-0383, U. S. A.

FIRST EDITION
First printing, 2000

Cover art and design: Lisa Novak
Illustrations: Carrie Westfall
Consulting editor: Richard Webster
Editing and book design: Christine Snow

Library of Congress Cataloging-in-Publication Data
Lin, Henry B.
  Chinese health care secrets : a natural lifestyle approach / Henry Lin.— 1st ed.
   p. cm.
  Includes bibliographical references and index.
  ISBN 1-56718-434-0
  1. Medicine, Chinese. I. Title.
R602.L55 2000
610'.951—dc21   99-045849

The practices, treatments, and methods described in this book should not be used as an alternative to professional medical diagnosis or treatment. The author and publisher of this book are not responsible in any manner whatsoever for any injury or negative effects which may occur through following the instructions and advice contained herein. It is recommended that before beginning any treatment or exercise program, you consult your medical professional to determine whether you should undertake this course of practice.

  Llewellyn Worldwide does not participate in, endorse, or have any authority or responsibility concerning private business transactions between our authors and the public.

  All mail addressed to the author is forwarded but the publisher cannot, unless specifically instructed by the author, give out an address or phone number.

Llewellyn Publications
A Division of Llewellyn Worldwide, Ltd.
P. O. Box 64383, Dept. K434-0
St. Paul, MN 55164-0383
www.llewellyn.com

Printed in the United States of America

Other Books by Henry Lin

What Your Face Reveals (1999)

Upcoming Books by Henry Lin

The Art and Science of Feng Shui (2000)

Contents

Introduction

Health care is an enormous business in the United States. In 1998, health care costs in the U. S. constituted 13.3 percent of the nation's Gross Domestic Product (GDP), which translates into over $1,121.4 billion nationwide, making it by far the most dominant economic driver in the country, well ahead of the second most dominant driver—computers and communications. Compared to Japan's health care costs which represents 6.8 percent of its GDP and 8.2 percent of Europe's, the U. S. has by far the most expensive health care system in the world.[1]

Yet the cost of health care is still increasing. Costs are expected to jump to 16.6 percent in 2002. According to the American Heart Association, heart disease alone is expected to cost the nation $274.2 billion in 1998, up 6 percent from 1997, or slightly over $1,000 per person per year.[2]

Has all this money helped the health of Americans? The answer is very disappointing. Let's take a look at the following grim facts:

- According to authoritative estimates, 58 million Americans have at least one type of heart disease,[3] which kills over 900,000 Americans each year and costs over $115 billion in medical treatment.

- About 37.7 million Americans have disabilities caused by a chronic condition or impairment.[4]

- Sixteen million Americans have diabetes, which costs this nation more than $92 billion annually in medical care.[5]

- Twelve million Americans are under medical care for cancer, which took more than 4.5 million American lives in the 1980s; in 1996 alone, about 1,252,000 new cancer cases were diagnosed, which did not include an estimated 800,000 skin cancer cases. In the same year, cancer killed 547,000 Americans or 1,500 people a day.[6]

- One out of every five American men will develop prostate cancer in their lifetime.[7]

- Each year, more than 182,000 American women are diagnosed with breast cancer.[8]

- About 16 million Americans suffer from asthma, which is becoming not only more prevalent, but also more severe, and costing about $5 billion each year.[9]

- Thirty-seven million Americans have arthritis, resulting each year in 45 million lost workdays and $35 billion in medical care and lost wages.[10]

- Twenty million Americans are affected by osteoporosis, causing 1.3 million bone fractures a year in people over forty-five years of age.[11]

- Over 40 million Americans have hypertension.[12]

- Thirty-four million American adults are obese,[13] which amounts to 35 percent of the adult population.

- Thirty-five million Americans suffer from allergies.[14]

- More than 30 million Americans have a mental illness.[15]

- Approximately 30,400 Americans take their own lives each year.[16]

- Cataracts affect 60 percent of Americans older than sixty.[17]

- Sixty million Americans suffer from chronic headaches.[18]

- Thirty million American men have chronic impotence problems.[19]

- Twenty percent of Americans have trouble falling asleep or staying asleep.[20]

- An estimated 1.5 million Americans have been infected with HIV.[21]

This puts into perspective the supposedly first-rate medical care that a wealthy country with leading-edge technology provides. In fact, Americans lead the world in wealth and technology, but also in degenerative diseases. Americans enjoy the benefits of computer-aided diagnosis, breakthroughs in biochemistry, and the highest standard of living in the world. However, Americans are simply not healthy. Occupational fatigue, depression, sexual dysfunction, and poor physical condition detract from the quality of almost everyone's life. Americans rate only 43rd in the world in terms of life expectancy. This is totally out of proportion to the amount of prosperity they enjoy. No wonder Marcia Angell, executive editor of *The New England Journal of Medicine*, regards the American health care system as "at once the most expensive and the most inadequate system in the developed world."[22]

Indeed, this nation is in the midst of a health care crisis that is leading more and more people to question the health care industry. Why is so much money spent each year on health care? How much does the health care system have to do with health? Is this system proactive or reactive? Should successful healing address and eradicate the cause of a disease, or simply suppress the symptoms? Is the current health care system addressing the issues that Americans face today? Where is this system heading?

Answers to these questions vary, but there is no question that the major killers of Americans are not battlefields, but their own environment—homes, workplaces, lifestyles—where they die from degenerative diseases such as heart disease, stroke, cancer, diabetes, and asthma. These are rightly termed "diseases of civilization." For more than 200 years, modernization has been working in a way that goes against nature. In an attempt to exploit nature in order to "benefit humans," industrialization constantly ignores the laws of nature. The exploding health problems we are faced with today are the inevitable consequences of this. It can be regarded as nature's vengeance on its violators.

If violation of natural laws is the root cause of most modern health problems, it stands to reason that the fundamental solution lies in returning to nature and reestablishing human-nature rapport. In fact, the most effective cures for these deadly diseases are—and ought—to be found in nature, rather than in a laboratory full of expensive, high-tech equipment. In this regard, the Chinese natural health care system has a decisive message for all humankind.

The keyword of this system is natural. By natural health care I mean a system of methods and tools used to promote health and cure diseases by completely natural means. There is no need for chemotherapy, medication, or even herbs.

The side effects of these treatments are well known. Tylenol, for example, one of the most popular and widely used medications in the U. S., with annual sales of $1.3 billion, has been attributed to hundreds of fatalities and serious liver damage.[23]

Herbs are not usually included in this system. Although the growing and processing is natural, most herbs are not suited for the human body. Consequently, they cannot be consumed regularly without side effects.

The term "natural" is used in a strict sense in this book. It refers only to the materials, methods, and activities that are considered a normal part of life, such as food, breathing, sleep, exercise, sex, environment, physical hygiene, and mental discipline.

The Chinese have tried to understand the human body and how and why diseases develop from time immemorial. Dr. Wan Laisheng, my late teacher, repeatedly told me: "There are five essentials of good health. They are diet, hygiene, rest, exercise, and environment. None of them is dispensable. All are required to ensure good health." Therefore, it is vital that we take charge of our own health by cultivating a healthy lifestyle and practice natural health principles. This is not only the first line of defense against diseases, it may very well be our last resort in terms of treatment, because modern health problems come from these basic activities of life.

Chinese natural health care is unique in that it is at once natural, preventative, root-seeking, holistic, and self-confident. It uses none of the artificial or chemical medications found in modern healing practices. Everything is completely natural and can be taken or practiced regularly on a daily basis. Indeed, it was considered the optimum way of life by the ancient Chinese.

The law of health is the law of nature. You cannot break the law of nature without damaging your own health. Food is a good example. When a Chinese patient sees a doctor, he or she will ask: "What kind of foods should I eat?" The Chinese have known for a long time that food can create disease, as well as treat disease. The right foods can trigger healing by themselves, and often do a better job than modern medicines. In fact, food is seen by the Chinese as both a source of nutrition and as a powerful medicine.

Secondly, the Chinese health care system is preventative in nature. The ancient Chinese considered the most effective cure to be prevention. In other words, not to let the disease develop in the first place, or to kill it as soon as it appears. In China the best doctors are also the best teachers who know how to prevent diseases. Optimum health comes from prevention rather than treatment of a disease. Just as a car will never be the same after an accident, neither will the body be the same after a serious illness. This is because the vital qi energy has been undermined.

Thirdly, the system addresses the causes of the disease. Mainstream health care seeks to suppress the symptoms of a disease, but Chinese natural health care addresses the root causes, while still taking care of the symptoms. There is a time and place for the Western approach toward disease, such as in life-threatening situations. However, these approaches are largely ineffective when used against degenerative and chronic diseases. For instance, the conventional medications for hypertension cannot correct the imbalance of energies that cause high blood pressure. Neither can antidepressants remove the root causes of depression.

By contrast, the Chinese natural healing system believes in eradicating the underlying causes of the disease. Consequently, when a Chinese doctor writes a prescription, he will always ensure that the major weight be given to the root cause of a disease, rather than the superficial symptoms.

Fourth, the system is holistic in that it treats the whole person rather than isolated portions of the body. Western culture and conventional medicine tends to compartmentalize things, focusing on only one aspect of the body at a time. In China, however, a holistic attitude is the norm. The Chinese see a human being as an organic whole, consisting of an interdependent mind, body, and spirit, as well as numerous cells. For the whole person to be healthy, the sum of its parts must be healthy.

In Chinese culture, man is seen as a trinity of spirit, mind, and body. Understandably, the Chinese health care system takes into account the interaction and interdependence of the physical, mental, and spiritual aspects of a patient. It tries to understand how the aspects affect and influence each other. Based on this understanding, a comprehensive and appropriate strategy of treatment is set up.

In the Western tradition, the body is separated from the mind. The Chinese natural health care system realizes that the human body not only has muscles and organs, but also has emotions and feelings that directly influence the well-being of the physical body, and vice versa. It emphasizes the close interdependence between mental well-being and physical health. The psychological and physiological aspects are as inseparable as light and dark. Physical health leads to mental well-being, which in turn enhances the immune system of the body. Chinese health care also takes into consideration the interactions of various internal organs.

Finally, the system is self-confident. It believes that the human body itself is a great healer, possessing the innate capacity to restore balance and heal itself. If we are capable of disturbing the organic equilibrium of the body, which the Chinese believe to be the cause of all diseases, we can also restore this equilibrium. In other words, healing is the result of a biological process undertaken by the body on its own behalf.

In the final analysis, healing comes from within. Chinese believe that most things get better by themselves, and indeed, most things are better by themselves in the absence of external interference. Human beings are no exception. The human body is a self-maintaining, self-repairing, and self-healing machine, just as long as we know how to build up, conserve, and control the qi energy in the body. This belief is in line with the Confucian teaching that "a superior man seeks help from himself, whereas a mean man seeks help from others." In fact, most Chinese people treat their diseases at home, using natural methods passed down from generation to generation. They go to see doctors at a hospital only when absolutely necessary.

Thus, the Chinese natural health care system is a philosophy of living. It advocates a lifestyle that will lead to optimal health in accordance with the laws of nature. At a time when business interests appear to override the moral conscience of health management organizations, and profit-seeking motives take priority over the welfare of people, it becomes all the more important that we learn this philosophy of living and make it a way of life. After all, health care is our business. Good health has little to do with money and cutting-edge technology, because it cannot be purchased. Rather, good health must be fought for and won through our own efforts in everyday activities.

Endnotes

1. "The World in 1998," *The Economist* 25: 81.

2. *Investor's Business Daily*, 3 January 1998.

3. *Investor's Business Daily*, 17 March 1999.

4. Wendy Wilcox, *Public Health Sourcebook*, (Detroit, MI: Omnigraphics, Inc., 1998), 3, 64.

5. *Public Health Sourcebook* (Detroit, MI: Omnigraphics, Inc., 1998), 57.

6. Allan R. Cook, *The New Cancer Sourcebook* (Detroit, MI: Omnigraphics, Inc., 1996), 4–5.

7. Allan R. Cook, *Men's Health Concerns Sourcebook*, (Detroit, MI: Omnigraphics, Inc., 1998), 128–129.

8. Mary Kane et al., *Sound Decisions* (Boston, MA: Mosby Consumer Health, 1995).

9. Linda M. Ross, *Allergies Sourcebook*, (Detroit, MI: Omnigraphics, Inc., 1997), 77.

10. Kate Lorig and James Fries, *The Arthritis Helpbook* (Massachusetts: Addison-Wesley Publishing Co., 1995).

11. Heather E. Aldred, *Women's Health Concern Sourcebook*, (Detroit, MI: Omnigraphics, Inc., 1997), 36.

12. Marvin Moser, *Lower Your Blood Pressure and Live Longer* (New York: The Berkley Publishing Group, 1991).

13. Dan R. Harris, *Fitness and Exercise Sourcebook*, (Detroit, MI: Omnigraphics, Inc., 1996), 57.

14. Allan R. Cook, *Environmentally Induced Disorders Sourcebook* (Detroit, MI: Omnigraphics, Inc., 1997), 40.

15. Donald F. Klein, *Understanding Depression: A Complete Guide to its Diagnosis and Treatment* (New York: Oxford University Press, 1993).

16. Cook, *Men's Health Concerns Sourcebook*, 1998.

17. Linda M. Ross, *Ophthalmic Disorders Sourcebook*, (Detroit, MI: Omnigraphics, Inc., 1997), 363.

18. Robert G. Ford, *Conquering Your Headaches: How to Get Rid of Your Headaches and on with Your Life* (International Headache Management, Inc., 1993).

19. Kane, *Sound Decisions*, 1995.

20. Rosalind Cartwright, *Crisis Dreaming: Using Your Dreams to Help Solve Your Problems* (New York: Harper Collins Publishers, 1993).

21. Kane, *Sound Decisions*, 1995.

22. *New England Journal of Medicine* (January 1999).

23. *Forbes*, December 1997.

Chapter 1

A Historical Overview of Chinese Natural Health Care

The theory and practice of natural health care has had a long history that dates back to the very beginning of Chinese civilization. Health care and longevity are amongst the most recurring themes in Chinese civilization. Everything from diet to medicine, sleeping to dressing, sex to exercises, housing to traveling, and religion to philosophy are discussed and studied endlessly. Oriental culture focuses on the study and improvement of human beings themselves. This is in contrast to Occidental culture which focuses on the study and understanding of the outside world in which we live.

The ancient Chinese were keenly aware of the value of good health, and made constant efforts to maintain and improve it. This is partly due to their obsession with immortality, a goal that is only possible when one enjoys good health and longevity. One of their earliest researches into health care created qigong, the Chinese breathing exercise that combines regulated breathing with meditation. Qigong was cited for its therapeutic value in *The Yellow*

1

Emperor's Classic of Internal Medicine, which is the oldest synthesis of traditional natural health care. This book is based on techniques used by the Yellow Emperor in promoting health and in preventing and treating disease.

The Yellow Emperor reigned over the northern part of China almost 5,000 years ago. His interest in natural health contributed enormously to Chinese civilization. He is said to have lived to the age of 111, and to have attained immortality after his physical death.

The Yellow Emperor had two famous advisers who taught him the art of breathing, dietary therapy, regulated sex, herbology, and the secrets of immortality. Qi Bo, a famous Taoist adept and the father of Chinese medicine, was one of his advisers. They had regular discussions on the essence of life, causes of diseases, ways to prevent and cure them, and techniques for longevity. It was these conversations that provided the information for the Yellow Emperor's book.

Qi Bo, as well as being an excellent doctor and the emperor's advisor, was also the father of massage therapy in China. He wrote ten books on the subject, claiming that appropriate pressure on specific parts of the body can promote health and prevent and cure disease. He states that there are fourteen meridians and collaterals spreading throughout the body. On these meridians and collaterals are hundreds of locations called acupoints, which are related to internal organs and the central nervous system. Through these meridians and acupoints, qi energy is dis-

tributed to various parts of the body, giving them vitality and immunity. As qi is the force on which life itself depends for its vitality and proper functioning, massaging these meridians, channels, and acupoints can bring about therapeutic results.

Another close friend of the Yellow Emperor was a woman known as the Plain Girl, who was one of the emperor's sexual partners. With her, the emperor learned the art of regulated sex. Their discussions and experiences were recorded in *The Classic of the Plain Girl,* which explains sexual yoga for health and longevity. Together they explored the secret of natural health through the regulated interflow of male and female essences during intercourse. The Yellow Emperor followed the unselfish advice of the Plain Girl and kept a harem of more than one thousand young women with whom he had regular intercourse in order to absorb their yin energy, which would promote and nourish his yang energy.

It has already been mentioned that one of the outstanding features of Chinese natural health care is that it is preventative in nature. Chinese doctors consider their first responsibility to be to educate their patients on how to avoid disease. The constant effort of prevention means that the entire body system is kept at a high level of health. Prevention can not only free you from disease, but can also promote your health without you realizing it. In fact, prevention of disease and the promotion of health are essentially the same process. Health means, first and foremost, absence of disease, so health is best promoted by keeping disease at bay. The significance of prevention is clearly stated in *The Yellow Emperor's Classics of Internal Medicine*:

> *To apply medicine to disease after it is already developed, or to suppress a revolt which is well expanded, is like digging a well when one already feels thirsty, or to forge weapons when a war has already started. Don't you think it is too late?*

In terms of prevention, the Chinese were the first to discover that regular exercise on a daily basis is essential to maintaining and promoting health. As early as 800 B.C., a method known as "daoyin" was developed for promoting and healing diseases by combining regulated breathing with soft body exercises. Daoyin was originally designed only for use in the palace. This means two things: first, only the emperor could hire those health experts to design health exercises in China and second, the royal family did not want to share this secret knowledge with the common society. Even so, it has had a large influence on the Chinese natural health care system. It marks the beginning of Chinese exercise therapy.

Confucius, the great Chinese sage, was born at about this time. He was a great educator who first claimed that education should know no social or ethnic bounds. Everybody—no matter how poor or humble he or she is—should be entitled to education. It is no exaggeration to say that he sowed the seed of democracy in human society. He was also greatly involved in natural

health care. For instance, he was one of the first people to discover the therapeutic effects of music. He believed that music was useful for maintaining a mind-body balance, and was therefore important for emotional, physical, physiological, and spiritual health. Because of this, he insisted that music should be part of the curriculum. Some of his students discovered that music could ease pain, reduce stress, and speed up the healing process. Confucius also paid great attention to the physical education of his students, insisting that this also be an essential part of his curriculum.

Toward the end of the second century A.D., an eminent doctor called Hua Tuo created a set of exercises known as five-animal play. This represented a huge advance in exercise therapy. Five-animal play consists of a series of exercises that imitate the movements of tigers, deer, bears, monkeys, and birds—in essence—promoting health by learning from nature. In introducing these exercises to his students, Hua Tuo said the following words:

> *Running water never gets stagnant, and a door-hinge never gets worm-eaten. For the same reason, by regularly exercising ourselves, we can maintain health and keep disease at bay. Regular exercise promotes blood and qi circulation, and thus keeps the body in high alert.*

Hua Tuo was also one of the first people to recognize the therapeutic effects of human urine on many kinds of diseases. He discovered that urine is a healthy substance containing nourishing compounds that are compatible with the body. Urine comes from the body and returns to the body, promoting its metabolic process and innate healing power. It can help restore the body's internal balance, bringing about healing in a magical way. Since urination is a function of the bladder, which is controlled and affected by the kidneys, the first application of urine was done to nourish the kidney yang energy through drinking one's own urine.

Hua suggested that urine drinking be considered part of the treatment for sexual dysfunction, including impotence, nocturnal emission, and incontinence. Later generations of Chinese natural therapists have developed Hua's theories into a separate doctrine called Urine Therapy, which has been used in China to help treat a wide range of diseases including asthma, hay fever, stomach ailments, bronchitis, pneumonia, tuberculosis, skin allergies, cancer (skin cancer in particular), and even AIDS. I am told that the results are encouraging and convincing. For most cases, you simply drink your own urine. My teacher, Dr. Wan Laisheng, considered the best urine to drink to be either the one released right after getting up in the morning, or the one released right after midnight.

NOTE: It is not recommended that you drink your urine often. This would eventually have the same effects as renal failure, returning all the toxins the kidney excreted back into the body.

Hua also made great contributions to acupressure and acupuncture. He discovered that the fingers have similar effects on the body as needles do, and are much easier, safer, and more convenient to use. Acupressure is a simpler, easier, and cheaper version of acupuncture that anyone can use. While acupressure and acupuncture can be considered twin methods in the Chinese natural health care system, acupressure is far more natural than acupuncture, which involves inserting needles to effect treatment.

Tragically, Hua was killed by the dictator Cao Cao in 220 A.D. shortly before his 100th birthday. Hua had been the dictator's private doctor, but did not want to devote his skills and talent purely to the dictator as was required. He wanted to help the common people, in particular the poor and helpless. However, it was not this that caused his tragic death. The dictator suffered from chronic headaches, which were diagnosed by Hua as being caused by the blocking of a qi channel in the nervous system. Hua suggested using acupuncture on the dictator's head to effect a cure. As one of the father's of Chinese acupuncture, Hua was totally confident of his skills. Unfortunately, the idea of metal needles being inserted into the dictator's head was interpreted as being murderous, and Hua was killed.

Hua's contributions to the Chinese natural health care system are monumental and decisive. His writings have been passed down from generation to generation, and widely practiced. His advice about the supreme importance of exercise to health and healing has been verified again and again, and has become one of the cornerstones of natural health care.

Another great contributor to the Chinese natural health care system was Dr. Zhang Zhongjing, who lived about 200 B.C. He refined the theory of the "three treasures"— essence, energy, and spirit—and used it to educate his patients on the natural ways of effecting treatment.

He also introduced into Chinese medicine a new method of diagnosis based on the theory of yin and yang and the five elements. His book, *On Febrile Diseases*, is considered one of the most important. In this book, Zhang proposed some purely dietary treatments for fevers, such as "Cinnamon Soup," which consists of cinnamon, ginger, jujubes, and other foods. These methods are still popular today.

Zhang Zhongjing was one of the first people to recognize the therapeutic effects of foods. He spent a great deal of time traveling around the country asking people how they treated their own diseases. This approach was much more productive than academic research or laboratory studies. The reason is simple. In those days, science was totally unknown, and professional doctors were rarely found. However, people became sick every now and again. Nonetheless, their diseases were cured, not by doctors, but by themselves, through very natural means. One of these means was food.

After years of study and the collection of much information, Zhang proposed the theory of dietary therapy as an important component of Chinese medicine. He had considerable success in using foods to heal many diseases, and can be considered one of the fathers of Chinese dietary therapy. Zhang Zhongjing classified foods into two major categories: one was for the nourishment of life energy, and the other for the healing of disease. Often, he found that these two functions were combined in the same foods.

The next person to have a major effect on Chinese natural health care was a Taoist adept named Kuo Han, who lived around the fourth century A.D. Kuo wrote more than 100 books on Taoism, many of which bear directly on various aspects of natural health care. For instance, he wrote profoundly on regulated breathing, physical hygiene, fitness exercises, longevity, and sexual discipline. Kuo practiced what he preached and looked like someone in his thirties when he was ninety years old.

During the reign of Emperor Liang Wu (c. 500 A.D.), Chinese health care took a large leap forward. At this time, Bodhidharma Dharma, an Indian Buddhist and founder of Zen Buddhism, came to China to spread the gospel of Buddhism. Dharma was the third child of an Indian king, Sughanda. He was a member of the respected Indian warrior caste, and spent his childhood in a Buddhist province in south India. He studied Buddhism and ultimately became venerated as the twenty-eighth reincarnation of Gautama Buddha, the founder of Buddhism.

Dharma settled down in the Hunan province of central China, and began teaching

Buddhism at the Sunsang Temple. It is interesting to note that the Sunsang Temple became more famous for its attainments in martial arts than for its authority on Buddhism. This is because Dharma was not only the patriarch of Chinese Buddhism, but was also the father of Chinese martial arts.

Dharma's students spent long hours every day reciting sutra, and Dharma became concerned about their lack of physical exercise. Consequently, he devised several sets of soft exercises to enable his students to remain strong and healthy. Not all of these exercises have survived. One set of exercises, known as The Classics of Washing the Braining, contained secrets about attaining immortality, and was hidden by jealous students.

Fortunately, his other exercises are still available. They include the famous yijinjing (methods of strengthening tendons) and Dharma's internal exercises, which helps to prevent and cure diseases. He also created Dharma's morning exercises, which are a special set of movements particularly suitable for the start of the day.

Many legendary feats have been associated with Dharma. For instance, he was reputed to have crossed the treacherous Yellow River with the help of a single reed. The most famous story about him concerns the nine years he spent in a small hut on top of the Sunsang Mountains. Every day he meditated in silence, facing a stone wall. After nine years the sun had clearly projected the contours of his body onto the stone wall he had faced. Ever since then, the phrases "facing the wall for nine years" and "facing the wall for ten years" have become idiomatic expressions in Chinese literature, encouraging people to achieve their goals through unbent persistence and arduous endurance.

Another breakthrough occurred at the hands of Dr. Sun Shimiao (590–692 A.D.), the leading doctor of the Tang dynasty, and a pioneer researcher in the field of dietary therapy. Dr. Sun explored all the traditional areas of medicine, but used dietary therapy as the first consideration in attempting a cure. He wrote:

> A truly good doctor first finds out the cause of a disease, and based on such finding, he first tries to treat it with foods. Only when foods fail to produce the desired result does he resort to medication. In terms of nourishment, medication is inferior to food, food is inferior to essence, essence is inferior to spirit.

Dr. Sun was one of the first to recognize how effective ordinary foods can be when prepared and used in the right way.

After six decades of study and research, Dr. Sun wrote his classic book, *The Priceless Recipes*. In thirty chapters, he explained the dietary treatments for many diseases. For instance, he recommended eating beef, pork, and lamb livers as a treatment for night blindness. This is because "the liver is associated with the eyes, and the animal livers can nourish and improve the human liver, which in turn contributes to the improvement of eyesight."

Dr. Sun also discovered that thyroid gland enlargement was caused by a lack of iodine. To cure this, he provided a dietary prescription made up of sea vegetation, such as kelp and sea moss, as well as fish. Other examples of his prescriptions include honey to help cure constipation, fatigue, insomnia, and impotence; wheat-germ porridge and calf and lamb liver for beri beri; perch to help patients recover after an operation or external wounds; and tofu to lower blood pressure and strengthen the digestive system. Consequently, the word "priceless" in the title of his book refers to the therapeutic values of his recommended foods, not their cost.

The Chinese have always known that foods can both promote and damage health, and thus leading to longevity or an early death. They have a proverb that proves this: "Into the mouth come diseases; out of the mouth comes disaster." Recent research indicates that diet is a major factor in many diseases, including osteoporosis, cancer, and heart attacks.

Chinese dietary therapy seeks to address three related issues: maintenance of health, prevention of disease, and the treatment of disease. The Chinese believe that food is the best medicine. Herbs should be used only when foods fail to effect a cure. Chinese diets are healthy because their cuisine principles were laid down by Taoist adepts and doctors, rather than cooks. (Cooks may be partially to blame because they are not necessarily health experts or nutritionists. Their job is to make dishes as delicious as possible. In so doing, they may have to use substances [such as sugar and fats] in excess, resulting in delicious but unhealthy foods.)

Thousands of years ago, the ancient Chinese worked out a number of dietary principles that are universally valid, and are consequently worthy of everyone's attention. For instance, the ancient Chinese suggested that we eat less fat and meat, but more fruits and vegetables. We should eat more raw than refined foods. We should balance the types of food we eat, eat a variety of foods, and not fill up more than 70 percent of the stomach's capacity at any meal. This is because we benefit the qi energy circulation and digestive systems by not overeating. We also should not eat food or soup that is too hot, avoid foods that have spoiled by being left out overnight, and eat a nutritious breakfast, a relatively heavy lunch, and a light dinner.

These precepts have been successfully used by the Chinese for hundreds of years. It is amazing that at the time these discoveries were made, vitamins were completely unknown. Just as surprising is the fact that the Chinese dietary health treatments that were developed 1,200 years ago are still just as valid today. This proves that their solutions are based more on acute insight and observation, than on philosophy. This is why they are so practical, effective, and priceless.

Although technology may change, the underlying truth, validity, and effectiveness of using ordinary foods to maintain natural health remain the same.

Dr. Sun also favored disciplined sexual activity to promote good health and longevity. He presented his case in these words:

One should not engage in sexual intercourse just to satisfy his lust. One should do his best to control his sexual desire so as to build up his vital essence. One should not let his passion go unchecked and lend himself to sexual extravagance merely to enjoy carnal pleasure. On the contrary, one must think of how one can benefit his health from sexual intercourse. This is the precious secret of the bedroom art.

Dr. Sun followed his own advice and was said to have acute hearing and eyesight at the age of ninety-five. He never stopped reading until his death at the age of 102.

The Yellow Emperor was one of the first people to seriously study the connection between one's sexual life and overall health. There has been a great deal of research into this aspect of Chinese natural health care ever since.

Mencius, the second generation Confucian sage, declared categorically: "Food and sex are natural necessities of life, in which we find the two greatest desires of human beings."

Significant research has discovered the inextricable link between a satisfying sexual life and good health and longevity. This is not surprising, as sex is the primal driving force of our existence. It is as basic to humankind as food and sleep. While diet and sleep make life possible, it is sex that ensures the continuation of the species. Sex is a hungry desire of both our bodies and psyches. Consequently, it is easy to understand the enormous effect sex has on our physical and mental health.

The Chinese did not study sex out of mere instinct or temporary pleasure. They regarded it as a human manifestation of the universal principle of yin and yang, and had come to the important understanding that one's sexual life had a significant impact on the person's health and longevity. They found out that there is a direct correlation between low sexual activity and depression, as well as between sexual inability and illness and aging. Sexual vitality is directly associated with overall health and longevity.

They also discovered that one's sexual vitality could be strengthened and maintained for a long period of time through regulated sex. Regulated sex consists of a number of interrelated skills and exercises, both mental and physical. Credit for this goes to the ancient Taoists who were the first to stress the importance of regulated sex as an effective method of natural health and healing.

One of the ancient Taoists sexual classics, *The Plain Girl*, explains how this came about. The Yellow Emperor and the Plain Girl, his sexual advisor, together explored the secrets of yin and yang, the arts of sexuality, its relationship to health and longevity, and its place in the natural health care system.

They were also aware that sex, like diet, is a two-edged sword. On the one hand, it can promote health and prolong life. It can even be used to cure diseases. Its benefits travel far beyond mere pleasure and fun. On the other hand, it can destroy health and shorten life. It all depends on how you practice it.

For example, excessive sex will seriously deplete the kidneys' energy, and affect the heart and nervous system. This is because the kidneys represent water, and the heart represents fire. Excess sex in the form of ejaculation drains the kidney water, which is needed for the balance of energy forces in the body. Automobile engines burn up if they are kept running without water. The human heart is affected in the same way if the kidneys are not in good condition. In Chinese philosophy, this is described as "water comes to the rescue of fire."

The kidney occupies a particularly important place in Chinese natural health care. It is considered not only an organ, but the source of life essence, and the regulator of sex hormones and energy. A healthy, strong kidney promotes growth, reproduction, and the immune system.

It is worth mentioning that the ancient Chinese were the first to think about genes and the genetic process concerning procreation. Although the concepts of genes and hormones were totally unknown to them, they found by a process of intuition, observation, and experience that the health of the parents, particularly the mother, had an enormous impact on the baby, and that this impact can be lifelong. This is because our primordial vital energy is inherited directly from our parents. This energy constitutes the initial foundation of one's health, which comes at birth and plays a significant role throughout life. This conforms with the theory of genes. Recent studies show that drinking alcohol and smoking cigarettes during pregnancy can have a disastrous impact on the baby. This is just one modern verification of the ancient Chinese theory on pregnancy and motherhood. In fact, Chinese fathers had strongly advised against drinking on the part of pregnant woman, for fear that this would cause health problems for the baby to be born.

Based on this understanding, the ancient Chinese devised a set of life rules for the pregnant mother to follow to provide the baby with as much strong primordial qi as possible. We have no choice over our ancestors, but we do over our descendents, and should make every effort to ensure that they receive the strongest genes possible to give them a good start in their lives.

This is both a theoretical and practical issue in the Chinese natural health care system. Children born with sufficient, strong, primordial qi energy have a stronger immunity, and better chance of enjoying good health and worldly success than those born with weak or insufficient primordial vital energy. It is the responsibility of parents, therefore, to see that their children are born with this physical advantage.

In this regard, we can turn to Dr. Hu Shicong (1205–1296) for advice. He was the royal doctor to Genghis Khan and his royal family for several decades. He set down the following rules for pregnant women and feeding mothers:[1]

> *Ancient Chinese sages set up the system of pregnancy education. According to this system, a pregnant woman should sit, stand, and sleep in right manners. She should not eat strange foods, not even foods that are good but cut in a strange way. She should not sit down on a biased seat, look at pornographic sights, nor listen to erotic and lustrous music. In the evening, she should hire a scholar to recite good poems and relate good stories to her. If she complies with these rules, her baby will be born with good appearance and superior intelligence. . . . a pregnant woman should avoid attending burial services, seeing disabled people, or even paupers. Instead, she should be encouraged to see good and healthy people, attend happy events, and view beautiful sights. . . . As a rule, a pregnant woman should not eat rabbit, otherwise her baby will be dumb. She should avoid eating goat, otherwise her baby will be born with some strange diseases. Eating infant chicken or dried fish during pregnancy will make the baby suffer from malignant boils later. . . . Eating the meat of ashes will make you difficult in childbirth. The same thing will happen if you consume too much ice cream.*

In ancient times, wealthy people almost always hired other women to feed their babies with human milk. These women are known as milk-mothers. Consequently, Dr. Hu also set down a set of regulations for milk-mothers:

> *The criteria for selecting a good milk-mother are: young, healthy, kind, generous, gentle, and reticent. Milk for the baby is like the food for an adult. Therefore, the diet of a milk-mother directly affects the health of her baby. . . . A milk-mother should avoid getting angry, for anger makes qi energy run the wrong way. If a baby is fed with milk while the mother is angry, the baby will become mad later. Alcohol triggers yang energy. Milking a baby after drinking wine will make the baby suffer from hot diseases later. Milking a baby right after sexual intercourse will make him weak and suffer from arthritis. Do not feed the baby while a milk-mother is too full or too hungry.*

What a detailed, stringent set of conduct codes for would-be mothers! No wonder some people make the comment that it is hard to be a Chinese woman.

Between the ninth and thirteenth centuries, exercise therapy experienced a giant leap forward and many new types of fitness exercise came into being. These include taich'i, baduanjin, xingyi, luohan, and many others. Throughout its history, Chinese natural health care has been closely associated with Chinese martial arts. As a matter of fact, all of the Chinese fitness exercises that are widely practiced today were first designed with a clear purpose and orientation for self-defense. Indeed, the supreme practice of the two are often combined in one and the same, as is the case of Hua Tuo, Dharma, Sun Shimiao, Zhang Shanfeng, and my late teacher, Dr. Wan Laisheng. All of them were excellent doctors in their own time, and were also first-rate masters of Chinese martial arts.

This is no mere coincidence. Martial arts, like natural health care, is a predominant topic in Chinese culture. In the final analysis, the ultimate goal of these two branches of human endeavors is the same—the attainment of Tao. Zhuang Tze, the second greatest Taoist sage after Lao Tze, remarked: "Martial arts are close to Tao." My teacher, Dr. Laisheng, used to tell me: "Chinese martial arts can serve three purposes at the same time. It can promote your health (*yang sheng*); it can defend you (*fan sheng*); and it can earn a living for you (*mou sheng*)." This special phenomenon might have been prompted in part by the fact that anyone involved in the art of defense will, inescapably, be prone to accidental injury. Therefore, it is essential for martial artists to know the art of self-healing themselves.

In his seven-decade long career as both a martial arts champion and a nationally famous traditional Chinese doctor, Dr. Laisheng developed a complete system of natural healing. This was based on both his first-hand knowledge gained by treating a huge number of patients, and also through the precious second-hand knowledge taught

to him by a dozen of the most famous martial artists and doctors of his time, some of whom were immortals themselves, i.e., they were more than 200 years of age when Wan met them.

In recent years, more and more Chinese are turning to traditional fitness exercises to help resolve their health problems, chronic and degenerative diseases in particular. Some of the exercises of this category are five-animal play, taich'i, qigong, baduanjin, and Dharma's internal exercises. When I practiced Dharma's morning exercises with dozens of fellow students under the guidance of grand master Dr. Laisheng, I felt a sense of joy and peace that is strong enough to deter diseases. In fact, these exercises produce therapeutic effects that are unmatched by the use of drugs.

Chinese clinical studies have shown that 90 percent of the medical cases under examination show a marked improvement or complete cure after six months to a year's practice of these natural healing exercises. These cases range from hypertension to diabetes, insomnia to fatigue, osteoporosis to neurasthenia, indigestion to constipation, arteriosclerosis to gastrointestinal disorders, dizziness to ear-ringing, arthritis to lumbago, pneumonia to cancer, toothaches to stomachaches, etc. It is hopeful that the Chinese natural healing system will be able to find an answer to the most difficult diseases, such as AIDS, as our understanding of the disease deepens.

In summary, research of the natural health care system in China has been intertwined with the entire process of Chinese civilization. It has permeated almost every aspect of life. The Chinese literally leave no stone unturned in their pursuit of health, for physical and mental well-being have had a higher priority than most other things in life for the Chinese. This mentality had continued until recently, when a market economy was introduced into the country. Nevertheless, tradition and civilization die hard. Organized mass training in taich'i, qigong, and other forms of fitness exercises show the continuation of the tradition. In fact, many hospitals and health care institutions in China use natural health care methods as integral parts of their holistic treatment strategy.

Endnotes

1. Hu Shichong, *Essentials of Healthy Diets* (Shanghai, China: The Commercial Press, 1948).

Chapter 2

Philosophy of Chinese Natural Health Care

As we have already mentioned, the Chinese natural health care system is a set of principles and practices based predominantly on the Taoist viewpoint regarding life and nature. This is a philosophy that goes back almost 5,000 years. It is both an art and a science of living. Taoist and Buddhist masters and adepts deserve most of the credit for the development and perfection of this system. These people were traditionally scholars, doctors, martial artists, and monks. It is no accident that such a profound and complex health care system should have been completed in their hands. One of the fundamental premises of Chinese civilization is the ability to explore every aspect of life for the sake of health, longevity, and immortality. This is not so much because the ancient Chinese were afraid of death. It was because they did not want to go through any more incarnations. They aspired to merge with nature and put an end to their individual cycles of reincarnation, which they believe almost everybody has to go through over and over again.

13

Another reason why the ancient Chinese were so concerned about natural health is that Tao—the Way of Nature—permeates the universe. Tao contains three major pillars of trinity: humans, earth, and heaven. The ancient Chinese considered the universe to be a process that works in exactly the same manner on the human body as it does on the rest of the universe. As a matter of fact, human beings are often considered microcosms of the universe. As Taoists understand it, there is much common ground between the way nature functions and the way we humans should live in order to be healthy and happy. It is no accident that Taoist principles lie at the very center of the Chinese natural health care system.

In the Chinese classics, Tao is treated as both the fountain and culmination of all knowledge, which is based on the theory of yin and yang and the five elements.

Yin and Yang

Taoism postulates that there are two primary forces constantly interplaying in the universe. One is the positive, active, male principle of yang, and the other is the negative, passive, female principle of yin. Strange to say, there is no conflict between these two opposing forces; instead, they are complementary to each other. Thus, the man complements the woman, and humankind is made complete; the darkness complements the brightness and a day is made complete; the action complements the idea and a pro-

ject is drawn to completion; human behavior complements the mandate of heaven and the universe is brought to completion, and so on. There is no limit to the number of opposites that together create a perfect whole. Humans and the universe are thus in harmony with each other when both follow the Tao—Nature's Way.

To the ancient Chinese, the existence of the universe depended primarily on the interplay of these two interacting forces or principles, yin and yang, each representing a constellation of qualities. It is from the combination and interaction of yin and yang, and of the five elements, that the myriad creatures are produced, including heaven, earth, and humans.

The principle of yang is conceived to be the principle and symbol of heaven. It is the positive or masculine force—inherent in everything active, proactive, warm, hard, bright, and steadfast. It corresponds to light, fire, day, sun, sky, masculinity, movement, exterior, boldness, action, gladness, and so on. Its characteristics are brightness, aggressiveness, positiveness, optimism, and so on.

The principle of yin, by contrast, is realized on the earth. It is the negative (not in any bad sense) or feminine principle—found in everything passive, cold, soft, wet, dark, secret, mysterious, dim, cloudy, and quiescent. It symbolizes darkness, water, night, moon, earth, femininity, stillness, interior, caution, inaction, melancholy, and so on. Its characteristics are dark, conservative, negative, passive, pessimistic, etc.

Through the eternal intercourse between yin and yang, all things have, and will, come into being. This includes heaven, which is predominantly yang; earth, which is predominantly yin, and human society, which is a combination of these two principles. In the same object, one principle or force may prevail at one time, but the opposite might prevail later. For example, a piece of wood that is cast into a fire changes character from yin to yang. As it stands, everything in the universe contains within itself these two primeval energy modes.

To further illustrate, let us consider the example of the Chinese lunar calendar, which uses these two basic principles of yin and yang to form the cardinal directions and the secession of four seasons. Thus, winter correlates to the north, when yin is at its zenith and yang is reborn. The winter solstice celebrates this event. Spring corresponds to the east and the color green. This is when nature resuscitates. Summer in its turn matches with the south when yang is at zenith and yin is reborn. Finally, autumn and the west correspond to the setting sun, when nature has finished its production and gets ready for its long winter hibernation.

The essential difference between the Chinese conception of yin and yang and other classic philosophical dualisms lies in the fact that the latter are involved in an eternal conflict, whereas yin and yang are basically in accord with one another despite their polarity. Both the feminine yin and the masculine yang are necessary to the order of the universe. Together in harmony they are always good. Moreover, each has the potential and possibility to be transformed into the other, as manifested in the famous eight trigrams of I-Ching, the Book of Changes. Of these eight trigrams, which are meaningfully arranged around a circle, without beginning or ending, only two are pure yin and pure yang, while all the rest contain the elements of both yin and yang. How can they work together, abandoning their disparate identities, to produce the miraculous order in nature? The answer lies in Tao, the Way of Nature, and the source of all harmonies.

Thus, the principles of yin and yang react in a never-ending cycle of growth and decline, as can be seen in the suppression and progression of the four seasons. At the same time, yin and yang join in a productive and harmonious union that gives birth to the five elements: water, fire, wood, metal, and earth. The great Confucian philosopher Zhou Tongyi of the Sung dynasty describes the above notion in his *Classics on Taiji* in the following fashion:

> *Wuji gives birth to taiji,*
> *Which moves and generates yang.*
> *Yang in turn gives birth to yin.*
> *Yang changes, yin unites,*
> *Creating water, fire, wood, metal and earth.*
> *The five elements bring about things in order,*
> *And the four seasons progress in sequence.*

Notice that the Chinese sages do not speak of creation, but of generation only. According to them, before heaven and earth existed, there was simply a primordial undifferentiated mass known as *wuji*, or literally, "nothing." Wuji seethed and churned, silent, isolated, standing alone, eternally evolving without fail, until eventually in the very center of this nebulous mass, a drop of primordial breath was formed, which is nothing but the now world-famous *taiji*, the Great Ultimate.

As the progression of the universe continued, yin and yang were formed. In due course, the five elements were produced which literally gave birth to everything we have now. Hence, the seasons and all the visible world are governed by the breaths and interactions of the five elements, which are spatial as well as temporal, material as well as spiritual in concept. The ancient Chinese see the whole universe as a state of constant flux, with everything interrelated and interdependent for existence on its own duality.

In modern physical terms, this is called a thermodynamic process. The microcosm begins with the simplest and most purposeful origin of life evolving from the macrocosm, then the body, mind, and soul all came into being through the process of balance and harmony, or in modern chemical terms, through metabolic process. Here, the dominant characteristics are balance and harmony, rather than struggle and competition. Balance and harmony are essential concepts that lie at the very center of the Chinese natural health care system as well as Chinese civilization.

One basic understanding of such principles is manifested in the view humans are microcosmic reflections of the universe. Corresponding to the macrotrinity of the universe consisting of heaven, earth, and man, human beings have body, mind, and soul to form a microtrinity. This concept of correspondence between macrocosm and microcosm can be shown as follows:

- Macrocosmic Trinity
  Heaven—universal or general balance
  Earth—social or relative balance
  Man —individual or particular balance

- Microcosmic Trinity
  Body—physical or physiological harmony
  Mind—mental or psychological harmony
  Soul—spiritual or aesthetic harmony

Together, these two sets of elements form a trinity of harmony, will, and purpose. It is important to remember that all six dimensions are interdependent and integrated as a unique way of thinking and practice in both the Chinese natural health care system and traditional Chinese philosophy.

To the ancient Chinese, the bond between man and nature is an organic and inseparable one. If man misbehaves, heaven is upset and earth does not prosper. Moreover, in Chinese thought, man does not occupy quite the ascendant role that he enjoys in Western philosophy, where he is viewed as the prime object of creation. To the Chinese, man is but a single, though vital, part of the complex nature in which he stands and lives. In the West, people have sought to conquer nature for their material ends. The Chinese, however, have aspired to attain harmony with nature in order to gain spiritual satisfaction and physical well-being. As the forces of nature can bring prosperity or disaster to man, so also can man disrupt the delicate balance of nature by his misbehavior. We only have to look at the environmental pollution of modern times to see this. Thus, heaven, earth, and man constitute a single, interdependent, indivisible unity which is governed by the cosmic law of Tao. To the ancient Chinese, no clear demarcation can be drawn between the supernatural world, the domain of nature, and that of man.

One example of the Chinese emphasis on the bond between man and nature is illustrated through its natural health care system which, when coming to diagnosis and treatment of a disease, will take serious consideration of climactic conditions that directly impact humans. Thus, not only are clothes adjusted to vary with weather and seasons, but diet and exercise types are also adjusted to accommodate the weather and season, too. In cold weather, the Chinese menus contain more ginger, garlic, peppers, and other foods of yang nature that serve to counterbalance the humidity and coldness.

In contrast, "cooling" yin-nature foods such as watermelon, pears, and towel gourd are common in the Chinese diet during the summer season. For the same reason, moisturizing yin-foods are recommended for dry climates in high altitudes, such as Tibet, but drying yang-foods are recommended for those living in humid areas with a lot of rainfall and high moisture.

Here, the predominant premise is if the sensitive organism of the human body is to function properly, man must do his part and conform to the law of nature. Unhappily, man tends to pursue his own headstrong purposes and follows his stupid ways of life. By meddling and interfering with the processes of nature and countering the rhythm of nature, he disarranges the cosmic order and breaks down the intricate machinery of macrocosm and microcosm, inviting natural calamities and health problems. The increasing frequency of disasters such as floods, acid rain and excess intrusion of ultraviolet rays from the sun, and the widespread occurrences of degenerative diseases on the part of modern man, bear convincing witnesses to the above-mentioned principle.

The Chinese believe it is from the willfulness and stubbornness of man that all the ills of society as well as of the body are engendered. If humankind were to live harmoniously with the environment, in a natural and simple way, devoid of ambition and aggression, the world would witness a spontaneous flourishing of good fellowship and individuals would enjoy healthy, happy, and long lives.

As we will find later, while exploring various aspects of the natural health care system in subsequent chapters, balance and harmony among opposites—be them man and nature, male and female, convention and tradition, or new and old—form the philosophical foundation of the Chinese natural health care system.

This steady preoccupation with the unity between man and his environment, and this veneration for nature, has endowed the Chinese culture, including its natural health care system, with color and pageantry, and imparted to its multifold observances an exuberance and gaiety characteristic of few other cultures and health care systems on earth. It also marks one of the most important differences between the Chinese way of thinking and that of the West. The incredible loneliness Americans experience in the Western culture results largely from the distrust of nature, characteristic of this culture. To the Western mind, nature is there to be exploited and made use of. For the Chinese, however, nature exists to be worked with, cooperated with, and imitated. The human being is seen as an integrated part of nature, affecting and affected by nature. Thus, human activities that damage nature will eventually come back to haunt us. The causes and effects of modern air pollution and global warming are strong cases in point.

Typically, the ancient Chinese regarded the human body as a reflection of the natural world. Interesting enough, they not only thought, but also spoke, of human health in terms of natural images. Thus, the flows of energy and fluids in the body are described in terms of channels and rivers, seas and reservoirs. For instance, in traditional Chinese medicine, a diagnosis might describe the body in terms of wind, heat, cold, dryness, and so on. Since human beings are microcosms of the universe, which in turn is the result of the interaction of yin and yang, the human being corresponds also to the primordial workings of yin and yang.

In a macroscopic sense, when yin and yang were first divided, yang being light went upwards and formed the heaven. Yin being heavy descended and formed the earth.

Again, if the microcosm of human beings are a reflection of the macrocosm of universe, the principles of yin and yang must be at work within the body of each of us, just as they are functioning in the universe. In terms of health, it is evident that the delicate biochemical balance which the Chinese call the yin-yang balance of the body can be disturbed by many factors, including diet, weather, aging, depression, disease, genetics, toxins, etc. Man's existence also corresponds to this distinction: the head is the heaven, the eyes are the sun and moon, and each part of the body, corresponding to the structure of the universe, is a spirit. The upper part of the body contains the yang spirits of the heavens, and the lower parts of the body hold the yin spirits of the earth. As well as this, we have in our body the heart, spleen, kidneys, liver, and lungs which each correspond to one of the five elements: fire, earth, water, wood, and metal.

Dietary components were also viewed from this perspective of yin-yang balance by the ancient Chinese. In his *Essentials for Eating and Drinking* (1367 A.D.), the famous Chinese doctor Jia Ming put forward the case in this way:

Food and drink are used to nurture life. But if one is not aware of the fact that the natures of foods may be opposed to each other, and consume them together at the same time, the balance of the internal organs will be disturbed and disastrous effects will result. Therefore, if we want to nurture our lives with food and drink, we must avoid such harmful combinations with great caution.

In terms of the human body and its structure, yin refers to the tissue of the organ, while yang refers to its activity. When yin is deficient, the organ does not have enough raw materials to function. In contrast, if yang is insufficient, the organ does not function in a healthy way as it should. For instance, a yin deficiency in the thyroid hormone levels, would eventually cause a yang deficiency in the thyroid, as its function becomes impaired by the lack of hormones. In similar token, poor thyroid function, a symptom of yang deficiency, would eventually result in a yin deficiency, as the gland's output of hormones decreased.

Thus, these two universal opposites are connected in a never-ending cycle of interaction and interdependence. This work goes on nonstop from womb to tomb. When a ruddy, healthy child is born, he is filled with the energy of primordial yang, just like the rising sun in the morning. The ancient Chinese regard this state of being as a purely yang body containing the source of primordial yang energy, or vital energy, that gives life to human beings. The three major schools of thought in China employ slightly different terms to describe this state of existence; it is described as "the Baby" in Confucianism, "the relics" in Buddhism, and "the Golden Pill" in Taoism. The terms vary, but they all convey great respect for this pure state of physical existence.

Qi Energy

In this regard we find a very fundamental premise of both the Chinese natural health care system and Chinese philosophy—the concept of qi, or the vital life energy that maintains life and enlivens all things. Qi is a bio-philosophical concept referring to the primary driving force of life. In traditional Chinese philosophy, qi energy is perceived to be a universal force permeating and penetrating all things.

In the case of human beings, qi falls into two major categories—prenatal qi and postnatal qi. As the terms imply, prenatal qi is what one receives from one's parents before being born, while postnatal qi is what one acquires after birth. Since the Chinese natural health care system is preoccupied with the concept of qi, it is easy to understand why the Chinese were the first to embark on the topic of genetics.

As has been mentioned before, Chinese natural health care provides a detailed list of rules regarding diet, rest, sex, physical hygiene, and emotional activities for a pregnant mother to ensure the health of her baby. The postnatal qi, on the other hand, is the qi energy one acquires after birth, through breathing and dietary intake. Prenatal qi is the basis and prime driving force of life, while postnatal qi is the material source of nutrition and body functioning.

Prenatal qi is classified into two types: the essential qi and the primordial qi. The essential qi is the essence of life a baby is endowed by his parents at the time of his birth. It is the material basis of his growth and development. The primordial qi is the qi the fetus received during his stay in the mother's womb. This primordial energy is generated at the moment when the father and the mother are engaged at the height of their intercourse, breathing life into the fetus in the womb. Both types of prenatal qi constitute the prime driving force of life which basically determines the baby's physique and immunity, as well as the functioning of his digestive, secretive, respiratory, and circulatory systems.

Likewise, one's postnatal qi is also divided into two types—heavenly qi and earthly qi. In the Chinese natural health care system, heavenly qi refers to the air one breathes, and earthly qi refers to the nutrition one gets from a proper diet.

While different types of qi have different origins, they are all vital to life and health. Moreover, they are complementary to and dependent upon each other. Thus, a baby gifted with strong prenatal qi has better appetite, digestion, and circulation than someone born with weak prenatal qi. But this is only a good head start. Health care is a continuous process of life. If a person does not follow a healthy lifestyle, he will soon run into trouble and be overwhelmed with diseases even if he is gifted with strong prenatal qi energy. On the contrary, if someone follows a healthy lifestyle, he will notice that his health keeps on improving and he will be free from health problems even though he was born with weak prenatal qi energy. Prenatal qi is the basis of postnatal qi, while postnatal qi is the continuation of prenatal qi.

The relation between prenatal qi and postnatal qi is exactly like that between one's IQ and diligence. High IQ is of course a blessing and preferable to low IQ, but it does not guarantee success in life. On the contrary, many successful people in the world are not typically highly intelligent. Indeed, they are of average intelligence, but they have achieved a lot in life thanks to their hard work and consistent efforts. History is full of such examples. Albert Einstein, for instance, was considered mediocre in school.

Thanks to the supplement of postnatal qi, the prenatal qi energy continues to grow and accumulate inside the body until puberty. After this, it starts to dissipate as one becomes sexually mature. The age when puberty starts, and more importantly, the rate and intensity of such dissipation, largely determine how long one is going to live. The important thing to know is that when the level of this primordial energy is significantly lowered, the entire body loses its vitality, and the immune system is weakened, opening the body to various diseases and possibly death.

Also, whenever there is a blockage of qi along its routes of travel within the body, known as meridians, illness occurs. This is because all life ultimately depends on qi for its proper function, and each cell in the body depends on qi for its vitality. Thus, blockage or disharmony of qi is believed to be at the root of most diseases. Again, these blockages and disharmonies are described in terms of yin and yang, which show up in organ dysfunction and mental disturbances. Thus, one of the primary tasks we must undertake to prevent disease and prolong life lies in promoting and conserving the qi energy, as well as allowing it to flow smoothly in the body.

As we grow in age and knowledge, the yang qi or vital life energy grows as well until it finally reaches its climax at puberty or maturity. During the course of life, we gather yin qi, but at the same time we slowly but steadily dispense with yang qi. As life goes on, yin increases, and yang gradually flows away.

The good news is that even after puberty and marriage, it is still possible to nourish and make up the loss of primordial life energy. In fact, it all depends on whether or not you follow a healthy lifestyle—to become a sage or a beast. Indeed, how to conserve and build up this vital energy throughout life is the focal point of the entire Chinese natural health care system. Almost all the skills and techniques illustrated in this book are pivoted around this topic, in the absence of which, the whole system will be reduced to insignificance.

The methods for nourishing and replenishing vital qi include proper diet, adequate rest, regulated sex, regulated breathing, fitness exercises, and environmental purity. Thus, as the energy generated from proper diet meets the energy provided by breathing exercises, they accumulate in the bloodstream to form vital energy to nourish the primordial energy that comes with birth. Similarly, as two healthy sexual partners make love under the guidance of Taoist sexual yoga, both benefit from the interflow of energy during intercourse, replenishing the primordial energy of both.

In passing, it is interesting to know that this bio-philosophical concept has been successfully applied to many other fields of human endeavor, including politics and feng shui, the Chinese geomancy. Thus, when a dynasty or regime is corrupted to the core and on the verge of collapse, it is said to have run out of its primordial qi energy. When a geographic site for construction is beautiful, open, commanding in sight, and protected on three sides (except the front side), it is said by feng shui masters to be strong in qi energy and will bring good luck and happiness to its residents.

Understandably, a healthy person has an abundance of qi energy flowing smoothly through the meridians, nourishing the internal organs. This abundance of qi energy and its smooth flow inside the body are reflected in a sanguine complexion, an overflow of energy that enables one to work for a long time with efficiency, and a strong immunity to diseases. With this in mind, it is easier to understand why Buddhist and Taoist adepts eat so little and yet are so energetic. This is because they have consciously and purposely stored up qi energy, and protected it with great jealousy. Consequently, the build-up of qi will be able to provide them with the energy needed for their activities in the absence of foods and sleep.

The modern discovery that the adrenal glands producing the mother hormone DHEA (dehydroepiandrosterone) are located on top of the kidneys corresponds beautifully to the ancient Chinese theory that kidneys store and promote the vital yang energy. Thus, the newly discovered DHEA is similar to the vital yang energy in traditional Chinese philosophical system. Just as the more yang energy one has, the healthier and more energetic one will be. Meanwhile, RNA produced by the thyroid gland seems to be a modern version of yin energy conceived by the Chinese.

The fluctuation in one's qi energy level will witness a dramatic turn at the end of one's physical life. As death approaches, the balance between yin and yang energy is no longer effective. As a result, man's breath, spirit, and seminal essence dissipate. Death is a natural result of this evolutionary process. It is a separation of the body and spirit, the yin and yang parts of the human being. This does not necessarily mean the end of life because even after the body dies, the spirit can survive. The concept of an eternal spirit is crucial to our understanding of the Chinese

effort to attain immortality, another interesting topic to be discussed later.

To the believers of Chinese ways of thinking, the totality of man is, therefore, composite, complementary, and holistic. The contrasting principles of yin and yang are the basis of this composition. The yin part that returns to the soil after death, i.e., the body, is known as waidan, or external elixir, in the system of Chinese natural health care. The yang part of the being that wanders upwards after death, i.e., the soul, is known as neidan, or internal elixir. Yin controls the internal tissues and lower parts of the whole body as well as individual organs, while yang manages the external surfaces and upper parts of the body and organs. Thus, yin takes care of the blood, while yang controls energy; yin governs the urination, while yang regulates drinking; yin takes care of exhalation, while yang governs inhalation, and so on.

Traditional Chinese medicine is another application of these principles. Typically, a Chinese doctor will employ a combination of yin-yang theory and the system of five elements to diagnose the cause of diseases and predict its development, and to formulate prescriptions accordingly. This is because traditional Chinese medicine regards any disease as a result of an imbalance between yin and yang. Understandably, all the descriptions and treatments designed are preoccupied with the restoration of yin-yang balance as the fundamental healing requirement.

Indeed, the striving for balance between man and its environment is central to Chinese culture as well as its natural health care system. The Chinese natural health care system advocates man living in complete harmony with nature, and maintaining a harmonious balance between yin and yang. That is why it pays such great attention to sexual relations which is, or should be, a classical example of yin-yang balance. The ancient Chinese held that sex plays a key role in the circulation of qi energy, and that regulated sexual intercourse guided by the principle of yin-yang balance contributes directly to the nourishment and strengthening of vital energy for humans, and to the harmony between man and universe. This is because man is of yang nature representing heaven, while woman is of yin nature representing earth. Sexual intercourse between man and woman thus constitutes a direct union and harmony between yin and yang, the image of heaven and earth. This is designed by nature.

Call it a trap of nature, if you want. The primary purpose of sexual relations is not to seek carnal pleasure, but to perpetuate the species and prolong one's life. Moreover, the happier the sexual experience, the greater will be the degree of balance and harmony, and the healthier it will be to both parties. This theory is very easy to verify through human experience. Clinical and social surveys find that the more harmonious and active the sexual relationship between the married couples, the healthier and longer they will live. In addition, the more harmonious their sexual relations, the healthier will be the babies born to them.

Since the totality of the human being is complementary and holistic, the trinity of spirit-mind-body constitutes another cornerstone of the Chinese natural health care system as well as traditional Chinese medicine. Through the functioning of vital qi energy, these three aspects of life are brought together in a complex nutshell, interacting and influencing each other. Thus, not only the physical status has the power to affect one's mental happiness; one's mental status can also impact on one's physical health. In order for the body to function optimally, the mind has to provide the necessary support. Indeed, the body is so at one with the mind that it is hard to treat them separately. Human existence is really an integrated entity—what affects one affects all. Furthermore, the ancient Chinese considered the power of the mind to be infinite, whereas that of the body is finite. Conclusion: so long as the mind is willing, the body will be strong. Hence the importance of a genuine knowledge of health completely devoid of commercial and political motives.

Understanding this is essential to the practice of natural health care. Health is largely a matter of the cumulative effect of the lifestyle we choose, rather than that of medical care or coverage. This is very similar to learning a language, which is not a matter of memorizing grammatical rules, but a matter of habit. It is the habit of thinking, speaking, and writing in that language that will make you a master of that language. One may have excellent mastery of all the grammatical rules of a language but still be unable to speak it. Similarly, one may have excellent, very expensive medical coverage but suffer from the worst health. Therefore, one of the keynotes in the Chinese natural health care theory is to urge people to cultivate a healthy lifestyle in terms of eating, sleeping, thinking, exercise, and sexual conduct, and to do this as early in life as possible.

This philosophy helps account for the mysterious fact that many Chinese feel happy although they are poor throughout their life. Yan Hui, the best student of Confucius, was reputed to always feel happy even though he often had trouble securing enough food for himself. His teacher always spoke of him with highest pride and respect. This shows that happiness is a mental status which can, and should be, achieved through proper mental discipline based on knowledge of life and nature. It has nothing to do with material gains or wealth. It does, however, have a great deal to do with one's health status.

Returning to the principle of trinity, we find that it has been emphasized throughout Chinese culture and natural health care for thousands of years, but has only recently been realized in the West. To think of humans in terms of trinity is a systematic way of thinking and problem-solving. This trinity exists for both the universe and the human being. Thus, the trinity of the universe is composed of heaven, earth, and mankind, while the trinity for a human being is made up of his mind, body, and the spirit. Just as it would be incomplete to talk about the universe without mentioning earth, it would be inadequate to talk about health care without considering mind, body, and spirit in a nutshell. Since the three aspects of a man are closely interconnected and interdependent on each other, any piecemeal approach will not achieve the optimum result. Thus, the ancient Chinese hold that to keep the physical body healthy, we need to keep the brain and its complex chemistry healthy as well. This unity of body, mind, and spirit underlies the theory and practice of Chinese natural health and natural healing, as well as Chinese medicine.

This way of thinking not only applies to the human being as a whole; it is also used in a more detailed way in human activities. Take sexual relations for instance. The ancient Chinese did not regard sex as a mere biological need. Rather, they saw it as a symphony made of physical, mental, and spiritual activities at the same time. They knew that sex has a lot to do with our physical, mental, as well as spiritual well-being. But to enjoy a good sex life, one must also enjoy good health, well-being, and spiritual awareness. Physical and emotional well-being promotes vitality and strengthens sexual ability.

The same systematic attitude is assumed by Chinese doctors. When they put together a prescription for kidney problems, they will also take into account the need for strengthening the spleen, lung, and heart, as well as liver. All these organs must work together as a team for the kidneys to function properly.

Three Treasures

Corresponding to the macrotrinity of universe, there is a microtrinity of life within each human being, i.e., essence, qi, and spirit. These three elements are known as the three treasures of life in the Chinese natural health care system, comparable to the three treasures of heaven—sun, moon, and stars—and the three treasures of earth—water, fire, and wind. Along with the macrotrinity of heaven, earth, and mankind, and the theories of yin and yang as well as the five elements, it forms the philosophical framework of the natural health care system.

The ancient Chinese hold that the three treasures are the fundamentals of life, accounting for life's generation, development, and changes. The three treasures are intimately linked to and dependent upon each other, although each has its own specific functions to perform. Essence is the material basis of life, qi is the driving force of life, and spirit is the commander of all life activities, guiding the transformation of essence into life energy and the circulation of qi around the body. In other words, essence is the source of qi and spirit, and qi is the link between essence and spirit. Affluence of essence will lead to abundance of qi energy, which in turn will generate high spirit. There can be no qi without essence, nor can there be spirit without qi. Just think of qi in its narrow sense of air or breath. Can there be spirit if one is out of breath?

The three treasures of life constituting the microtrinity in humans represent the three different levels of human existence: the physical, energetic, and spiritual. Essence is the physical cream of life which embraces the concept of sperm, blood, enzyme, saliva, and hormones. Qi is the driving force of life, which is made up of the prenatal qi stored in kidneys, and the postnatal qi coming from breathing and diet. Spirit governs the mental and emotional activities of life. Together, they form the basis of the existence, development and changes of life. Promoting the three treasures means promoting health and self-healing. Thus, we see one of the fundamental beliefs in the Chinese natural health care system, i.e., that immunity and health restoration ability are inherent in the human body in the form of the three treasures. This belief is unambiguously stated in *The Yellow Emperor's Classics of Internal Medicine*:

Take life easy and throw away your desires, and true qi will follow your command. If you can keep essence and spirit within your body, how can disease happen?

Essence is the first treasure in this micro trinity which, in a narrower sense, refers to sperm or male hormones in the man, and ova or female hormones in the woman. There is a close relationship between essence and overall health. For one thing, our immunity to disease depends primarily on our essence. That explains why one is more vulnerable to cold or flu after sexual intercourse, and why indulgence in carnal desires almost always results in various diseases. Expense in essence means a lowering of immunity power; excess expense in essence spells disease and death.

That is why the ancient Chinese advised people to jealously guard their essence if health and longevity were sought after.

It is significant to note the intimate connection between essence and immunity, or essence and health, which was held firmly by the ancient Chinese and verified again and again by numerous clinical cases. This connection shows that immunity is a natural factor generated inside one's own body, not given by others. The human body is the greatest health promoter and natural healer if we know how to take care of it. In other words, health and healing can be achieved by ourselves, in a natural way. Our body is capable of self-healing, and we can become our own health care providers, if we know how to preserve and enhance our immune system. This is an active set of billions of white blood cells spreading out throughout the body, all with just two goals: to recognize external factors of disease; and to respond to the threat of disease.

The second treasure in the trinity of human life is called qi, or life energy. The whole life ultimately depends on qi for its existence, and all vital organs of the body ultimately rely on qi for their proper and effective functioning. Qi literally means the air or breath, but refers to a much broader category of life energy in Chinese culture. It assumes a variety of forms, such as primordial qi, blood qi, protective qi, and nourishing qi. Different forms of qi come from different sources and serve different purposes. Some come from birth, such as the primordial qi; others from essence, still others from food, water, and breathing. All kinds of qi, however, are closed related to one another. They are also closely linked with essence and spirit, the other two pillars of the life trinity.

Qi determines our energy level, sexual vitality, work efficiency, physical courage and personality, and the length of life. Those people full of qi will have a sanguine complexion, high work efficiency, better endurance, strong immunity, and great courage. They look younger and live longer than those of their same age but with lower qi level.

As with other elements essential to health, qi level in the body normally declines with age as a matter of natural course. That is why, for one thing, the older one gets, the more timid one becomes. This subtle relation between qi level and personality has been well explored by Chinese sages. Mencius, for one, was very proud of his ability to build up a strong qi reserve. He once remarked: "I am very good in conserving my strong qi." On another occasion, talking of a brave historical figure who dared to challenge even his emperor, Mencius made this comment: "It is a rare thing that one is born with such strong qi. He should learn to treasure and preserve it throughout his life." This is exactly what Confucius had accomplished. Commenting on himself as an elderly man, he proudly declared: "Wealth cannot corrupt me; poverty cannot transform me; force cannot bend me." What a strong personality! What a marvelous reserve of qi!

Significantly, Confucius made an insightful observation on the relations between qi level and age on the one hand, and personality and orientation on the other. He declared in all solemnity: "Young people should guard against carnal desires because their blood qi is at an unstable and fluctuating state. Middle-agers should guard against physical fighting because their blood qi is at its peak, and elders should guard against material avarice because their blood qi is already weak." I believe anyone old enough will be able to verify with his or her own personal experience this Confucian truth declared more than 2,000 years ago. I have always regarded Confucius as the father of psychology. Judging by his own words, I think it is fair to say that Confucius has opened up a promising field of human study called physio-psychology. It will be of great significance to go deeper into this field and uncover more relationships among qi energy, personality, and age.

It remains a challenge to modern science to prove it, although many scientists have already come to the understanding that qi is not something fictitious; (many scientists believe in God, but they can't prove that either) it is a biophysical substance similar to electricity. Qi is to life what electricity is to the flashlight—the more abundant the electricity, the brighter the flashlight. A flashlight not in use does not mean the absence of electricity. It is simply conserved and stored for future use. The same holds for qi. The more of it one has, the more energetic and

healthy one will be. But constant use of qi without rest and replenishment will cause it to run out of supply, and usher in the end of life itself. For this reason, the ancient Chinese advised us to build up more energy than we consume so that we will never run out of qi. This is achieved by means of various methods of natural health care, such as diet, sleep, proper exercise (especially the breathing exercise qigong), mental peace and discipline, physical hygiene, regulated sex, and environmental awareness, all of which will be discussed in great detail later.

The third treasure in the life trinity is spirit or, in modern scientific terms, the health of the cerebral cortex. Typically, in the Chinese health care system, spirit is considered the commander of all life functions, and is therefore of supreme importance in the trinity. This belief is reflected in a famous Chinese saying: "Nourishing essence is more important than nourishing blood; nourishing qi is more important than nourishing essence; nourishing spirit is more important than nourishing essence." This insistence on the mind-body connection and the superiority of the mind marks a major departure of Chinese philosophical thinking from its Western counterpart.

In a general sense, the entire Chinese natural health care system is concerned about fostering and promoting the three treasures. Thus, a healthy diet and regulated sex are aimed at fostering the essence; breathing exercises are designed to promote the qi energy; and rest and sleep are meant to conserve and restore the spirit. Essence, sexual essence in particular, is considered the basis of the prenatal life. It is a very precious substance which will give birth to new lives if put onto others, and will nourish oneself if kept inside the body. Qi is the driving force of the functioning of internal organs, and that of the circulation of blood. Short of qi, yin and yang will lose their balance, blood will cease to circulate around the body, and various organs will function abnormally. Spirit is the command of essence and qi. It guides the activities of the body. If one's spirit is dull, one will be short of qi and essence. It is a common observation and life experience that when one is in depression or low in spirit, one's breath is short and shallow—short of qi, and one will have poor digestion leading to shortage of essence.

Therefore, in traditional Chinese medicine, the principle of mutual dependence and relative importance among the three treasures is widely followed in both diagnosis and treatment. Thus, when a traditional Chinese doctor diagnoses a patient, he would first look at the patient's face and measure the spiritual level of the patient. If the patient is diagnosed with having his spirit flying out of the body, it is a signal of the severest case and often forebodes imminent death. This diagnosis of spirit on the part of the Chinese doctor is, of course, more an art than a science. It is an art rooted in the soil of rich clinical experience and a profound understanding of Chinese philosophy. Only when the doctor believes that the patient's

spirit is still good will he proceed to take measures in order to build up the qi energy and essence of the patient.

It is interesting to note that the same principle governing the relations among the three treasures of life has also been applied to many other fields of human endeavor in traditional China. Thus, in physiognomy, the Chinese art of face reading, a master face reader will always look first at the eyes of his client to make sure that the spirit is still around. If the client's spirit is found to be exceptionally low or almost destroyed, the master will strongly advise the client to stay home for fear that severe disaster or imminent death is projected. If the worst comes to the worst, staying home can at least give the impression of dying a natural death, the lesser of the two evils.

What keeps us healthy, after all? What makes the difference between health and sickness? In the parlance of modern science, many diseases are caused by viruses and bacteria. While nobody is living in a virus-free environment, why do some become sick while others escape unscathed? According to the theory of the Chinese natural health care system, it is the vital energy, or primordial qi energy, inside our body that determines our immunity power and therefore our health status. The relationship between the two is a direct one. In other words, the higher the reserve of vital energy, the stronger the person's immunity will be. It is the vital energy that helps us fight against bacteria, viruses, and harmful materials that enter our body.

The stronger the vital energy, the more effective and victorious will be our immune system. As part of the vital energy weaponry, antibodies, lymph nodes, white blood cells, and hormones each play a role in maintaining and restoring health health once the body is afflicted with disease.

In modern terms, the three treasures of life can be thought of as the equivalent of immunity, which is based on the vitality of billions of white blood cells. White blood cells serve two basic functions: to recognize germ invaders, and to fight the invaders once identified. When bacteria enter your body, specialized cells called neutrophils rush to the scene to virtually wipe out the invaders. Other cells soon come by to clean up the job. When viruses attack your body, your immune system dispatches antibodies to tackle the invaders. Without an immune system, even the mildest infection would be lethal, as is the case of AIDS today. But the effective functioning of your immune system depends directly on the strength and vitality of these cells. In parallel terms, the fuller the vital qi, the more active and vital the white blood cells, and therefore the stronger the immunity. A strong immune system gives you good protection against bacteria and viruses. That is exactly why people who constantly nourish and conserve the vital qi have a much lower number of health problems than those who waste the precious qi.

Cause and Effect

Another principle underpinning the Chinese natural health care system is that of cause and effect. The Chinese always go a long way in finding out the root cause of a problem, and focus their attention and solutions there. In terms of medicine, they always want to know the "why's" of the disease before they contemplate on the "how's" and "what's." Even when a patient has severe symptoms, a Chinese doctor still sees to it that the prescription and treatment address the root cause of the disease first while trying his best to alleviate the symptoms. This principle goes even farther and deeper in natural health than in traditional Chinese medicine, if only because the natural health care system is preventive in the first place. Prevention of diseases, or proactive, rather than passive, treatment of disease form the cornerstone of natural health care.

What are the causes of diseases? According to the ancient Chinese, the causes of disease can be summarized into two categories: external and internal. Externally speaking, there are six disease-causing factors including wind, cold, heat, moisture, dryness, and fire. Excessive exposure to these factors will trigger diseases. Therefore, these factors are called the "six external triggers of disease" in Chinese tradition.

Internally speaking, man is an emotional living entity. If there is an abrupt change or excess expression of emotions, such as joy, anger, worry, grief, fear, and fright, one's health will be damaged and disease will occur. Therefore, these seven kinds of emotion are called the "seven emotional triggers of disease," as contrasted with the six external triggers of disease. If external triggers work together with emotional triggers of disease, the damage to the health will be very serious.

The question still remains why people exposed to the same level of external triggers do not all become sick. The answer lies in the immunity power of individuals, which is closely associated with the vital qi energy level of each individual. Since the vital qi energy level is largely a function of our lifestyle including diet, sleep, exercise, and especially sexual life on the male side, it all boils down to the issue of ejaculation frequency in the final analysis. Those people who ejaculate cautiously and rarely are much less vulnerable to disease than those who squander away their precious sperm. In other words, they have stronger immunity than others.

Five Elements

Yet another important concept intimately linked to the Chinese system of natural health care is that of the five elements, i.e., water, fire, wood, metal, and earth, in that order. Even the order itself is significant, which starts with the element of water. For one thing, it coincides with the proven scientific theory that the prerequisite of life on any planet in the universe is water. For the Chinese sages, the five elements are the basic components and raw materials of the universe, human beings included. That is why the art of Chinese fortunetelling classifies individuals into five elements based on one's day and time of birth, as well as on one's facial structure and physical shape.

In the Chinese natural health care system and traditional Chinese medicine, major bodily organs and parts have been classified according to the five elements. Thus, kidneys correspond to water, regulating the storage of nutrition and use of energy; the heart corresponds to fire, representing consciousness and spirit; the liver corresponds to wood, manufacturing blood and governing emotional response to outside environments; the lungs correspond to metal, regulating respiration and maintaining cybernetic balance; and the spleen corresponds to earth, distributing nutrition throughout the body and giving it strength and vigor. In addition, water governs the kidneys, anus, bladder, and bones; fire governs the heart, small intestine, and arteries; wood governs the liver, eyes, gallbladder, nails, and ligaments; metal governs the lungs, mouth, skin, hair, and large intestine; earth governs the spleen, stomach, nose, and muscles. Even the five fingers of the hand are classified in terms of these five elements. Thus, the ring finger corresponds to water, the middle finger to fire, the small finger to wood, the index finger to metal, and the thumb to earth. Even one's emotional states are classified according to the five elements theory. For instance, anger is considered a wood emotion, joy a fire emotion, sorrow a metal emotion, fear a water emotion, and melancholy a metal emotion.

In clinical application, the interrelations among the internal organs are understood on the basis of mutual production and containment among the five elements. Thus, kidneys (water) nourish the liver (wood), the liver (wood) feeds the heart (fire), the heart (fire) warms the spleen (earth), the spleen (earth) supplements the lungs (metal), and the lungs (metal) strengthen the kidneys (water). On the containment side, a healthy liver (wood) can regulate the spleen (earth); a strong spleen can absorb the extra water in the kidneys; strong kidneys can prevent the fire of the heart from burning the lungs (metal), and so on.

It is significant to point out that the interaction between the heart and kidneys is of special importance to the Chinese natural health care system. This special interaction is known as *shui-huo-ji-ji* (water and fire are in perfect harmony), or "the communion between the heart and kidneys," the disturbance of which will lead to various ailments including nocturnal emission, night sweating, insomnia, and chronic fatigue. Thus, through the mutual production and containment of internal organs, the entire human body forms a superb complex system with the ability to maintain and heal itself.

It is only natural that the theory of the five elements has been extended into the area of diet due to the all-around importance of diet in human health. The ancient Chinese had established a framework in which the tastes of food and drink are related to different organs of the body, and therefore to health and healing. Thus, sweet belongs to the earth element, and is consequently related to the spleen and affects it directly. Similarly, bitter belongs to the fire element, and relates to and affects the heart. Sour belongs to the wood element and relates to and affects the liver. Pungent belongs to the metal element and relates to and affects the lungs. Finally, salty belongs to the water element and relates to and affects the kidneys. This correlation between tastes and internal organs finds direct application in the healing process. For instance, patients with kidney disease should be especially careful in the amount of salt they use, for salt directly impacts on the kidneys. Likewise, patients with liver disease should guard against the consumption of sour foods and drinks.

It is of significance to note that this relationship between tastes and internal organs has been one of the guiding principles used in discovering the medical effects of various herbs. Thus, herbs that taste sweet are judged to have medical effects on the spleen and therefore are used to heal related diseases. In the same way, herbs that taste salty are judged to have medical effects on the kidneys and are used to heal kidney diseases.

The preoccupation of Chinese philosophy with the five elements is further shown in the following amazing discovery which relates sounds to the five elements, and consequently to the internal organs. In Chinese musical theory, there are five major sound families corresponding respectively to the five elements. Thus, the Gong family sounds correspond to earth, the Shang family sounds correspond to wood, the Jiao family sounds to fire, the Zhi family sounds to metal, and the Yu family sounds to water. Since different sounds are related to different elements, which in turn correspond to five major internal organs, the discovery of this delicate connection has been successfully employed in the design and development of sound therapy, which is described in appendix 2 on sound qigong. For instance, making the sound "Gong" while exhaling in a qigong exercise can promote digestion and relieve stomach ailments and ulcers. (Gong is related to earth, which stands for the spleen and stomach in traditional Chinese medicine.)

Since the relationships among the five basic elements is at once mutually productive and mutually destructive, an ailment in one organ will negatively affect one or more related organs. Similarly, the strengthening of one organ can promote the health of other organs. Thus, a deficiency in the kidney will lead to liver and heart problems, because kidneys stand for water, the deficiency of which will cause the withering of the wood—liver. For the opposite reason, a deficiency of water will allow the fire to go rampant without check. Since fire is the organ of the heart, we will see heart problems as a result of kidney disease. The same principle applies to other organs based on the productive and destructive relationships among the five elements. The important thing is to maintain a delicate balance among all organs in order to keep healthy and prevent diseases. It is this essential understanding that forms the basis of herbal descriptions on the part of Chinese doctors.

With the above philosophical concepts in mind, it is easy to understand why the Chinese always try to adapt individual lifestyles to the laws of the universe, rather than the other way round as is often the case in the West. Thus, the ancient Chinese ask us to adjust our diet, clothing, time of sleep, and even emotional status in accordance with the four seasons. In fact, the whole fabric of traditional Chinese social values is geared in many ways toward appreciation and imitation of the underlying forces at play in the universe, or the Tao of nature. By contrast, people in the West try to force nature to adjust to human needs. Thus, airconditioning is widely used in everyday life to change nature, to make people comfortable. The side effects of the widespread use of airconditioning are still revealing themselves. Just by looking at their antinature characteristics one can predict the existence of such effects of technology. Another example is the prevalence of automobiles. America is known as a country on wheels, which replace the natural functions of the feet and pollute the air.

To sum up, the entire Chinese natural health care system is concerned about man-nature balance, about cultivating a healthy lifestyle including the daily contents of diet, sleep, exercise, sex, and thinking; and about conserving and building up the all-important qi energy reserve inside the body. Indeed, qi lies at the very core of disease prevention and the self-healing process. The ancient Chinese knew early in their civilization that there are as many ways and levels to conserve and nourish qi as there are to dissipate and waste it—physical, mental, psychical, dietary, sexual, and environmental. This understanding gave them a holistic perspective on health problems focused on vital energy, or immunity. Thus, when warning people against catching a cold in winter, a Chinese natural health system doctor will ask people to conserve their semen and put on more clothes. Obviously, they did not see cold as the fault of weather alone. Rather, the afflicted have as much, if not more, to blame for themselves. This is because they themselves do not make an effort to conserve and nourish their vital qi, or their immune system in the first place. Thus, for thousands of years, preventing and treating diseases have gone side by side in the Chinese natural health care system under the guidance of the same set of principles. When we talk about a holistic approach towards natural health in the following, we are exploring treatment of diseases at the same time.

Chapter 3

Natural Health Secrets
of Diet

M encius, a great Chinese sage who lived more than 2,100 years ago, declared that the greatest desires of human beings are food and sex, in that order. Actually, these are the two most basic desires of all life forms including humans. Compared to sex, the need for food is even more urgent and fundamental. Diet serves two functions: to ensure physical survival and to seek satisfaction. Unfortunately, these two basic functions do not always agree with each other. Instead, they often conflict, and our health depends on how we handle that conflict.

The fact is that we are what and how we eat. If we eat fresh, healthy foods, we will be healthy. However, if we eat unhealthy foods, or eat good foods in an improper way, we are bound to experience problems with our health. For instance, it is estimated that diet is a factor in 30 to 40 percent of all cancers that develop in men and in 60 percent of all cancers that occur in women.[1] Unfortunately, many people are not aware of this powerful truth or just don't listen.

Our lives depend on a good diet so that our bodies can grow and function properly. From a nutritional point of view, the main sources of energy are carbohydrates, such as starches, which are broken down to sugars, and fats, which are converted into fatty acids. Proteins are necessary, not only as energy sources, but as building blocks that are reconstructed with the amino acids derived from proteins. In addition to these macronutrients, the body also requires minerals and vitamins for certain metabolic processes.

As the Chinese see it, food is medicine in itself, and the best medicine at that. The Chinese developed the theory of dietary therapy, which serves three purposes: to promote health, to prevent disease, and to kill disease. It is a popular Chinese belief that eating while you are hungry is medicine in itself, and not eating when you are not hungry is also medicine. The Chinese also believe that nourishment from herbs is not nearly as good as nourishment from foods. Obviously, our choice of diet deserves careful study.

I purposely put diet on the very top of my discussion list for another reason: I believe that food is our first line of defense against diseases. As the ancient Chinese proverb says, "Into the mouth come diseases; out of mouth springs disaster." While the second half of this sentence needs to be understood in the context of a feudal, dictatorial society, the first half of the sentence is universally true. Thus, our mouths are our first line of defense against disease, if not disaster.

As we know, the mouth is one of our major routes of contact with our environment. If you are not careful about what, when, how, and how much you eat, you are bound to run into trouble. For instance, the foods we eat may be rotten, poisonous, or contain harmful preservatives and additives to make it taste and smell better; chemicals may be altered as a result of heating, salting, freezing, and other processes; it may become contaminated by bacteria, fungi, and other organisms that can produce health-damaging metabolites; it may be polluted by chemicals and other man-made pollutants in its course of growth. Eventually, all these chemicals enter the body through the mouth and perform their dirty work there.

As if to confirm the wisdom of the ancient Chinese, an increasing number of modern Western studies are pointing to diet as the dominant or major cause of various illnesses, including cancer and heart disease. For instance, there is an established relationship between high sugar consumption and diabetes,[2] between intense use of salt and hypertension, and between the amount of fat intake and the occurrence of cancer, specifically colon cancer. The outstanding characteristics of the typical American diet are convenience and taste. Convenient and refined foods are vastly different from raw foods; such a diet is nutrient-poor. Because these diets have been depleted of nutrients, and loaded with potentially dangerous chemical materials, our health has suffered greatly as a result.

America is the wealthiest and best-educated nation on earth. However, the way most Americans live and eat almost ensures the occurrence of a large amount of degenerative diseases. Americans eat too much animal protein, too much fat, too much salt, and too much sugar. The typical American diet consists of 12 percent protein, 42 percent fat, 22 percent complex carbohydrates, and 24 percent refined sugar.[3] This is considerably less healthier than what the U.S. government recommends: 12 percent protein, 48 percent complex carbohydrates, 30 percent fat and only 10 percent sugar.[4] In countries where people eat substantially less fat, sugar, salt, and animal protein, the occurrence of such diseases is minimal. In China, for instance, heart disease, hypertension, breast cancer, and obesity are rare in comparison to their frequency in America. Even in Japan, the second wealthiest nation in the world, which retains its distinct Chinese cultural background, the frequency of the above-mentioned diseases is much lower than in America. The fact is that the Japanese have an average daily intake of 2,600 calories, the lowest of any industrialized nation, compared to an average of 3,400 calories in the U.S.[5]

Sugar

Packaged foods are extremely popular in America, but they often contain hidden sugar and fat to improve their taste. Sugar has many vices. It not only depresses the immune system (mostly in diabetics), it promotes dental cavities, and also weakens the effect of other nutrients such as calcium, magnesium, and vitamin B and also hinders with body's absorption of other nutrients it need. This is because sugar contains a lot of calories but is stripped of all vitamins, minerals, and fiber. What is left are pure calories. If your diet contains too much sugar, you will get a lot of calories from sugar but not enough of the other nutrients you need. Meanwhile, too much sugar can ruin your teeth, weaken the immune system, and make you fat. It is important, therefore, to reduce your sugar intake to a minimum.

Sugary foods can also affect the body's metabolic rate. The sugar boost happens only for a short time. After that, you sink into a slump. To recover, you take in more sugar to boost your energy. Thus you find yourself in a vicious eating cycle. With your appetite yearning for more and more rich, fat, and sugary foods, your metabolism becomes more and more sluggish. It is just impossible for the body to keep up with the accumulation of calories. It cannot burn the calories as fast and efficiently as it should. The result is that the food you eat is not so readily used as fuel; instead, it keeps piling up as fat. Carrying it around as excess weight makes you even more tired. Eventually, the self-perpetuating cycle handicaps any efforts to relieve obesity.

By contrast, raw fruits and vegetables contain plenty of vitamins, minerals, and compounds which can prevent cancer in different parts of the body. I believe they can even prevent AIDS. After all, AIDS is a problem of the immune system, and these nutrients are well known to be potent supporters of our immune system. Research has shown that vegetables like bok choy, broccoli, cauliflower, turnip, kale, and cabbage have the ability to prevent problems with the prostate, lungs, bladder, colon, esophagus, and breasts. The same effect can be achieved by eating fruits such as apricots, grapes, oranges, pineapples, watermelon, and strawberries. To obtain the optimum effect, these vegetables and fruits are best consumed in their fresh, raw form.

Fat

Then there is the all-pervasive fat in the American diet. Most Americans consume about 40 percent of their total calories in the form of fat—well above the 25 to 30 percent fat consumption considered desirable.[6] Fat, saturated fat in particular, is one of the worst factors in our diet. An excessive intake of saturated fat is the major cause of obesity, heart disease, and strokes. This is because fat interferes with normal digestion and builds up cholesterol in our body. Obesity alone is no laughing matter. About 34 million American adults are struggling with this problem, let alone a fast-growing number of kids joining the obese group each year.[7]

The ideal body weight for a woman ranges from 101 to 130 pounds, adding three pounds per inch above five feet and one inch. The ideal body weight for a man ranges from 105 to 134 pounds, adding three pounds per inch above five feet and one inch.[8] Unfortunately, American diets almost always fail to keep the weight off, because they are too hard to adhere to, and do little to promote metabolism and bowel movements. Traditional Chinese diets, on the other hand, contain a lot of plant elements and natural foods which greatly help metabolism, energy buildup, water retention, and bowel movements. The American Heart Association says, for good health, less than 30 percent of the calories you take in each day should come from fat. My recommendation is that you get no more than 20 percent of your calories from fat. This means you make up the calories you need every day by taking in more complex high-fiber foods, for instance, vegetables.

The prevalent obesity in this country should be a major concern. This is not a mere issue of appearance; it compounds many health problems. Overweight people put increased stress on their hearts, muscles, and bones and find breathing more difficult. Indeed, obesity can lead to a variety of degenerative diseases such as diabetes, hypertension, cardiovascular diseases, and cancer. Researchers have found that the risk of death from heart attack is twice as high for an obese person as for someone whose weight is normal. Also, the risk of death from diabetes is three times as high, and from hypertension, twice as high. There is also a high correlation between the mortality rates of breast and prostate cancers and the amount of animal fat intake in the diet. Statistics show clearly that obese people are short-lived people.

An international study shows that death rates from cancer are the highest in northern European countries where saturated animal fat is heavily consumed. The lowest mortality rates of these diseases are found in Asian countries such as China and Japan, where the average daily intake of saturated animal fat is the lowest. Moderate mortality rates of cancer are found in South American countries where the consumption of animal fat lies between that of the northern European countries and Asian nations. There is also an abundance of evidence pointing to the association between diets rich in animal fats and the high rate of gastrointestinal cancer (except stomach cancer). This is because diets high in animal fat promote the growth of hormone-producing bacteria in the large intestine. Saturated fat also raises the cholesterol levels in the blood, and cholesterol is the precursor of all hormones. High cholesterol also causes blood clotting which leads to heart attacks.

Regular high-fat diets disturb the hormone function in the body. While this is true for both sexes, its adverse effects are much more apparent in women than in men. The following biological changes are observed in women who eat a high-fat diet as compared to those who do not: menopause occurs about four years later than normal; menstru-

al periods are further apart, heavier, longer, and more painful; puberty or maturity comes earlier (twelve years old versus fifteen years old), and increased chances of breast cancer. Dr. Paul Kuehn, former president of the New England Cancer Society and chairman of the Cancer Commission for New England of the American College of Surgeons, also finds from his own practice of treating more than 8,000 breast cancer patients that more than half of them were overweight. This suggests to him that fat consumption does play a role in breast cancer, and that decreasing fat in the diet certainly won't hurt anybody.[9]

A recent clinical study suggests that dietary changes can reduce blood pressure as effectively as drug treatment, and it achieves the same result without any side effects. In a study sponsored by the National Heart, Lung and Blood Institute, people put on a low-fat diet that included ten daily servings of fresh fruit and vegetable, plus two servings of calcium-rich dairy products, had shown their systolic and diastolic readings reduced by 5.5 mm and 3.0 mm, respectively. Those afflicted with hypertension showed a reduction that was twice as big. A similar study conducted on Yi people in Yunnan province of China came to the same conclusion. The study shows that Yi people never developed hypertension as long as they stayed with their traditional diet of rice, a little meat, and a lot of fruits and vegetables.

How We Eat

While most of us know that fatty foods and overeating can make us obese, few people know that even the manner in which we consumes food can determine whether we become obese or not. One of the principles regarding diet in the Chinese natural health system requires that we eat slowly and chew thoroughly. This is not only essential for good digestion and longevity, but is also essential to prevent obesity and other diseases. This is because when food enters the body, the level of blood sugar in the body rises. As the blood sugar level reaches a certain point, the central nervous system sends out a signal to the stomach to stop, preventing us from overeating.

On the other hand, if you gobble up your food, the stomach does not have enough time to respond to the stop signal being sent to it. Naturally, this leads to overeating. A survey shows that obese people take an average of ten minutes to finish a meal, while thin people spend an average of fifteen minutes. An experiment based on these findings shows that after twenty weeks of slow eating, obese people lost an average of ten pounds; a very convincing result, indeed.

Equally, if not more, important is the fact that by chewing thoroughly we generate more saliva in our mouth. This is one of the most vital digestive enzymes. The more we have, the better our digestion and nutritional supply is. It is not what we eat that make us healthy, and still how much we eat. It is how much we digest that determines our health. This is because our body needs the right nutrients for the supply of energy and metabolic process. A strong digestive function will ensure that such nutrients are absorbed by the body through diet. Besides, the more thoroughly you chew the food, the more delicious it tastes.

Of course, the vice of red meat does not lie solely in the fat it contains. There is much more to it than that. For a long time, the Chinese have believed that animals, like humans, are born with feelings, including fear and horror, anger, and hatred which, when released, will poison the meat we eat. Moreover, they have the ability to extract revenge in a subtle way against their human killers. This revenge comes in various forms; people who have killed a large number of animals have often died in a variety of strange or violent ways.

A well-documented Chinese story illustrates this. Many years ago, there was a premier in the Sung dynasty who enjoyed an extravagant life style. This included killing one lamb each day for the enjoyment of himself and his family. He succeeded in doing this for 300 days in a row, ever since he became the premier. Suddenly, an unexpected disaster fell upon him and his family. On the 298th day of his premiership, he went to see the emperor as usual, but the bottom of his garment became mysteriously loose in the presence of the emperor. This was considered a gross disrespect for the son of heaven in ancient China. Fortunately, the emperor forgave him since this was the first time. The premier was extremely frightened, and he kowtowed again and again for the royal generosity. He returned home and told his wife the story. Both made it a point that he should check his bottom three times before going to work in the morning. He did, looking into the mirror again and again before leaving the house.

Shortly after his morning conference with the emperor began, the bottom of his costume became loose again in the presence of the emperor. This did not escape the sharp eyes of the emperor whose mind was still fresh from yesterday's episode. This time his majesty got angry. He did not say a single word but stood up and walked out of the court. The conference ended abruptly in a tense atmosphere.

The premier went home terrified and trembling, almost to the point of mental collapse. After receiving a barrage of consolation and encouragement from his wife, he decided to wear a brand new garment the next day, and check for a full hour in the mirror before going to offer his humble apology to the emperor. The emperor's anger seemed to have abated after a night's sleep. He received the premier calmly, and went directly into the urgent issues facing the country, leaving the premier literally no time to offer his well-prepared apology. Things went smoothly for two hours before, all of a sudden, the hat on premier's head fell to the ground. This was considered an even graver disrespect for his Majesty, which put the tolerance of the emperor to the limit. Without hesitation, he ordered the immediate execution of his premier.

The moral of this tragedy, according to some historians, is that the spirits of the 300 lambs killed and consumed by the premier were eventually working out their vengeance. While there is no scientific proof of this morality story, modern science does confirm part of the belief held by the Chinese for thousands of years that animals possess similar feelings as humans. They can experience the same emotion of horror, anger, and hatred when being killed, and that such feelings will automatically release a huge amount of poisonous elements into the body. When such meat is consumed by human beings, poisons find their way into the body and damage the metabolic process of body cells, leading to various diseases including cancer. A case in point is the fact that Inuits use red meat as their main staple food. Due to the geographic environment in which they live, they do not have reasonable access to vegetables and fruits. As a result, their average life span is only twenty-seven years, way below the world average.

The situation has been worsened as a result of modern commercialism. In addition to the traditional problems of red meats, animals are now fed large amounts of hormones. It is estimated that at least 17 million pounds of hormones are fed to animals each year in the United States to boost the production of meat and increase profits. These animals are eventually consumed by the public. Consuming animals fed with such chemicals is virtually the same as eating hormones directly. How can our systems handle large quantities of pollutants such as hormones? In fact, red meat is one of the major sources of dietary pollution. It is one of the primary causes of the development of malign tumors in the body.[10] Besides, it can contribute to a number of degenerative diseases such as fatigue, aging, indigestion, obesity, and so on.

Protein

How about protein? While a necessary source of life energy, it can be harmful to our health if it comes from the wrong sources and is consumed in too great an amount. An excess intake of protein puts enormous stress on the kidneys and causes rapid and, in many cases irreplaceable, loss of calcium from the bones. Countries that consume the most animal protein show the highest rates of bone fractures and osteoporosis. In contrast, countries like China and Japan where people eat less animal protein and smoked foods, osteoporosis rates are considerably lower.

A number of studies show that when the animal protein in the diet is replaced by vegetable protein, cholesterol levels decline as a result. While the acceptable level of protein for a healthy adult is 50 grams a day, the average American takes in six to ten times that amount. Worse still, many population studies show that diets high in animal protein are also related to a higher rate of breast cancer and a higher incidence of premature death. In a landmark study completed in the early 90s, scientists from Cornell and the Beijing School of Preventive Medicine showed that eating a diet low in protein dramatically reduces the risk of breast cancer, heart disease, colon cancer, diabetes, and several other life-threatening diseases.[11] Unfortunately, many people today still believe that only animal meat can provide good quality protein, and that we need plenty of protein each day to live and stay well. This is simply not true. Just look at horses, oxen, and elephants. Are they not more powerful and energetic than human beings? What do they consume? Grass and water (including morning dews) and nothing else.

The ancient Chinese knew that all we need in terms of nutrition are grains, vegetables, fruits, clean water, and fresh air, plus sufficient sunlight. These items contain all the nutrients from nature needed for the maintenance of life and the replenishment of vital energy. Nutrients come from the earth, sunlight, air, and water. Vegetarians are the most direct beneficiaries of nutrition provided by nature.

Indeed, you do not need to worry about protein, as long as you eat fruits, nuts, seeds, vegetables, and whole grain, because these foods contain enough protein, and the best protein at that. Both nutritional and clinical studies conducted in China show that vegetarians have the most wholesome diet. The rate of heart disease among them is the lowest, and their chances of developing cancer is much lower than that of people who eat meat. In addition, vegetarians enjoy good digestion, smooth bowel movements, sound sleep, high spirits, and strong immunity. It is an established fact that fruits and vegetables promote bowel movements, which in turn contribute to better sleep and therefore high spirits. Better sleep and high spirits will strengthen our immune system. However, too much animal protein in the diet will, according to Dr. Art Mollen, sap the immune system and promote the formation of free radicals, a class of compounds implicated in the aging process. Moreover, excess intake of meat is directly related to higher rates of cancer and heart diseases. For instance, New Zealand has one of the highest rates of cancer and heart disease in the world, presumably because New Zealanders consume plenty of sheep. So also are Australians and Canadians who consume a lot of beef and chicken. By contrast, those mountaineers living in the Urals and Pamirs who have little animal meat to consume enjoy an average lifespan of over 100 years.[12] That is why Dr. Sun Yatsen, the father of Chinese Republic and a professionally trained Western doctor, clearly told us: "It is a universally acknowledged fact that vegetarian diets are the secret to longer life."[13] Therefore, eating less protein will enable you to lose weight and lower your blood pressure and cholesterol levels, while enhancing your immunity and slowing the aging process.[13] This may explain why vege-

tarians tend to enjoy longer average lifespan than nonvegetarians.

Yes, our body needs proteins, fats, cholesterol, and complex carbohydrates. However, as we habitually use refined, high-fat, and sugary foods, the insulin switch is turned on and its opposite hormone, glucagon, does not have a chance to interfere and work for our health. Glucagon can speed up the transformation of fat into energy and thus make us slim and energetic. When it does not function properly, we experience additional problems such as water retention and insomnia.

Cholesterol

Cholesterol is perhaps the most talked about aspect of nutrition nowadays. Cholesterol is the precursor of all sex hormones in the body. It was isolated in the eighteenth century and was first seriously studied by a German scientist named Windhaus. It is a waxy substance that occurs naturally in all parts of the body. It travels in the blood in packages called lipoproteins. In fact, cholesterol is something everyone needs in order to make many hormones and vitamin D, to produce bile acid, and to process the fats one takes in. There are two kinds of cholesterol. One is known as high-density lipoproteins (HDL), which is helpful to our health. The other type is called low-density lipoproteins (LDL), the bad cholesterol. LDL comes into our body mainly through consuming saturated fatty foods.

A normal body will produce enough cholesterol to meet its daily needs. However, an average American consumes anywhere from 300 milligrams to 400 milligrams of cholesterol a day, more than double the amount our body needs. It is now well known that excess cholesterol stored in our body can cause various heart disorders. Cholesterol is not soluble in the blood, and therefore can easily be deposited if there is an excess amount of it in the bloodstream. When there is too much cholesterol in the blood, the excess cholesterol piles up in the artery walls, narrowing the passages that supply vital blood to the heart, and slowing or even blocking the flow of the blood. If a blood clot forms in the narrowed artery, a heart attack or even death can occur.

Why do some people have too much cholesterol? Poor diet is one of the major reasons. Saturated fat and red meat can raise the cholesterol level significantly, and only one high-fat meal a day is enough to expose you to a greater risk of high cholesterol. Indeed, living on a fatty, salty diet can have a variety of nasty consequences, including obesity, impotence, and heart disease.

On the contrary, low-fat foods such as fruits and vegetables have favorable effects on the cholesterol makeup of the body. For one thing, such foods contain a large amount of vitamin C. A study of 827 people by the USDA and the National Institutes of Health examined their subjects' vitamin C intake and cholesterol profiles. Researchers found that people with high levels of vitamin C in their blood also had high levels of HDL, the helpful cholesterol that lowers the risk of heart attack.

Fiber

Another devastating characteristic of processed foods is the shortage of fiber. Fiber is hardly ever absorbed by the body, and only passes through our body, leaving it in a form basically the same as when it entered. But it is essential in maintaining the colon and modulating blood sugar. The normal Chinese diet has always been high in fiber, and the digestive system evolves to depend on this nutrition for its proper function. Moreover, fiber in the diet binds cholesterol and helps eliminate it from the body. Fiber also helps to prevent heart disease, hypertension, and obesity.

Fiber deficiency is a result of a refined food diet, which inevitably leads to the following physiognomic consequences:

- Obesity: Fiber contains no calories, and therefore does not lead to obesity. Moreover, it can even prevent the body's indiscriminate absorption of dietary fats by literally taking some of them away with it as it exits the body, just as river water takes away some of the sand as it flows down the basin. In the absence of fiber, all the fats one takes in will stay in the body, leading to obesity and hypertension.

- Constipation: Fiber helps bowel motions because it absorbs water, making the feces soft and enabling them to move down the large intestine more easily. A shortage of fiber slows down the bowel movement, leading to difficulty in motion.

- Coronary artery disease: Since the primary function of fiber is to provide stool bulk by absorbing water and speeding up the process of bowel movement, it is able to keep cholesterol out of the blood by inhibiting its absorption in the intestine. Thus, a shortage of fiber could increase the risk of cholesterol-induced coronary artery disease.

- Colon cancer: Since fiber can speed up the passage of potential carcinogens through the large intestine, it reduces the chance of their staying in the colon and developing into local malign tumors.

- Diabetes: A shortage of fiber in the diet disturbs the production of insulin by the pancreas. This leaves excess sugar in the blood system.

- Diverticular disease: Constipation resulting from lack of fiber will cause ruptures of the walls of the large intestine after repeated laboring at bathroom, thus leading to hemorrhoids and diverticulosis.

A nasty consequence of processed foods is that they can clog up the colon (including the large intestine and rectum). Researchers have found that wastes piled up inside the body for more than two days will generate poisonous materials, which are blamed for many forms of diseases, such as insomnia, impotence, indigestion, and depression. If you are already sick, slowing down bowel movements is bound to aggravate your situation. This is one way in which a body full of refined foods becomes a breeding ground for diseases.

The ill function of our "disposal system" can trigger off a chain reaction in various organs and body systems, such as the liver, the kidneys, the lymph, the lungs, and the circulatory system. For example, if the liver is damaged by bowel dysfunction or inaction, the blood becomes polluted. This allows alien substances to have a chance to alter the cell's structure. This change may even set the stage for cancer. Therefore, Chinese doctors always check their patients' record of bowel movements before making a diagnosis and writing a prescription.

To maintain smooth, regular bowel movements, we must supply our body with a large quantity and variety of fiber-rich foods such as fresh vegetables, fruits, nuts, and wholesome grains. Another health benefit of eating a variety of foods is that it ensures you get all the nutrients you need to fight disease. Complex carbohydrate foods contain plenty of fiber, which is the indigestible residue of food that passes through the entire bowel and is then eliminated in the stool. That is why carbohydrates are rarely stored as fat, even if eaten to excess. In that case, the excess is generally burned up in wasteful metabolic reactions that tend to increase the body's metabolic rate. This is a healthy indicator. In other words, the thermal effect of carbohydrates is much higher than the thermal effect of fats, animal fats in particular.

Colon cancer alone is no joking matter in this country. Colon cancer strikes 130,000 Americans each year.[15] The rarely told story is that this cancer is completely preventable. According to Dr. David Alberts, director of the cancer prevention and control program at the Arizona Cancer Center in Tucson, colon cancer is one of the most preventable cancers (next only to lung cancer). "If people take steps to prevent colon cancer, we could virtually wipe the disease out," Alberts said. Researchers have long observed that Chinese people who eat a diet low in fat and high in vegetables, fruits, and wholesome grains have only one-tenth of the chance of dying from colon cancer that Americans do. By contrast, high-fat diets that contain little fiber from naturally grown products can promote the development of colon cancer.

The key difference between these two types of diets lies—from the viewpoint of colon cancer—in a substance known as insoluble fiber, found mostly in fruits, vegetables, and whole grains. Insoluble fiber, so-called because it passes through the body virtually undigested and intact, promotes the buildup of water in stools, which in turn reduces the time food stays in the colon, facilitates bowel movements, and thus prevents the development of colon cancer. The longer digested food stays in the colon, the greater the chance that bacteria will grow and release toxic chemicals, including fecal bile acid.

The prevention of colon cancer and other related diseases lies, therefore, in a simple lifestyle change from a high-fat, refined food diet to a low-fat, high-fiber diet combined with proper exercise. A colon-cancer preventive diet consists of six to ten servings of fruits and vegetables a day, and at least one portion of wholesome grains, plus plenty of water and fruit juice. Of special importance is breakfast, which should consist of whole-grain cereal and fruits only. In fact, such a healthy diet is not only important to preventing colon disease, but vital to good overall health. It was found that a diet high in fruits and vegetables almost always reduces the risk of cancers of the lung, colon, pancreas, stomach, bladder, cervix, ovary, and endometrium.[16] People who eat the most of these foods have half the cancer risk of people who eat the least. For every vegetable and fruit contains hundreds of phytochemicals, many of which are potent cancer fighters.

Phytochemicals are what give fruits and vegetables their flavor and color. They are a plant's immune system, combating disease and the disastrous effects of ultraviolet rays and air and water pollution. Scientists have discovered that they can do the same for humans if we take them in sufficient quantities. A phytochemical reduces free radical-generating oxidation and reduces the cytotoxic effects of low-density lipoproteins, or the bad cholesterol. In humans, phytochemicals help prevent heart attack, cancer, stroke, hypertension, high cholesterol, and arthritis. A 1993 study showed that phytochemicals can protect DNA. He also found that such nutrients reduce the incidence, number, and size of mammary tumors in rats.

Complex carbohydrate foods contain, besides phytochemicals, multiple nutrients such as potassium and antioxidant vitamins. Potassium is an aging fighter. Antioxidant vitamins contained in tomatoes or green vegetables can boost immunity, slow the corrosion of aging cell membranes, and protect your heart. By eating mainly vegetables and fruits, you bathe yourself in cancer-fighting phytochemicals and bone-saving calcium.

Also fatally lacking in refined foods are some vital metabolic catalysts called enzymes. Most of our comfort foods are sadly enzyme-deficient, a fact which is held accountable for the widespread cases of arthritis, indigestion, and premature aging in America. This issue of enzymes is present not only in the foods themselves; it has a lot to do with the way they are prepared as well. It has been found that food microwaved, irradiated, canned, frozen, or overcooked is also enzyme-deficient.

We are very much prisoners of our own culture and tradition. This can be a good or a bad thing, depending on which culture you are born into. In Asian countries, the diet is primarily whole grains, vegetables, fruits, and sea foods. Sea vegetables like seaweed and kelp all contain rich trace minerals and calcium not available in vegetables grown in the ground. These nutrients are shown to have marvelous preventative and curing effects on many kinds of diseases such as

bronchitis and even cancer. In Western society, however, the mainstream diet is eggs, red meat, dairy products, and refined foods. Typical American diets, for instance, get 40 percent of their calories from fat, and 70 percent of protein from red meat. A comparative study of general health levels between Eastern and Western peoples can tell us, even in the absence of more rigorous scientific proof, that the Asian diet is much healthier than its Occidental counterpart.

It is important that diets become a major part of a cultural exchange. For the sake of our own health, we must be ready to give up comfort foods in favor of natural, fresh foods, especially vegetables, fruits, beans, and whole grains. We should make these foods the heart of most meals. This is the surest way to get plenty of vitamins, fiber, protein, folic acid, and antioxidants—the building materials of a strong body defense system against hypertension, cancer, heart disease, and other modernization diseases.

Salt

Salt is another major contributing factor to many chronic diseases. For the sake of taste and flavor we have a tendency to add too much salt to our diet. The refined foods we get from grocery stores are overloaded with sugar and salt. Salt has no vitamins, no minerals, no protein, no fiber, no nutrients of any kind. Salt robs calcium from the body and attacks the mucous lining throughout the entire gastrointestinal tracts. An excess intake of salt has been shown to be closely related to hypertension, neurasthenia, constipation, kidney diseases, edema, swollen tissues, and gastric cancer. This is because too much salt in the body retains fluid, increasing the blood pressure, and predisposing the person to problems such as swelling of the legs. Meanwhile, the heart has to work harder with the increased amount of blood volume. A high gastric cancer rate has been discovered in Japan where fish is often preserved in salt.

Excess salt intake is especially damaging to the kidneys. In traditional Chinese medicine, salt is thought to work directly on the kidneys. Unfortunately, Americans on average have the highest daily salt intake in the world. Although opinions differ as to how much salt is enough per person per day, the average amount is thought to be one gram per day. Americans, on average, consume at least twenty times that amount. This excess is due to the high amount of salt hidden in our diet, such as in breads, cheese, ham, bacon, and numerous staple foods. In contrast, the ancient Chinese who sought immortality lived in the mountains and consumed no salt at all. They lived on fresh fruits and berries. They were very healthy, and had never heard of the many degenerative diseases we have now.

Food Energies

Another significant discovery by the ancient Chinese is that different foods possess different energies, and thus impact the human body in different ways. Foods were divided into two categories by means of the universal polarities yin and yang: warm and cold.

Warm and hot foods, for instance, are considered to possess yang characteristics and are capable of warming up the body, stimulating sexual vitality, and facilitating blood circulation. These foods are excellent for the winter season and are particularly good for patients afflicted with cold or yin diseases. Goat, ginger, dates, pepper, garlic, wine, lichee and longon (Chinese fruits), and chicken all fall into this category. Thus, when a person suffers from cold diseases, it is important that he or she takes in foods that are warm and hot in nature, to counter the effect of these diseases.

Yin foods are cold and can nourish the kidneys and calm the spirit as well as the organs. They are therefore good for the summer months. They are particularly good for patients with "hot" diseases such as insomnia, constipation, nosebleeds, and blurred eyesight.

The ancient Chinese hold that people themselves are born with different energy types. Some are clearly biased towards yin, others towards yang, while others fit somewhere inbetween. This classification of energy types with regard to human beings is completely independent of gender. However, it has a lot to do with the food one eats. The dietary principle working here is one of balance and harmony. Thus, for those biased towards yin, more "warm" or yang foods should be consumed to keep the balance between yin and yang. Similarly, those born of yang-biased energy type should consume more "cool" or yin foods to keep the balance. Those who are born in the middle of the yin-yang spectrum are especially blessed as they fare equally well with yin and yang foods, and are allowed by nature to enjoy a greater variety of foods.

Besides the individual's body energy type, the ancient Chinese also regarded climate and the seasons as important considerations in determining which types of food should be made the major dietary components. Since the Chinese philosophy holds that man is a microcosm of the universe and must live in sync with his macroenvironment to maintain good health, the kind of food he eats should be in sync with the four seasons. This is known as the principle of "eating in season" in the Chinese natural health care system. In other words, the system recommends an adherence to a diet that is appropriate to the season.

Winter is considered a season of conservation and rest in preparation for the coming spring. In this cold environment, one should eat more warm and hot yang-foods, such as mutton and pepper, so as to strengthen the internal yang energy and overcome the cold, yin weather. For exactly

the opposite reason, one is advised to eat more cool, yin-natured foods, such as pears, honey, wax gourd, watermelon, and sea vegetables in the summer to block the hot, yang weather in the environment.

In spring, one should eat more foods with a sweet taste, such as dates, beets, and sweet potatoes, in order to nourish the liver. This is because the spring season stands for wood in the theory of the five elements, and thus corresponds to the liver. (Refer to chapter two for discussion of the five elements.) In a similar fashion, in autumn one should eat more juicy, oily foods, such as fruits, pure water, and juice, as well as vegetable oils. This is because autumn is a dry, windy season that requires a greater intake of water and oil to lubricate the internal organs of the body.

This delicate classification of foods and their compatibility with individuals is a characteristic of Chinese dietary culture that contrasts sharply with the indiscriminate use of foods here in the States.

Caffeine

Other dietary components that are popular in America are coffee and commercial soft drinks. Coffee has been the Western counterpart of tea for hundreds of years, while commercial soft drinks have, in the past two decades, taken away part of the market traditionally monopolized by coffee. Today, at least half of all Americans drink coffee, and almost 60 percent consume soft drinks.

Caffeine is basically an addictive drug that can cause headaches, irritability, muscle twitching, and rapid heart rate. It interferes with a peaceful sleep, and can be conducive to cancers of the prostate, bladder, and the pancreas.

As expected, the harm that caffeine can do to our health is much greater for children than for adults. This is because caffeine stays in the body of a child longer than in that of an adult. For instance, it takes about five hours for an adult body to clear the amount of caffeine contained in a cup of coffee, but it takes twenty hours for a teenage body to process the same amount of caffeine. Caffeine is also more harmful to women than men. A number of studies have shown the negative effects that caffeine consumption by pregnant women has on their unborn babies. These effects include prenatal death, delivery complications, lower birth weight, as well as infertility.

Tea

The Chinese did not drink coffee until the end of nineteenth century when the influence of the West began. Instead, they have a long tradition of generously and regularly consuming tea. For them, it is almost a way of life. While both coffee and tea contain caffeine, there are some important differences between the two. For one thing, tea contains less caffeine than coffee. More importantly, tea—green tea in particular—contains healthy enzymes that are beneficial to your health. Green tea also has a number of therapeutic functions that are absent in coffee. First, it cleanses the internal organs, especially the stomach and intestines. As such, it has the ability to prevent and cure stomach and intestinal ailments, including cancers in these portions of the body. Second, tea can prevent the oxidization of cholesterol in the body, thus preventing arteriosclerosis and heart diseases.

The most exciting news about tea is the recent discovery of catechins—the most powerful antioxidants generously contained in tea. Lester Mitscher, a chemist at the University of Kansas, reported in 1997 that catechin is 100 times more powerful than vitamin C and twenty-five times more effective than vitamin E in halting oxygen damage to DNA. Earlier in 1992, Dr. Hasan Mukhtar of Case Western Reserve University showed that mice that were given green tea and exposed to chemical carcinogens or ultraviolet light developed an astonishing 90 percent fewer tumors than those that were not given tea. When exposed to catechins, Mukhtar says, malignant cancer cells commit "suicide" while normal cells aren't affected. According to him, the difference may have to do with an "antioxidant-responsive" gene that is especially active in cancer cells. According to Jerry Jankun, a tumor biologist at the Medical College of Ohio, even after cancer starts, catechins can help stop it from spreading by blocking an enzyme that tumors use to grow new capillaries.[17]

However, the medical benefits of tea catechins are not limited to fighting cancer. Studies in Japan indicate that catechins have an anticlotting effect on the blood and also lower blood lipids without reducing HDL, the so-called "good" cholesterol. Researchers were at first puzzled over the fact that the heart disease rate is so low in Japan, compared to most other industrialized nations, especially as the smoking rate in Japan is higher. Eventually, they found the secret, which lies in the fact that the Japanese, like the Chinese, are heavy drinkers of tea. A fifteen-year study of men in the Netherlands concluded that those who drank more than four cups of green tea a day were 69 percent less likely than others to suffer a stroke. Studies of mice in Japan suggest that catechins also help protect tissues from sun damage, cigarette smoke, air pollutants, and radiation. Some bacteria seem susceptible to catechins as well. Asian studies have shown that green tea inhibits bad breath, gum disease, and tooth decay in laboratory rats.[18]

While both black tea and green tea contain catechins, green tea is far more beneficial to our health. This is because black tea leaves have to be fermented to promote flavor. This production process destroys a lot of the catechins. By contrast, green tea leaves are not fermented and are therefore healthier. To catch the full benefit of tea, one should drink at least three cups a day.

Smoking

Another fierce enemy of our health is cigarette smoking. Though not a dietary factor, cigarettes are listed here because they are mainly consumed through the mouth like foods. The first alarming fact about cigarettes is that it has a stranglehold on about 50 million Americans. As is universally known today, cigarettes contain nicotine, which is an extremely addictive substance. (In fact, more addictive than cocaine.) People smoke for different reasons, but mainly for pleasure and to avoid unpleasant situations or feelings. For many smokers, cigarettes are antidepressive and help them concentrate, remember, and think more quickly. For such short-term benefits, they are consciously willing to trade their health and even their lives. This alone shows how addictive a substance nicotine is.

According to an expert estimation, 50 million Americans are smoking, a bad habit which is responsible for one out of every five American deaths, killing over 400,000 people in the U.S. each year and costing $50 billion annually in medical expenses alone.[19] This does not take into account the loss of income due to illness and premature death as a result of smoking. Smoking is unequivocally linked to lung cancer, responsible for an estimated 97 percent of all lung cancers in men and 74 percent of those in women.[20] Almost all lung cancer patients reported that they have been long-term, heavy cigarette smokers. This is because the membranes lining the lungs can absorb cancer-producing chemicals from the tobacco when deeply inhaled. The protective mechanisms by which the lungs rid themselves of impurities are first paralyzed and then destroyed by tobacco smoke. Prolonged exposure to the smoke causes changes in the lung cells that signal the early development of cancer. Deaths from lung cancer are about six times more frequent among men who smoke regularly than among nonsmokers.

Lung cancer is just the first in a long list of smoking-related health problems. Tobacco is a far bigger villain than most of us could ever imagine. Besides lung cancer, smoking is the single most important cause of cancer of the lungs, kidneys, mouth, throat, bladder, breast, cervix, larynx, nose, and esophagus. Nationwide surveys found the following sobering facts about smoking:[21]

- Smoking causes 40 percent of all cases of bladder cancer, accounting for more than 4,000 new cases annually.

- Up to one-third of all cases of cervical cancer are directly attributed to smoking, accounting for 7,000 new cases a year.

- Women who smoke have a 75 percent higher chance of developing breast cancer than nonsmokers.

- Smoking causes 40 percent of all cases of kidney cancer.

- People who smoke a pack of cigarettes a day are twenty-five times more likely to develop laryngeal cancer.

- Smoking at least doubles the risk of gastrointestinal cancer.

- Smoking causes the vast majority of all cancers of the mouth, lips, cheek, tongue, salivary glands, and tonsils.

- Smoking accounts for 80 percent of all cases of esophageal cancer, leading to 15,000 American deaths each year.

- Smoking is responsible for the vast majority of deaths from throat cancer which kills about 4,000 Americans a year.

According to a report presented by the World Health Organization, it is estimated that in the next twenty-five years, deaths related to smoking will total 8.4 million.

Since smoking decreases the body's absorption of insulin, it is conducive to diabetes and exacerbates the damage to small blood vessels in the ears, eyes, and feet of diabetics. Meanwhile, carbon monoxide and other poisonous gases in tobacco smoke replace oxygen in the blood cells, promote coronary spasms, and cause accumulation of clot-producing platelets, exposing smokers to a much higher risk of heart disease. Smoking also interferes with the blood in a way that makes blood fats more apt to stick to artery walls. If you are also overweight, the chances are that you have an overabundance of these fats for smoking to work its ill effects on.

Smoking is also found to double the risk of strokes, and the risk is almost ten times greater for women than for men. Premature aging also has a lot to do with smoking. Constant exposure to tobacco smoke prematurely wrinkles the facial skin and yellows the teeth and fingernails. According to Dr. Peter Proctor, a dermatologist and research pharmacologist in Houston, tobacco smoke damages the linings of blood vessels, which produce less nitric oxide, and this might inhibit hair growth and "age" hair follicles prematurely.

Even if you are not a smoker, passive smoking, or secondhand smoke, can have disastrous health hazards, too. A report published in *USA Today* and *The New York Times* carries the results of a survey on secondhand smoking conducted by researchers at the Harvard School of Medicine.[22] The survey started in 1982 and involved 32,046 women. The conclusion of the survey is frightening: secondhand smoke almost doubles the risk of heart disease. The available evidence also indicates that chronic exposure to passive smoke increases the risk of heart disease by at least 30 percent among nonsmokers.

Another study found that couples with at least one member who smokes are three times more likely to have trouble conceiving than nonsmoking couples. This is because tobacco smoke interferes with the implantation of a fertilized egg within the uterus. It reduces the quantity of sperm cells in a man's semen and increases the number of abnormal sperm cells and a man's risk of penile cancer. After conception, smoking women are more likely to miscarry or deliver prematurely than nonsmoking women. Some researchers have come to the conclusion that toxins in the bloodstream of pregnant smokers pass through the placenta to the fetus, sowing the seeds for future cancer. Youngsters with smoking parents have six times as many respiratory infections as the children of nonsmoking parents. Children of smokers face an increased risk of coughing, asthma, chronic bronchitis, and pneumonia. These children also face a higher risk of middle ear infections. There is even evidence to suggest that smoking fathers may contribute to the risk of having stillborn or malformed babies.

The real vice is, of course, the nicotine that cigarettes contain. Nicotine in any form has a negative effect on small blood vessels. Nicotine damages the tiny particles in the blood called platelets, which in turn become garbage, contributing to the build-up of plaque inside the artery walls. Nicotine also stimulates the production of chemical substances called catecholamines, which are known to increase the heart rate, blood pressure, and the oxygen needs of the heart. These effects may have serious consequences in a heart already short of adequate nourishment, because blood vessels are being narrowed by nicotine-created plaque. As if this is not enough, nicotine further infuses the blood with carbon monoxide. This thickens the blood, reducing its ability to transport oxygen, and causes clotting in arteries that have been narrowed by plaque.

Nicotine also has a pronounced effect on the stomach, causing ulcers. Nicotine tends to reduce the bicarbonate output of the pancreas, thus creating the kind of acid conditions on which ulcers thrive. As far as the effects of cigarettes on the brain, they are also negative; smoking impairs both short-term and long-term memory.

Does smoking have anything to do with your sexual vitality? The answer is a definite yes. Cigarette smoking may make you look or feel sexy, but its effects are just the opposite—sexually dampening. For one thing, heavy smoking in men has been found to reduce male hormone levels, and inactivate, and even destroy, sperm. Chronic smoking lowers men's testosterone levels, reduces their sexual vitality, and leads to impotence and sterility. In fact, many people suffering from impotence are heavy smokers. If you stop smoking for just a couple of weeks you will notice a marked difference in your sexual performance.

Researchers at the Boston University School of Medicine examined the medical histories and penile X-rays of 195 impotent men, whose average age was thirty-five. All of them had blockages in their penile arteries. The smokers all had significantly worse blockages than the nonsmokers. The longer a man smoked, the greater was the clogging of the penile arteries. Since the arteries in the penis are responsible for male potency, the conclusion is inescapable: smoking can cause impotence at an early age. The study also found that smoking aggravates penile artery blockage in men who have experienced groin trauma resulting from accidents, such as falling off a bike.

The intensity of smoking (meaning the number of packs per day), coupled with the length of time one has been smoking, largely determines the risk of developing lung and nasal cancer and emphysema. It is estimated that every pack of cigarettes smoked takes away two hours of life. Smokers of a pack or more of cigarettes a day are two times as likely to die from lung cancer, bronchitis, emphysema, or heart disease, and take as much as nine precious years away from their lives as a result. If you smoke ten cigarettes each and every day, your risk of death from lung cancer will be at least three times as high as that of a nonsmoker. Your risk of dying from pneumonia will also be at least three times as high, and your risk of dying from a stroke will be at least twice as high as that of a nonsmoker.

Today smoking is recognized as one of the major threats to the health of people around the world. It not only poses a serious threat to the smokers, but also to those "passive smokers" who happen to be in close contact with smokers.

For women, the risks from smoking are even higher. Smoking increases the chance of lung cancer in women by twelve times. Another study finds that women receive a higher nicotine level than men when smoking the same amount of cigarettes. It also poses some gender-specific threats to women and their children. For instance, smoking lowers the rate of estrogen production in women. As a result, smoking women reach menopause at an average of 1.74 years earlier than nonsmoking women.[23] Smoking is also conducive to infertility.

Smoking is intimately linked to infant mortality, low birth weight, and other physical and mental impairments. Indeed, cigarette smoking is the largest known risk factor for low birth weight because it retards fetus growth. Smoking women are about twice as likely to deliver an underweight baby than nonsmoking women. The Surgeon General has reported that cigarette smoking during pregnancy is associated with fetal growth retardation and infant death. Smoking during pregnancy has been linked to 20 to 30 percent lower birth weight, an average of 142 grams lighter than those born to nonsmoking mothers. About 30 percent of all low birth weight cases can be avoided if mothers do not smoke during pregnancy. Studies show that women who quit smoking during their pregnancy had a lower rate of low birth weight.

Of course, the health benefits of stopping smoking, or better still, not smoking in the first place, goes far beyond infant birth weight. For instance, when people stop smoking, their risk of lung cancer and heart disease dramatically decreases. Evidence shows that ten years after quitting smoking, the heart and lung tissues of some ex-smokers can be restored to their original vitality, greatly reducing the risk of death from heart disease and lung cancer. Of course, the earlier one stops smoking the better.

Alcohol

Another enemy of our health that creeps into our body through the mouth is alcohol. Alcohol directly affects our liver, heart, and respiratory and nervous systems. It adds pressure to the liver, causes clogging of the blood vessels, and inhibits the body's ability to burn fat, because the liver, which normally burns fat, is too busy processing the alcohol. Consequently, the fat gets stored—around the waists of men and in the hips and thighs of women. This is why regular, heavy drinking alone can make you overweight. Another significant reason why regular drinking can make you obese is because most alcoholic drinks contain a lot of calories.

Regular alcohol users also run the risk of developing cirrhosis of the liver, acute pancreatitis, inflammation of the esophagus, diabetes, exacerbation of peptic ulcers, hormonal deficiencies, gastrointestinal disorders, liver cancer, ulcers, stomach bleeding, stool bleeding, hemorrhoids, kidney stones, amenorrhea (failure to menstruate), hypertension, and stroke. Researchers find that the risk of death from cirrhosis for someone who drinks three times a week is ten times as high as that of a nondrinker. Also, the risk of death from a car accident is twice as high for a drinker as it is for a nondrinker.

Alcohol depresses the respiratory system and the muscles, a double whammy that can severely inhibit the ability to breathe. Excessive drinking also leads to mental depression. Many people have started drinking because they want to forget their worries and relieve stress. Unfortunately, the effect is just the opposite. Alcohol may temporarily make you oblivious to your problems, but down the road, it is likely to make you even more stressed when the effects of the alcohol have gone. The ancient Chinese wrote about this situation in this way: "Using alcohol to depress the depression will make you all the more stressful, just like cutting flowing water with a knife cannot stop the water from flowing." Thus, an alcoholic locks himself up in a vicious cycle of destruction.

As with tobacco, alcohol consumption presents a greater health risk for women than for men. The fact is that women usually get intoxicated faster than men even if they have consumed the same amount of alcohol. There are several reasons for this. First, women generally weigh less than men do, so the same amount of alcohol is concentrated in a smaller body mass. Second, women typically have a higher percentage of body fat and less body water than men. Since alcohol dissolves much more easily in water than in fat, the difference in body composition means that when alcohol enters a woman's body, it stays there longer and has a more lasting effect. Third, there is an enzyme in the stomach (alcohol dehydrogenase) that metabolizes alcohol before it gets into the bloodstream, and that enzyme is about four times as active in men than in women. So even if a man and a woman weigh the same, have the same proportion of body fat and drink the same amount of wine, more pure alcohol is likely to reach a woman's blood system than a man's.

Heavy alcohol consumption by women is also shown to be associated with breast cancer and reproductive problems. This is largely because alcohol increases the estrogen levels along with other numerous effects on hormone production in the body. Women who heavily consume alcohol have been found to have a 39 percent lower level of dehydroepiandrosterone, the mother of all hormones—a precursor of testosterone, which is the most potent naturally occurring androgen—and the source of human immune power, 65 percent higher testosterone level, and 23 percent lower progesterone level.[24]

In men, like smoking, alcohol consumption has been shown to be a direct cause of impotence. Excess alcohol decreases the body's ability to produce testosterone, a hormone that has a tremendous effect on fitness, sexual vitality, and body composition including muscles, bones, and blood. Dr. Susan Rake, author of *The Hormone of Desire: The Truth about Sexuality, Menopause, and Testosterone*, holds that without testosterone, sexual desire, sexual pleasure, and sexual function are all compromised. Dr. Rake cites a Massachusetts male aging study in which almost 2,000 men experienced a decline of testosterone accompanied with various degrees of sexual dysfunction. Therefore, heavy drinkers are more likely to lose their sexual desire, and become impotent and sterile.

Before we shift our topic to other dietary components, a few words of justice must be said about wine and other alcoholic products. Poetically referred to as the "substance in the cup" in China, alcohol has been one of the greatest of human fascinations for thousands of years. As such, it must possess some merits in itself. In fact, alcohol does not speak all that poorly for itself if one knows how to take advantage of it, rather than being taken advantage of by it.

For one thing, alcohol has been a constant source of inspiration for literary people. It is well known that many of the greatest poets in the world composed their best poems after drinking. (Alexander Pushkin, the founder of modern Russian literature, and Li Po and Du Fu, two of the greatest poets in China's history, are good examples.) Today, this inspirational effect of alcohol has extended its application into the commercial world. In China, at least, it is almost a prerequisite for commercial success, because almost all major commercial deals are signed at dinner tables full of wine.

As has been mentioned before, many people take to drinking because of depression. There is a famous Chinese saying that says, "Use alcohol to kill worry." Worry is a fact of life. As long as people have desires and needs to satisfy, they are bound to run into worries. This is especially the case with modern humans. Drinking can make us temporarily forget about the stresses in our lives. Moderate drinking can reduce stress and anxiety levels, and induce feelings of relaxation and con-

viviality. This is because a moderate amount of alcohol has an anxiety-relieving, mood-elevating effect. A moderate amount of drinking means a small glass of wine a day.

Alcohol—on the condition that it is taken moderately—has a therapeutic effect on various ailments such as stomach ailments, arthritis, rheumatism, and injuries from falls, fractures, contusions, and strains. Alcohol relieves fractures and strains mainly through its ability to promote blood circulation in the body, especially to the injured part of the body, where blood is clotted or extravagated. Alcohol also appears to encourage the development of high-density lipoproteins (HDL), the good cholesterol, because it can keep the bad cholesterol (LDL) from accumulating on artery walls.

Researchers at the University of Pittsburgh found that moderate drinking by postmenopausal women increases their estrogen levels, which may in turn reduce their risk of developing heart disease and arthritis. Nearly a dozen major studies in several countries have linked moderate drinking to a lower occurrence of heart attack caused by blood clots. For instance, researchers have come to the conclusion that red wine deserves the credit for the low rate of heart disease in France, even though the French are among the heaviest consumers of red meat. The reason, they said, is because red wine can prevent cholesterol from oxidization, thus reducing the risk of arteriosclerosis. Here, as elsewhere, the golden rule is moderation.

Another study found that a moderate intake of up to three glasses of red wine a day can help stave off coronary heart disease by dilating small blood vessels and increasing the blood flow to the tissues. It is also found that beer, with lower than 5 percent alcohol content, contains multiple nutrients necessary for health, such as protein, calcium, and riboflavin. Beer has also a benign cooling and regulating effect on the body. A Japanese scientist discovered that beer is a great promoter of urination, even greater than water. It also facilitates the production of stomach hormones and the release of stomach acid, thus promoting digestion and enhancing appetite. Beer can also prevent and treat hypertension and kidney diseases.

Grape wine possesses similar good medical values. It has been found that moderate consumption of grape wine can enhance the body's ability to absorb zinc from the diet. Zinc is a vital mineral for digestion and sperm production. That explains why moderate, regular consumption of grape wine can promote our appetite and sexual vitality. Again, moderate consumption is considered about one glass a day.

The beneficial effects of moderate drinking on heart attacks is also well documented. For instance, Arthur L. Klatsky, an M.D. at the Kaiser-Permanente Medical Center in Oakland, California, conducted a study on 120,000 people and found that those who drank moderately were 30 percent less likely to suffer heart attacks than were nondrinkers. Independent of age, sex, or prior

related disease, even people who drank six drinks a day had fewer heart attacks than teetotalers.[25]

Dr. Klatsky's findings are confirmed by Dr. Thomas Truelson and his colleagues at the Institute of Preventive Medicine in Copenhagen. Dr. Truelson did a sixteen-year study of more than 13,000 people. He found that those who drank between one to six glasses of wine had a 34 percent lower risk of stroke than those who never or hardly ever drank wine. This is because wine, especially red wine, contains plant compounds called tannins, flavonoids, and polyphenols, which can act as antioxidants and help stop fat from sticking to artery walls and clogging them.[26]

The latest scientific studies have revealed some encouraging benefits of moderate, regular alcoholic consumption. According to one report a few drinks a day can keep many diseases at bay. These vary from preventing ulcers and heart disease to protecting your eyes and mind from the ravages of age.[27] A recent study in Germany on 900 people found that those who had one or two drinks a day were 75 percent less likely to suffer from stomach ulcers. Moderate drinking of wine was associated with lower mortality, including heart disease and cancer.[28]

However, all scientists agree that the key to benefiting from drinking alcohol is moderation, defined as one to two glasses of wine or beer a day. There is a definite line between beneficial drinking and harmful alcoholism. Too much is as bad as too little—this is the essence of Confucianism.

Water

Finally, I want to say something about water. All too often, we tend to forget and neglect the significance of this omnipresent dietary component, because it is too cheap to merit our attention. It is good to keep in mind that water is contained in almost all dietary forms. In addition, we drink water in pure form every day. Water is simply indispensable to life.

No wonder that in Chinese philosophy, water comes first in order in the five basic elements of universe. Actually, the human body itself, like the earth, is largely made of this substance. Between 55 and 68 percent of the total mass of our bodies is made of water. Perhaps you do not know that even bones consist of one-third water. Muscle tone cannot be kept without adequate water either, for three-quarters of muscles are water. This is all designed by nature and therefore must be maintained in order to be healthy.

Violation of this natural law can have serious health consequences. In an extreme case, such as losing one-tenth of the water in our body, a condition known as dehydration, can result in death. Even a smaller loss of water will disturb the proper functioning of the body, causing many health problems. For example, when our water reserve falls below 1 percent of its norm, we feel thirsty. A loss of 6 percent of our water reserve will lead to fainting. Consequently, it is essential that we take in plenty of water every day to keep our body in good shape. Water is not only necessary for life. It can also help prevent many kinds of diseases, such as constipation, infection, and kidney problems.

The fact is that almost every fluid connected with life and living things is based on water. Human cells must have water to live and function. Dry out a living cell and it will stop working. Water in our body is used and consumed for multiple purposes: to help regulate the body's temperature, to digest food, to wash away bodily wastes, and to moisten the lungs and skin. Food cannot be digested without water. Water is needed in the process of hydrolysis in which proteins, starches, and fats are turned into nutrients that body cells can take. Not only the intestines, but also the kidneys, bladder, skin, and lungs depend on water to get rid of toxins. In particular, the kidneys use water quickly, and have a heavier dependence on our timely replenishment of water for their functioning.

The percentage of water in blood plasma is 90 percent. In a sense, losing water means losing blood. In addition, water keeps the body temperature at a normal level. This is essential in summer and dry seasons. It serves as a coolant for the body engine. Under very hot or dry conditions, the body can lose up to a quart of water through sweating alone. Water is also necessary for transporting nutrients, lubricating joints, and eliminating wastes in the body. Even the smallest deficit of water can make you sick. In fact, dehydration is a hidden, yet common, cause of fatigue and premature aging.

Indeed, water is an even more important and urgent daily necessity than food. We can survive for about two weeks without eating anything, but we can survive for no more than five days without drinking water. Although an individual's biological needs vary as to the timing of drinking water, the ancient Chinese have some golden advice for us. They suggest that we drink a cup of water as soon as we get up in the morning but considerably—at least fifteen minutes—before breakfast. This practice, especially when followed with religious consistency for years, will bear marvelously favorable effects on your health.

The ancient Chinese hold that this cup of water, called Holy Morning Water in ancient Chinese classics, is necessary to wash away the yin-qi (deadly spirit) that has accumulated in the body during sleep. With the extra yin-qi washed away, yang-qi (the lively spirit) begins to produce itself until a new balance is struck between the yin and the yang. As a result, we will feel doubly invigorated during the day.

Another direct benefit of drinking a cup of water first thing in the morning is that it serves to remind the body's biological clock that it is time for a bowel movement. It boosts our appetite and digestion functions. This effect is most obvious when we combine the drinking of water with morning exercises. Morning exercises cause the water we drink to flow more vigorously in the body, literally washing our bowels and internal organs, and eliminating dirty compounds through urination and perspiration.

The ancient Chinese also recommended that we drink plenty of water between, but not too close to, meals. Make sure that there is enough lapse of time between when you drink water and when you take meals. The reason for this practice is that while indispensable to the body and health, water can dilute our digestive enzymes. As a consequence of this dilution, there will not be enough concentration of enzymes to digest the food we eat. Consequently, we may suffer from indigestion and eventually suffer from diseases of the stomach.

Quantity

For the sake of health, we not only need to keep a close eye on what we eat, but also on how much we eat. Since eating is a pleasant experience, we have a tendency to enjoy it too much. All too often, the desire of the mouth exceeds the real need of body. The mouth is a very poor judge of the nutritional need of the body; it only knows tastes. Another driving factor of overeating in America is the temptation to dine out. It is estimated that about 10 percent of all Americans eat virtually all their meals outside of the home. The bad thing about this practice is that, besides the problem of food hygiene, the meals almost always are big and heavy.

Modern surveys and research find that overeating can lead to hypertension, fatigue, bowel and liver toxicity, heart attack, and even cancer, in addition to obesity. The most immediate effect of overeating is the added pressure on our stomach and digestive system. It is easy to overwork the stomach and digestive system by putting too much in their systems. Both our stomach and digestive systems have a limited capacity. They simply cannot take the extra workload for too long without trouble and punishment.

Just like our bodies and minds, our digestive systems need rest and relaxation for maintenance and long-term efficiency. Neglecting this damages and lowers the function of the digestive system. Once our digestive system is in trouble, all other parts of our body will be hurt as a consequence, because the nutrition needed for the proper functioning of our body must go through the digestive system first before it can be used by the body.

Thousands of years ago, the ancient Chinese knew that overeating could damage our health. In the Chinese natural health care system, there is a binding principle regarding the amount of eating. It is to eat only until you are 70 to 80 percent full—when you feel that you are no longer hungry. The body reacts to an excessive food load by punishing the eater with various ailments.

It is also understood that each human body has a biological clock that reminds us when we are hungry and really in need of food. You do not need to worry about lack of nutrition; your body will let you know in time. In case of overeating, however, our bio-

logical clock gets dull, and we just have no way of knowing how much food we have taken in until it is too late.

The Chinese fathers told us that a normal person should eat no more than three meals a day, including a high-quality breakfast full of nutrition, a lunch that is the heaviest of all in terms of quantity, and a dinner that is the lightest of all in terms of quantity.

After a long night's sleep without food, our digestive system is in high gear. It is the optimal time for digestion, and we want to provide our body with the best foods at this time. Our body is in dire need of nutritional supplies to restore the glucose reserves to an appropriate level. Our brain cells get their energy supply mainly from glucose, which is derived entirely from food.

Our body also requires that we provide it with high-quality energy sources to meet the challenge of a new day. If we do not eat breakfast like many busy or lazy people do these days, or eat a poor breakfast in terms of quality and quantity, we will have a deficiency of glucose, making us tired, moody, and dizzy. If we fast for too long, we reduce the amount of digestive enzymes in the body, which leads to digestion and stomach problems. Therefore, breakfast is the most essential meal of the day.

At lunch time, after half a day's work—or play—most of the foods we have taken in as breakfast have been digested and used. There is another half day ahead of us. This requires that we take a relatively heavy meal at lunch. After work in the evening, our body is ready for rest and sleep, and our digestive system is in its lowest gear. Therefore, dinner should be light, otherwise food will get stagnant in the body and our sleep will be disturbed.

To prevent overeating, it is best to dine at home, eat sparingly, and chew thoroughly. Occasional fasting is another natural health technique that is recommended by the ancient Chinese. This is especially useful when you eat too much. It is a helpful and healthy practice to stop eating for one or two meals, so that your body can fully digest what you have taken in without additional burden. This is an effective natural means to cure indigestion and prevent obesity. Sometimes, I fast for a whole day as I feel that my stomach has enough work to do and I do not need additional nutrition for the time being. Not eating at all under such circumstances does not interfere with my normal work. Quite the contrary, I feel the better for it—physically and mentally. Not only do the minor ailments that are due to overeating completely disappear, but I emerge from a day's fasting with renewed vigor and spirit for my work.

Enzymes

Another dietary factor that has a significant impact on our health is the way we prepare foods. This is because the supply of dietary enzymes we get depends on the way we prepare the food. For one thing, fresh, natural foods contain rich enzymes, upon which depends almost all of our bodily functions.

However, if we use high temperatures to prepare and preserve foods, we destroy most of the vitamins. Therefore most of the comfort foods we find in stores today are enzyme deficient. This artificial depletion of dietary enzymes is, according to Dr. Howell, "one of the paramount causes of premature aging and early death and the underlying cause of almost all degenerative disease."[29]

Why are enzymes so vital to health? Enzymes are biochemical catalysts secreted by the pancreas and other organs and glands. These catalysts are indispensable for the proper functioning of human body. Some of them help in digestion and are therefore called digestive enzymes. Others enter the bloodstream to clear the blood of dead cells, dangerous microbes, and poisonous toxins, and still others are used to aid in metabolism and immunity. As such, they are vital to your overall health and well-being.

True, every one of us is born with a certain level of enzyme reserves. This should be looked upon as a strategic reserve and a precious substance, because our productivity of enzymes is very limited. Therefore, they should be used only as a last resort. So if we do not take in enough enzymes in our diet, the body automatically turns to the reserve for help. The consequence is that you are in danger of running out of the vital supply of enzymes. Once the enzyme level is low, digestion is affected, immunity runs low, and the body gets dirty as a result, leading to various health diseases. Therefore, you should eat fresh fruit and vegetables in their original form as people in ancient times did. Raw foods are the best source of enzymes. At least, you should not overcook them in the sense of both intensity of heat and length of time, nor overfreeze them.

Feelings

Equally true is the fact that a merry state of mind promotes digestion, whereas a stressful mind hampers digestion, and an angry mind will turn nutritious foods into poisons. This fact tends to be ignored by most people, but the Chinese natural health system considers it to be a crucial factor of dietary hygiene. Dr. Sun Shimiao, for instance, clearly warns his patients against eating while in a stressful and worrisome mood. Therefore, make sure that you come to the dinner table in a happy mood. If you are distressed or angry, do not eat immediately. Rather, calm down for several minutes with deep breathing, or by watching a light television program before you commit yourself to eating.

Much has been said about the significance of food and our diet on our health. To sum up this chapter on diet, I would like to provide the following checklists of do's and don'ts in terms of dietary health.

List of Dietary Do's

- Eat oatmeal or rice congee for breakfast. This is helpful because shortly after waking up, the stomach is not ready for heavier, more nutritious food. Oatmeal or rice congee can bring the stomach to its optimal functioning level and generate saliva, a vital substance in digestion and in maintaining overall health.

- Eat a heavy (but not too heavy) breakfast but a light dinner. The breakfast should be nutritional with sufficient vitamins, proteins, fiber, and other nutrients.

- Reduce significantly the sugar and salt in your diet.

- Reduce the fat in your diet.

- Build your meals around grains, rice, wholesome wheat products, potatoes, beans, and vegetables.

- Eat simple foods in their natural and raw forms.

- Eat at least two servings of fresh fruit each day.

- Eat one egg every day. Eggs contain multiple nutrients and are helpful to many kinds of diseases. It is best to eat your eggs boiled or poached. Frying the egg exposes the cholesterol to heat and oxygen, thus damaging the cholesterol by oxidizing it.

- Opt for fish instead of red meat. Fish is a high-protein, low-fat food.

- Eat one or two apples a day.

- Drink plenty of water each day, making sure to drink a glass right after you get up in the morning and before breakfast. Water taken on an empty stomach cleanses the bowels and causes them to move properly. Eighty percent of the body is made up of water. Drinking insufficient water on a regular basis dehydrates the body and the mind.

- Drink 10 ounces of orange juice each day.

- Drink at least two cups of green tea daily.

- Drink three spoonfuls of soup before each meal.

- Use skim milk and dairy products.

- Skip sugared cereals and select whole grains.

- Be cheerful while you are eating.

- Stop eating when you are 70 to 80 percent full.

- Chew seven times before you swallow.

- Take a spoonful of vinegar each day after your meal to aid in digestion.

- Use organic olive and vegetable oils instead of animal-based oils.

- Include garlic as a regular part of your daily diet. Garlic has been shown to have a number of therapeutic effects, the best being its ability to boost immunity.

List of Dietary Don'ts

- Don't smoke.

- Don't drink more than one alcoholic beverage a day.

- Don't drink alcohol on an empty stomach. If you must drink, do it after you have already taken some food.

- Avoid fried foods.

- Do not eat more than one serving of red meat per week.

- Don't eat poultry and meats produced with hormones to boost growth.

- Unless advised by doctors to the contrary, don't eat between three meals a day.

- Limit your intake of convenient and fast foods such as vacuum-packed or frozen precooked meals ready for the microwave oven, instant mashed potatoes and hot cereals, envelopes of soup, dessert, and sauce mixes. For these foods are high in fat and calories.

- Avoid microwaved or frozen foods.

- Don't eat foods while they are hot.

- Don't eat to the full capacity of your stomach.

- Don't eat while you are angry.

- Don't eat while you are deeply depressed or stressed.

- Don't talk while you are eating. Rather, concentrate your mind on the foods you are eating.

- Don't eat too quickly.

- Don't overcook foods, especially vegetables. You want to preserve the vitamins in them.

- Try not to use canned food. This is because in the process of preparing for canned food, a lot of the nutrients in the food are lost or destroyed.

- Don't wash rice too much before cooking.

Endnotes

1. John F. Potter, *How to Improve Your Odds Against Cancer* (Hollywood, FL: Frederick Fell Publishers, 1988).

2. According to Dr. Leonard A. Cohen, head of the section of nutritional endocrinology, the American Health Foundation, sugar causes the pancreas to produce a large amount of insulin very rapidly, which can have a harmful effect on the pancreas. *Healing Unlimited* (New York, NY: Boardroom Classics, 1995), 75.

3. Ibid., 80.

4. Ibid.

5. Hirotomo Ochi, *East Meets West: Super Nutrition from Japan* (Japan: Ishi Press International, 1989).

6. Bandaru S. Reddy and Leonard A. Cohen, *Diet, Nutrition and Cancer: A Critical Evaluation* (Burlington, NJ: Franklin Electronic Publishers, 1986).

7. Dan R. Harris, *Fitness and Exercise Sourcebook* (Detroit, MI: Omnigraphics, Inc., 1996), 57.

8. *The Merck Manual of Medical Information*, (Doylestown, PA: Merck Research Laboratories, 1997), 647.

9. Paul Kuehn, *Breast Care Options for the 1990s* (South Windsor, CT: Newmark Publishing Company).

10. R. Sinha and N. Rothman, "Role of Well-done, Grilled Red Meat, Heterocyclic Amines in the Etiology of Human Cancer," *Cancer Letters* (September 1, 1999): 189–94. M. J. Hill, "Meat and Colo-Rectal Cancer," *Proceedings of the Nutrition Society* 58, no. 2 (May 1999): 261–4.

11. *Healing Unlimited*, 29.

12. Editors of Tianhua Publishing Company, *The Vegetarian Diet, Health and Longevity* (Taipei, Taiwan: Tianhua Publishing Company, 1986).

13. Ibid.

14. *Healing Unlimited*, 297–9.

15. *Time*, 12 April 1999.

16. M. R. Forman et al., "The Effect of Dietary Intake of Fruits and Vegetables on the Odds Ratio of Lung Cancer Among Yunnan Tin Miners," *International Journal of Epidemiology* 21, no. 3 (June 1992): 437–41. W. Zheng et al., "Diet and Other Risk Factors for Laryngeal Cancer in Shanghai, China," *American Journal of Epidemiology* 136, no. 2 (July 15, 1992): 178–91.

17. Glenn Garelik, "Call Green Tea the Cure-all of Cure-alls," *Investor's Business Daily*, 28 September 1998.

18. Ibid.

19. *Public Health Sourcebook* (Detroit, MI: Omnigraphics, Inc., 1998), 57.

20. *American Scientist*, July/August 1981.

21. *Healing Unlimited*, 263–264.

22. *USA Today*, 20 May 1997.

23. S. M. McKinlay et al., "Smoking and Age at Menopause in Women," *Annals of Internal Medicine* 103, no. 3 (September 1985): 350–6.

24. M. Valimaki, "Pituitary-gonadal Hormones and Adrenal Androgens in Noncirrhotic Female Alcoholics After Cessation of Alcoholic Intake," *European Journal of Clinical Investigation*, 20, no. 2 (April 1990): 177–81.

25. *Annals of Internal Medicine* (August 1981).

26. "More Good News for Wine Drinkers—It Stops Stroke," *Reuters Limited*, 4 December 1998.

27. John Carpi, *Investor's Business Daily*, 19 January 1998.

28. S. C. Renaud et al., "Wine, Beer and Mortality in Middle-aged Men from Eastern France," *Archives of Internal Medicine* 159, no. 16 (September 13, 1999): 1864–70.

29. Edward Howell et al., *Enzyme nutrition: the food enzyme concept* (Garden City Park, NY: Avery Publishing Group, 1986).

Chapter 4

Natural Health Secrets of Sleep and Rest

The human body is an organic entity. In the same way that a machine needs to be looked after to work properly and to last, the human body needs proper maintenance to function effectively and to remain in good condition throughout its life. To ensure this, the body needs sufficient sleep and relaxation to balance the periods of work and study. While our diet supplies part of the energy consumed by the body, the rest needs to be provided by sleep. Sleep is needed by most people to restore the yin-yang balance of the body, and to replenish the energy and spirit consumed. Ignoring or neglecting this truth can lead to major health problems. This is a binding law of nature. That is why Confucius encouraged his students to learn from King Wen and King Wu. These important sages of ancient China taught people to alternate between study and relaxation, work and sleep.

The ancient Chinese used the movement of the sun to illustrate this law of nature. The sun rises in the morning and retires at night to rest. We humans should follow this rule, too. On average, human beings spend one third of their lifetime in bed. There is nothing surprising about this. Simply because we are human beings, we need regular sleep and relaxation. This replenishes our energy so that life can continue and our health is maintained. This is because energy that is consumed without timely replenishment immediately weakens our immune systems.

According to modern medical theory, viruses are to blame for our illness. The relevant question is why do they make us sick at certain times, but not at other times? Why do some people get sick, but others, while living in the same environment with equal exposure to viruses, do not? The answer lies in our own immunity. I think all of us have experienced the fact that when we are physically or mental exhausted, we are much more vulnerable to disease. In fact, most people catch colds and the flu when they are fatigued.

Sleep is vital to health and life; a rat denied of sleep will die.[1] To keep our immunity at a high level all the time, we need sufficient sleep and rest each and every day. Modern studies show that restful sleep preserves our sexuality (both male and female), relieves stress and depression, enhances our work productivity, and increases our happiness.

On the other hand, a chronic lack of sleep can weaken our immune system, raise our blood pressure, short-circuit our growth, dampen our sexuality, make us more stressful, lower our work efficiency, and increase the risk of accidents. Statistics show that insomniacs are two and a half times more likely to have car accidents than other drivers, because sleep loss affects concentration. Insomnia can also increase the risk of major depression. There is a misconception that if we eat well and take in more foods rich in protein, we can reduce our need for sleep. It is true that high-protein foods can boost our energy for a short while. However, our bodies still need rest, and the best way to do that is to sleep. Nothing can take the place of sleep.

Understandably, as sleep comprises such a significant part of life, it has been studied intensively. The ancient Chinese were pioneers in this field. Their tireless study and careful observation of the subject of sleep and its relationship to overall health resulted in rich literature on the art and science of sleep. There is a popular belief that sleep is sleep, and that it makes no difference how we sleep or when we go to bed. The ancient Chinese thought otherwise. They discovered that when and how we sleep can have a tremendous effect on our health over time.

First of all, there is the issue of the proper amount of sleep. It is the general rule of nature that we all need approximately eight hours of sleep each day for the body to recover from work and energy consumption. Typically, insufficient sleep will cause a shortage of energy and lower the spirit. As a consequence, the body will draw on its "strategic reserve" of vital energy to cope with the daily needs. If one lets this situation carry on for too long, the eventual result will be a total nervous and physical breakdown.

Unfortunately, people constantly violate this law of nature. This might be one of the biggest health problems in America. According to a survey conducted by the National Commission on Sleep Disorders Research, an estimated 60 million Americans are chronically sleep-deprived. On average, Americans sleep 20 percent less than their ancestors did a century ago. How much does lost sleep cost us? The same research organization estimated it to be about $46 billion a year. This astronomical figure is largely made up of the disastrous consequences resulting from insufficient sleep; these include the space shuttle Challenger explosion, nuclear plant disasters such as Chernobyl, plane crashes, and numerous car accidents.

While insufficient sleep is bad for our health and work, excessive sleep is not good either. The Chinese natural health care system holds that if one sleeps too much, excess stale air is stored up in the body. As a result, the natural balance between yin and yang is disrupted, leading to various health problems. The ancient Chinese also taught us that lying in bed for too long hurts one's vital qi energy and bone system. This should come as no surprise, because too much time in bed means a lack of physical exercise, which in turn causes indigestion and poor circulation of qi and blood. That explains why those who sleep too much have low spirits, weak appetites, weak lungs, and suffer from bone and muscle pain.

We see the ancient Chinese adage working here as well—too much can be as bad as too little. In geometrical parlance, the art of sleep lies in finding out the "golden mean" of the appropriate amount of sleep one needs. Individuals vary, but the golden rule of eight hours seems to be a universal truth.

This high proportion of our very limited lifespan spent on such a seemingly "unproductive" activity as sleep sounds like a tremendous waste of human resources. It makes us wonder how much more we could accomplish if we only needed half that amount of sleep. General George Patton, for one, was a strong advocator of less sleep. He advised his men to reduce the amount of sleep because they would get plenty of sleep after death. To him, sleep was something those of weak character do while heroes remain on guard.

In terms of sleep, just a handful of people, like George Patton, are exceptions to the rule of human biology. Napoleon Bonaparte, Winston Churchill, China's Chou En-lai, Margaret Thatcher, and Bill Clinton are other examples. It is said that Napoleon would sometimes remain awake for several days in the heat of his military campaigns. However, he would make it up by sleeping for twenty-four hours after the victory.

Winston Churchill usually slept no more than five hours a day and found that was quite sufficient for him. For most of his later life, China's Chou En-lai slept for an average of four hours a night, yet possessed great energy and unrivaled efficiency during his twenty-seven-year career as China's premier. Margaret Thatcher sleeps for only four hours a night, and Bill Clinton averages five to six hours a night.[2]

Without a doubt, these are people whom history labels as great leaders. Presumably, there are genetic factors in their favor. However, most of us need about eight hours of sleep each and every day to keep ourselves fit and to enable our bodies to function properly. The short-term gains of work accomplished by reducing the amount of sleep are compensated by a loss in health and career advancement later in life. Almost everybody has experienced the reduction in mental ability, including memory, analytical power, concentration, imagination, and creativity by being overtired.

Again, variations exist among individuals as to exactly how many hours of sleep one needs. There are heavy sleepers and light sleepers, and those who fall in between. Several factors account for the differences. Age, for instance, is a major factor. Children under fifteen usually need nine to ten hours of sleep each day, while elderly people usually need about six hours of sleep each day. Health is another factor that determines the amount of sleep we need. As a general rule, the healthier one is, the less sleep one needs as compared to other people of the same age. Yet another important factor is the effect of our diet on sleep. A better diet and good nutrition can compensate for part of the lost sleep one normally needs.

Then, there is the issue of timing for sleep. We all have biological clocks that keep us on a daily cycle. The ancient Chinese held that the biological clock inside the human body normally works in accordance with the clock of nature. As the day breaks, the sun (standing for the yang polar) rises, and the yang energy in our body also becomes active. As the sun sets, the yang energy inside the body begins to recede after a day's work.

The moral is, therefore, that we should keep our living hours in sync with nature, getting up when the sun rises and going to bed when it sets. This way we ensure the conservation and replenishment of the vital energy in our body. The ageless golden rule is "early to bed and early to rise which makes you happy, healthy, and wise." However, we can easily put our biological clocks out of sync with nature if we stay up late and rise late, or if we follow an irregular sleeping schedule.

While the general rule in Chinese regimens advocates a healthy lifestyle of early to bed and early to rise, the term "early" is only vaguely defined. Again, your biological clock seems to have the final say. Young people tend to have slower clocks, which is why they are night owls and find it hard to get up in the morning. As we advance in age, our clocks speed up. As a general rule, "early" in the Chinese natural health care system means before 10:00 P.M. in the evening and no later than 6:00 A.M. in the morning, with exactly eight hours included. Of course, this may vary with the individual's time schedule and physical needs. Usually the clock tells us it is time to go to bed when our energy level reaches a point where replenishment in the form of sleep and rest becomes necessary.

This biological clock is closely tied to an individual's metabolic rhythm. To follow its "ticking" is the principle of Tao and therefore is to the benefit of your health. To ignore it is against Tao and therefore is asking for trouble. Studies show that people feel happier if they sleep in sync with their biological clock.

Our biological clock seems to be less effective when it comes to getting up in the morning. Unless you are in the habit of getting up early in the morning, the chances are that you will stay in bed long after you should be up. Therefore, we should cultivate a habit of keeping regular bed hours, including Saturday and Sunday. Once a habit is formed, it is very hard to break, so it is desirable to learn a healthy lifestyle as early in life as possible. That is why, in China, the training for martial artists and most other artists starts very early in their lives.

Besides the effect of our individual biological clocks, the Chinese natural health care system contains a refined set of rules governing the timing of going to bed and getting up. This set of rules is based on the relationship between nature—especially the succession of the four seasons—and humans.

This set of rules advises us to go to bed early and to rise early in the springtime; to go to bed later than usual but still rise early with the sun in the summer; and in autumn, to go to bed early and rise early. The only exception is winter. At this time of year we are advised to go to bed early and to rise late, once the sun is high in the sky. The reason we are advised to go to bed late in summer is because if we go to bed early, the heat of the season will penetrate our bodies while we are not on guard. This can cause health problems known as "hot diseases" in Chinese medicine. We are advised to stay in bed longer than usual during the winter season for the exact opposite reason. If we rise before the sun, we have to cope with the cold when we are least prepared to do so, having just got out of a warm bed. This leads to "cold diseases" and drains our energy reserves.

More important than the amount of time we spend in bed is the quality of sleep we enjoy. In the final analysis, it is the quality, not the quantity, of sleep that really counts, although one can affect the other. Indeed, the quality of sleep itself is an important barometer of our health.

There are three criteria by which the quality of sleep can be judged. First, the time it takes for you to fall asleep, including after going to bed and after waking up in the night. Second, the depth and profundity of sleep, i.e., how sensitive you are to noises and disturbances. Third, the number and frequency of dreams that you have during a night's sleep.

Naturally, the sooner you fall asleep, the better the quality of your sleep will be, and vice versa. The inability to fall asleep after lying in bed for more than half an hour is a disease known as insomnia. This can lead to many other physical and mental ailments if it lasts for more than a week. Likewise, the less sensitive you are to external noises or disturbances in your sleep, the higher will be your quality of sleep, because your sleep is deep and profound. Conversely, the more dreams you have during sleep, the lower the quality of rest you receive.

Dreams are a subconscious mental activity that takes place during sleep. They show that your mind is still working while your body is at rest. In that sense, dreams can be called thieves of sleep. One of the main reasons why some people sleep less than others, but wake up in better spirits and with more strength than people who have slept longer, is that they enjoy a higher quality of sleep. This more than makes up for the deficiency in quantity. In other words, dreams are bad from a health viewpoint. The less dreaming we do, the better health we will enjoy.

The Chinese natural health care system holds that there is an intimate relationship between diet and sleep. In other words, what we eat, when we eat, and how much we eat all affect the quality of our sleep. In fact, unhealthy habits, such as overeating or an excess consumption of spicy foods are major causes of insomnia. Stimulants, such as coffee, tea, and alcohol, also affect our sleep.

This conclusion is based on the Chinese understanding that overeating disturbs the proper function of the stomach and spleen. In traditional Chinese medicine, the spleen and the stomach are considered organs of the same family. Together, they govern your digestive functions. Moreover, the spleen is considered to be more important than the stomach in traditional Chinese medicine, which uses the element of earth to represent the pleen in the five element system. Consequently, the clear qi cannot move up to the brain and the stale qi cannot move down to the lower part of the body. This creates unease and restlessness of the mind.

The following foods are conducive to sleep: milk, chicken, peanuts, fish, lotus seeds, bananas, grapes, dates, and honey. We should still keep in mind that even healthy foods should not be overconsumed at dinnertime, as they will affect the quality of our sleep.

Of course, this is not to suggest that hunger is good for sleep. Hunger lowers the blood sugar and thus interferes with sleep. (Actually, low blood sugar stimulates the hunger center in the brain, but the reason why I put it this way is because I believe that it is food and nutrition that determine the blood sugar level in your body in the first place.) Hunger makes our stomachs growl and even ache. Nobody can sleep well under such conditions.

In addition to dietary advice, the Chinese natural health care system offers the following to improve the quality of your sleep:

- Take a warm bath before going to bed. The Chinese experience shows that a warm—not hot—bath taken at bedtime can relax our bodies and minds, elevate our body temperatures, and make us feel sleepy. Besides, the very sense of a clean body leads to better sleep, especially for many hygiene-conscious people.

- Soak your feet in warm water for five to ten minutes immediately before going to bed. This practice was highly recommended by the ancient Chinese as an important measure of natural health and healing. Its therapeutic effects have been well proven. The benefits include warming the body, especially in winter, so that you can sleep comfortably; diverting the blood from the brain to the lower parts of the body, so that one can have a valuable sound sleep; helping to prevent and cure arthritis and other related feet and back ailments; promoting blood circulation; nourishing the kidneys; and replenishing the vital energy. It can also help people suffering from impotence.
  NOTE: People suffering from high blood pressure are not advised to follow this rule. The Chinese believe that soaking your feet in hot water increases blood circulation, which in turn increases blood pressure.

- Keep regular hours as to when to go to bed and when to get up. Such a schedule helps align your biological clock with its natural cycle. As a result, you fall asleep more easily and get up when you should. You should keep to this schedule and not break it on the weekends.

- Ensure that there is enough air and ventilation in the bedroom. If necessary, open a window to let fresh air in. This is good for your heart and brain. Recently, when one of the longest-lived Americans was asked about her secrets of health and longevity, she replied that she always kept one window in her bedroom open, even while sleeping.

- Do not go to bed with an empty stomach. Hunger spoils a good sleep in two ways: it lowers the blood sugar level, and makes your stomach growl and feel sore.

- Neither should you go to bed with a full stomach, that is, immediately after dinner. It not only lowers the quality of sleep, but also creates other health problems, such as stomach ailments and heart disease.

- Restrict the intake of caffeinated products, such as coffee, tea, chocolate, and commercial soft drinks, especially in the late afternoon.

- Turn off the light in your bedroom, as well as televisions and radios. Darkness and quiet are usually conducive to a fast, sound sleep.

- Do not cover your head while sleeping, not even in the winter. By covering your head while sleeping, you deny yourself the benefit of fresher and more air you need for your health.

- Keep the room temperature cool. This promotes a better sleep, and strengthens our immune system during the deepest hours of sleep. The ancient Chinese believed that there is a positive correlation between room temperature and mind temperature. Cool temperature in the bedroom is helpful for falling asleep and sleeping better. The fact that most people sleep better during winter than they do in summer demonstrates this.

- Ensure that your bed is comfortable. This means that your bed should have a good quality, firm mattress that supports the spine and does not allow the body to sag in the middle of the bed.

- Do not go to bed with an active mind. Deep thinking can do this, as can stress and strong feelings or emotions, such as anger and jealousy. Your brain, like your body, needs time to cool off. Involved thinking keeps the mind active long after the project is over, interfering with your sleep. To enjoy a good night's sleep, stop all serious thinking at least a half an hour before bedtime. If the mind is still in an excited state, go for a walk to relax your mind first.

- Cultivate a habit of practicing qigong every day before going to sleep. This helps your mind relax. (See the appendices.)

- Massage your body at bedtime, either by self-massage, as described in Dharma's internal exercises in appendix 5, or ask others to do it for you, if necessary.

- Do some physical exercise every day, especially in the afternoon. While regular physical exercise induces deeper sleep, an afternoon exercise session can improve sleep quality and quantity. In one recent trial at Stanford University, people with moderate insomnia fell asleep twice as fast and slept an hour longer once they began taking a brisk walk.[3] However, do not exert yourself too much, least of all before bedtime. That is counter-productive. Chinese soft exercises are excellent for improving sleep quality, because they are peaceful and leisurely, and can calm your mind and train your body, without exerting yourself. Again, a short walk outside immediately before going to bed can be helpful to fall asleep.

- Take pleasure in sex. In many cases, nothing works better for a high quality sleep than mutually satisfactory sex at bedtime. Sex not only makes one comfortably relaxed, it also releases certain hormones that are conducive to deeper sleep.

When you wake up in the morning, do not jump out of the bed right away, even if you are running late and have an important appointment. It is better to stay in bed for a few more minutes, opening your eyes until you are mentally and physically prepared to get up. This practice was advocated by the ancient Chinese on the grounds that getting up abruptly in the morning will hurt your vital qi. They also believed it could induce heart disease and the common cold. This is because the human body and mind both need a period of transition from one status to another, so that internal qi can be preserved and the yin-yang balance maintained. Also, it is commonsense that if you jump out of the bed immediately after you wake up, especially during the winter, your immune system is still dormant. It is not fully ready yet to fight the external cold weather.

In this regard, my teacher Dr. Wan Laisheng taught me some special skills. One of these is to bend both legs against the chest inside the bedding before getting up in the morning. The way to do this is to grasp the knees against the chest and stretch the legs as far as you can towards the head, preferably reaching beyond it. Another skill is to massage your body beneath the bedding for a few minutes. Yet another method is to rotate your eyeballs for a while to make you fully awake and alert.

It has been a long-standing tradition in China for people to take a short nap after lunch. Almost everyone, from emperors to presidents to common citizens, follows this tradition with religious enthusiasm. Being too busy for a nap is no excuse. Indeed, you may even be considered with suspicion if you break the tradition and walk around in broad daylight while others are in bed.

If you visit China, you will notice a period of silence at the peak of the day, which usually lasts about one to two hours. This is the Chinese time for a nap. During that period of time, all businesses come to a standstill. Foreigners used to laugh at this Chinese tradition. However, shortly after they come to China, they usually take up the practice. This is not so much a matter of doing in China as

the Chinese do as that of enjoying life to a fuller degree. It really gives you pleasure, relaxation, and renewed energy to continue the "battle of life" in the latter part of the day. You will find the productivity of work increases, and you will be in a better spirit to work late into the night if necessary.

Modern scientists have discovered that the habit of taking a short nap after lunch has great therapeutic value on certain diseases. Most significant is the discovery that such a habit can reduce the chances of getting heart diseases by 30 percent. This is because a nap after half a day's work serves to replenish our energy, maintain our body, and reestablish the balance between the body and the mind, especially the balance of hormones associated with the function of heart. The Chinese know that in a sense, the human body works like a light bulb. The more you take care of it by letting it rest every once in a while, the longer it will last and the better it will serve your purpose. The Chinese love to say: "Time lost on grinding the ax will be more than compensated in cutting trees later."

On the contrary, if you work all day long without a break, you will damage your health by drawing heavily on the strategic reserves of your body. Therefore, it is highly advisable to take a nap for about an hour after lunch. This habit is especially helpful during the summer time when energy consumption is the highest. You will feel the difference in spirit and energy levels after taking a nap. The enhanced spirit will sustain you well into the evening. However, do not nap immediately after lunch, wait fifteen minutes or so. Instead, relax for a while or walk half a mile before you take a nap.

To the ancient Chinese, the manner of sleep is another important issue in natural health care. One secret they discovered was that when it comes to sleeping, the solos do it the best. Wu Pu, the student of Hua Tuo, when asked by the emperor as to his secret of health and longevity, replied: "I sleep all by myself." People sleep better when they sleep by themselves. If two people sleep together in the same bed, they will affect each other by any movement they make. Another important discovery is that the most health-inducive manner of sleep is that of a dog. My teacher, Dr. Wan Laisheng, used to tell me: "I do not know what Tao is; all I know is to sleep like a dog." (In this context, Tao refers to the Chinese natural health care system.)

How, then, do dogs sleep? Just take a while to observe their sleep and you will come up with the answer. The good thing is that dogs, unlike human beings, are very uniform and consistent in their sleeping manner. As a rule, they all habitually turn to their sides while sleeping. To sleep like a dog means turning to the side in your sleep. Specifically, if you are a male, you sleep better on your right side. If you are a female, the left side will be better for you. Of course, we use both sides alternately during the entire course of sleep.

According to the ancient Chinese, it is easier to conserve the qi energy in the body by sleeping on the side. The Chinese sages hold that while we are awake there is a natural mechanism inside our body that serves as a "lock" and prevents qi energy from leaking. While we are asleep, however, we lose our consciousness and give up the check on the energy gate. Consequently, qi energy and vital essence find it easier to leak out. By sleeping on our sides we can fasten the lock, preventing vital energy from escaping.

For the male, the invisible lock for vital qi energy resides in the right kidney while for the female it is found in the left kidney. By turning to the right side, a man automatically tightens up the lock on the energy gate. In the same way, a female will do better to conserve her vital qi by turning to her left side. Secondly, the heart of a male is located more to the left of the chest, while that of a female is located more to the right of the chest. By turning to the right side a man relieves the pressure on his heart, allowing it the maximum freedom to perform its function while the body is at rest. This enhances the function of the heart. The same thing happens to a woman when she turns to her left side to sleep. Thus we see that our sleeping manner has a lot to do with our health.

The Chinese natural health care system recommends the following sleep postures tailored toward special medical cases. For instance, it is advisable for people who have had a stroke to lie on their backs with their heads higher than the trunk. The same posture is recommended for patients with asthma. For those suffering from stomach illness, the right posture is to turn to the left side to limit the amount of stomach acid flowing back into the eating tube. For hypertension sufferers, the recommended posture is to place the head in a position about 15 centimeters higher than the rest of the body. For those inflicted with serious heart diseases, the right posture is to lie with the head considerably higher than the body, and avoid turning to the left side. Similarly, hepatitis sufferers should turn to their right sides while sleeping, to promote the nourishment of the liver by the arteries. Other positions, such as turning to the left or lying on the back put the liver above the abdominal arteries, thus interfering with the proper functioning of the latter.

For all its biological necessity to life, sleep is not the only form of rest. Rest means freedom from activity and worry, as well as peace of mind and soul. It does not necessarily mean lying down in bed. Actually, many Chinese have been known to enjoy excellent health and extraordinary longevity with little sleep. However, they spent a lot of time sitting meditating and practicing qigong.

Meditation, with the mind concentrated in that part of the lower abdomen known as dantian, and eventually becoming void, serves a similar purpose as sleep. Indeed, it may be a better alternative for some people. For one thing, meditation and qigong ensure that no nocturnal emission occurs. However, most of us are not trained to stand the ordeal of long hours of meditation. Nonetheless, we can learn from "professional" meditators and benefit by imitating their practice. Simply close your eyes and take deep breaths for three minutes after every half an hour of work. Think of dantian and forget about everything for a short time. This replenishes your energy, drive away fatigue, increase your work efficiency, and prevent diseases.

How can this simple action be able to put diseases at bay? The answer is that our immune power is weakened when we allow our qi energy to be used up without adequate, timely replenishment. Meditation, or even closing our eyes for a while, can help replenish us with vital qi energy needed for the maintaining of immunity. It is during the deepest phases of sleep that our immune system is strengthened and recharged. A study done at the University of California in San Diego showed that after missing five hours of sleep, a healthy man produced fewer disease-fighting immune cells. Another study performed by Eve van Cauter, an endocrinologist at the University of Chicago, provided similar results. She found that it is only during sleep—dreamless sleep—that the body restores its physical plant, repairing skin, building bone and muscle, and preparing itself for the battles of the day to come. In other words, a good night's sleep is needed to restore our energy and immune system to a sufficient level.

Quality sleep may also be the ultimate anti-aging therapy. It repairs organs, bones, tissue, and skin. Besides, regular, sufficient sleep brings about many other health benefits: it increases the rate of pleasurable brain waves, it decreases blood pressure and muscle pain, builds and repairs our body machine, and makes us safe from the external environment by closing the potential "openings"— lowered immunity—where diseases may otherwise enter.

The time spent on meditation is as effective to health as time spent on sleep. If you can carry on working without rest, you are not a human being. The greatest beauty of meditation with the eyes closed is that it is easy to do, and can be done as often as needed. You do not have to take off your clothes. You do not need a bed. You can do it any-

where, and anytime you want. A car performs better and lasts longer with frequent maintenance. In the same way, a human body that rests every now and again functions more effectively and lives longer, too.

Endnotes

1. *Health*, September 1997, 108.

2. *Health*, July/August 1996, 75.

3. *Health*, September 1997, 115.

Chapter 5

Natural Health Secrets of Physical Hygiene

If health means the absence of toxins and waste, it stands to reason that we must keep ourselves clean internally and externally in order to be healthy. In fact, a large number of diseases are caused by the neglect of physical hygiene. A dirty body does not necessarily mean a body covered with mud or dirt. It also means the internal body and how important it is to keep it clean. Physical hygiene means, among other things, building up a strong base of qi energy. Such a base automates much of the internal cleaning job. As a result, a bowel movement becomes a regular, natural process without pain or difficulty. A strong qi energy means that urination, breathing, and sweating all function automatically.

Every day we eat food, drink fluids, and breathe air. All of these materials enter our body. Some of them become nutrients and are used by the body for energy, but most need to be eliminated from the body in a regular, timely manner. It is alarming to think that all these materials may be contaminated before they enter our bodies. This makes it even more important that we clean our bodies on a regular basis.

How regularly should we clean our bodies? Again, the ancient Chinese looked to nature for the answer. They found that the cycle of nature is twenty-four hours, with sunrise and sunset, day and night, work and sleep, yin and yang, alternating and replacing each other to complete a day. As microcosms of nature, we humans need to function in a similar manner in order to be healthy. This means, among other things, to get rid of the waste matter inside our bodies, and to clean our body externally, every twenty-four hours. This takes the form of bowel movements, bathing or showering, brushing our teeth, and other related activities.

There are four basic areas of the human body involved in this internal cleansing. They are the bowels, lungs, kidneys, and skin. The bowels get rid of the wastes in the colon resulting from what we eat. The lungs drive out the stale air in the body resulting from breathing. The kidneys clean the body through urination, and the skin drives poisons out of the body by sweating through numerous pores.

In order for these cleaning organs to work effectively, however, the body needs a sufficient supply of vital qi energy. For instance, it takes a large amount of qi energy in the body to digest the foods we eat, to pass liquids through the two million filters of the human kidneys, to prepare nutrients for the billions of body cells, to bring in oxygen to purify the five to eight quarts of blood in our body, to expel carbon dioxide, to throw off body poisons from the skin in the form of sweating, and to get rid of solid wastes through bowel movements.

To understand the vital importance of qi energy, just consider the case of constipation. Many ill people have trouble moving their bowels. One common reason is because their qi energy levels are low as a result of a long or severe disease, and there is not enough driving force to move the bowels regularly. It is interesting to note that diarrhea, a seemingly opposite phenomenon to constipation, has its root cause in weak qi energy, also. When qi is weak, the body is not able to digest food properly. This can explain why some patients with chronic diseases have some form of a movement problem, be it constipation or diarrhea.

Thus, we see the vital importance of qi energy. Just as gasoline is the driving force of automobiles, qi is the fuel of life and the driving force of various body organs. Indeed, qi is the very basis of our vitality and immunity. It plays a key role in the body's healing process.

In addition to the internal cleaning process, we have a number of external cleaning jobs that need to be done regularly. The following is a list of actions we need to perform on a daily basis to be healthy and happy. Many of these actions may sound like commonsense advice taught to children at school. All the same, we should review these actions on a regular basis, all the way through life.

Hand-washing is one of the most important, simple hygienic measures people can adopt in order to stay healthy. Wash your hands frequently with soap, especially when you first come home, before meals, and after bowel movements. The rationale for this is self-evident, because our hands carry a lot of bacteria. To eliminate these before they can enter our bodies, we need to wash our hands with soap.

Brushing your teeth at least once a day is another important habit. Brush your teeth after dinner and/or at bedtime and cultivate a habit of rinsing your mouth with water after getting up in the morning and after every meal. Two rows of bright teeth are an important mark of good health. They add luster to your appearance and increase your attractiveness.

Remember that prenatal qi energy requires a constant supplement from postnatal qi energy for us to remain fit and healthy. Postnatal qi energy relies on the proper digestion of healthy foods, which in turn depends on strong teeth and a healthy stomach to get the job done. Toothaches and tooth decay are often the consequences of ignorance and neglect of dental hygiene, and are often associated with indigestion, malnutrition, and constipation.

In brushing the teeth, pay great attention to the kind of toothbrush you use, and the manner in which you brush the teeth. These measures are meant to protect our teeth, and to prevent the enamel covering the teeth surface from wearing out. As a matter of principle, the Chinese natural health care system recommends that we use soft toothbrushes only. The best toothbrushes are those made of animal hairs. It is hard to find such toothbrushes in the market nowadays. Instead, we have soft toothbrushes made of other materials so it isn't necessary to have one made of animal hair. To further protect your teeth, you must soften the toothbrush in warm water for a minute before brushing.

Not only do we need to brush our teeth regularly, but we also need to learn the right way to brush them. This seemingly insignificant factor plays a large part in the health of our teeth. Most people brush their teeth horizontally, from side to side. This practice is harmful to the teeth, and destroys the tooth enamel. Tooth enamel has a greater chance of being destroyed when brushed from side to side rather than up and down.

It also depends on how hard you brush. Although enamel is one of the hardest substances, nothing can stand the constant brushing over a long period of time. As the Chinese proverb says, "A constant drop of water will penetrate a rock." According to Michele Darby, the author of *Dental Hygiene Theory and Practice*, improper toothbrushing, including horizontal scrubbing and excessive pressure can cause tooth trauma, which in turn can result in tooth abrasion, the wearing away of the tooth surface.[1]

Based on Dr. Darby's observation, if you constantly brush your teeth in a horizontal manner with a hard toothbrush and too much force, your teeth will gradually decay.

Toothbrush trauma initially results in gingival abrasion, and eventually in gingival recession, gingival clefts, or festooning of the gingiva.[2]

Indeed, our teeth are essential tools for the protection of our health. Damage resulting from unhealthy brushing habits is not limited to your teeth. It can also extend to your heart. Recent scientific studies show that the way we brush our teeth has a lot to do with the health of our heart. This is because blood flows from the teeth to the heart. In other words, if the blood is infected by unhealthy teeth, the heart can be in danger.

Another essential element of physical hygiene is to have a bowel movement once a day, preferably shortly after you get up in the morning and before breakfast. This habit of moving the bowels at regular intervals helps your health and healing enormously.

As we know, regular and smooth bowel movements are necessary to get rid of the bodily wastes. Such wastes can generate poisons inside the body if they are not removed in a timely manner. This can lead to many health problems such as headaches, insomnia, indigestion, loss of appetite, constipation, ulcer, hemorrhoids, and even intestinal cancer. Therefore, we need to eliminate such wastes to keep our bodies clean and healthy. (Refer to the listing for constipation in chapter 14, "Special Solutions for Special Problems," if you are have difficulty moving your bowels.)

Other important steps for good physical hygiene include the following:

- Take a bath at least once a day to clean your skin and promote the blood circulation in your body. Skin is the largest eliminative organ in the entire body, and contains 96 million pores. Most body poisons are expelled through these pores. Every day we excrete a great deal of sweat, sebum, and dirt that accumulates on the skin during the course of the day. It is important to clean your skin regularly to ensure that it functions smoothly and efficiently. Taking a bath is the best way to achieve this purpose. A warm bath is highly beneficial to your health. Quite apart from its cleansing function, a warm bath can soothe pain, relax nerves, relieve fatigue, promote blood and qi circulation, and improve sleep.

- The typical American practice is to take a shower in the morning. However, I would recommend taking a warm bath before going to bed in the evening. First, it helps the circulation of blood in the body, as this slows down while we are lying in bed. Secondly, it effectively improves the quality of sleep.

- Shampoo your hair every morning. This not only keeps your hair in good health, but enhances your spirit as you prepare for a new day's challenge. This means that you will function more efficiently during the day.

- It is also important to urinate completely and take a warm bath after sexual intercourse. This hygienic practice can prevent many difficulties in the future such as prostate problems, urinary dysfunction, and sexually transmitted diseases.

- Attend to your fingernails once a week. Fingernails harbor bacteria. Looking after your fingernails reduces the risk of bacteria getting into your mouth while eating.

- Everybody in the family should have his or her own towel, comb, and toothbrush. Do not share these daily necessities with each other. They also need to be cleaned or changed frequently.

- Keep your home well ventilated. Allow plenty of fresh air to circulate in the rooms where you work and sleep. This boosts your spirit and helps blood circulation. Our hearts and minds need fresh air to function properly. Also, germs tend to live longer in stale, poorly ventilated environments.

- Keep your home and work environments well lit. Sunlight is free and kills many kinds of bacteria. Chinese patients of pneumonia are advised to sit in sunlight for some time everyday, because it is believed that sunlight can even kill the bacteria that causes pneumonia. Also, clean your house on a regular basis. The bathroom, basement, and laundry room can collect mold and mildew. This produces a sharp, musty smell, which can cause allergies and other ailments.

- Germs love the warm dampness of a bathroom. Colds can also be transferred in the bathroom. One particular concern is the toilet. Every time we flush it, we send germs and bacteria onto other bathroom surfaces. Consequently, it is a good habit to close the toilet lid before flushing.

- The kitchen is probably the most contaminated place in the house. Food-borne bacteria can come into the kitchen every time you bring home the weekly shopping. The USDA estimates that half of the approximately 80 million cases of food-caused illnesses originate in family kitchens, not restaurants. It is important to keep raw meats and poultry separate from other foods and to use separate cutting boards for meats and vegetables. You should also wash your hands frequently while preparing such foods.

Thus, a general knowledge and daily practice of hygiene are indispensable to our health and to keeping diseases at bay. Some of the recommendations listed here may sound obvious, but it is important to keep them in mind and incorporate them regularly into our lifestyle. As human knowledge increases, we will be able to know more about how diseases occur in our environment and nip them in the bud, so to speak.

Endnotes

1. Michele L. Darby, *Dental Hygiene Theory and Practice* (W.B. Saunders Company, 1995), 445.

2. Ibid.

Chapter 6

Natural Health Secrets of Mental Hygiene

Most people know that a sound mind dwells in a healthy body. For all its truth and wisdom, this statement only gives us a one-sided picture. The other side of the story reads: "A sound body depends on a healthy mind." In fact, the mind and body are two faces of the same coin—the whole person. They are inseparable from and indispensable to each other. Together, they make a healthy person. Only when we take care of both sides of our lives can we hope to enjoy really good health. Modern research in the field of psychoneuro-immunology verifies what the Chinese have known for thousands of years—that our mentality and emotions have a direct effect on our immune systems, and therefore upon our physical health.

Unfortunately, not all of us know this truth. People in the West tend to be preoccupied with the physical, tangible aspect of life that they often neglect the significance of the mind. Typically, Western science is built on the Cartesian split between the body and mind. This split is so deeply ingrained that most Westerners take it for granted.

It is often assumed in Western society that the patient's mental state is not important; that the mind is subjective, irresponsible, and a negligible factor in health care, while the body is physical, tangible, measurable, and therefore, all important. Sadly, some Western doctors rely on technological equipment, and willingly become slaves to, rather than masters of, this equipment. To them, only visible things are important; anything invisible or intangible is nonexistent and unimportant. Consequently, it is no wonder that some doctors are unable to make a diagnosis without the help of modern equipment.

The ancient Chinese, however, never lost sight of the close interconnection and interdependence between the body and mind. Guided by the powerful, omnipresent theory of yin and yang, which lies at the very core of Chinese culture and its natural health care system, the Chinese were able to arrive at this conclusion thousands of years before the terms "psychology" and "science" were even heard of. To them, this is just one classical example of the universal yin-yang balance. Here, the body stands for the visible yang while the mind represents the invisible yin. To them, the mind and the body are a complete and inseparable ensemble. Thus, our emotional and mental states play a significant part in our vulnerability to, and recovery from, disease.

A healthy mind is indispensable to the proper functioning of the body. If the mind is not in a healthy state, the body will be in trouble, too. The Chinese natural health care system sees no essential difference between mental and physical ailments. Thus, a mental dysfunction will lead to a physical disease, and is often a reflection of some physical disease.

On the other hand, a physical disease will lead to mental dysfunction, resulting in depression, worry, and fear. The ancient Chinese understood how virtually all illnesses start with the mind. In fact, anything in our mind is readily reflected in our cells. Thus, a low spirit has a negative, depressing effect on body cells and organs, disturbing their proper functioning and lowering their immunity.

When we nourish our mind, we nourish our body at the same time. For life to go on normally and for any healing to take place, the body must be able to provide the raw materials or building blocks. But raw materials alone are not enough. Equally essential is a positive and healthy attitude toward one's health problems. The more positive our outlook and mental state is, the better our health is and the healing process will be fast and trouble-free. In fact, this insistence on the inseparable link between the mind and body is one of the greatest contributions the ancient Chinese have made to health care. Only by linking together these two aspects of human life can we hope to get a full picture of human beings and their health problems.

The ancient Chinese classified the emotional activities of humans into seven categories: joy, anger, brooding, sorrow, fear, surprise, and melancholy. They categorized these seven emotions as the internal causes of disease. This contrasts with the external causes of diseases such as diet, trauma, and weather changes.

In *The Yellow Emperor's Classics of Internal Medicine*, it is clearly stated that all kinds of diseases have their origins either in weather changes, emotional fluctuations, or in diet. The ancient Chinese also discovered that any excess outburst of emotions, be it anger or joy, have a negative impact on our health because it drains qi energy from the body. For example, they believe that excessive anger hurts the liver, excessive sorrow hurts the lungs, excessive fear hurts the kidneys, excessive worry damages the spleen, and excessive joy and fright hurt the heart and kidneys.

If different emotions can hurt different internal organs, then such emotions can be symptoms of diseases in the corresponding organs. Thus, being quick to anger is diagnosed to be a disease of the liver; a tendency to be fearful is a sign of qi energy deficiency in kidneys; a tendency to worry is diagnosed to be a disease of the spleen; a tendency to be joyful is a disease of the heart; while being overly sorrowful is a disease of the lungs. This is another contribution the Chinese have made to the science of medical diagnosis. Generally, effective treatment for a disease is not possible without taking into account the methods of coping with mental depression, which is frequently the root cause of physical illness.

Of the seven emotions, anger is the greatest enemy of health. In *The Classics of Magic Fly*, another early text in the Chinese health care system, it is said that "in excess anger, one's qi energy and blood circulation in the body can be completely blocked. There is no cure for the disease of being susceptive to anger." In fact, anger has been shown to have a close link with kidney and heart diseases, and especially cancer. This is because anger, pent-up anger in particular, is a form of chronic stress. Dr. Hans Selye, an endocrinologist and director of the Institute of Experimental Medicine and Surgery at the University of Montreal, discovered that anger frequently produces hormonal imbalances and suppresses the immune system. Since hormones are vital to body functions, such an imbalance can lead to high blood pressure and damage the kidneys and the heart. Since our immune system is responsible for engulfing and destroying cancerous cells, a suppressed immune system makes us more vulnerable to the development of cancers in our body.[1]

In the five element system of Chinese medicine, it is believed that the liver belongs to wood, and wood should be allowed to grow freely, without hindrance. In other words, the qi of the liver should be allowed to flow smoothly if health is desired. However, anger and stress serve just the opposite purpose; they hinder liver qi energy from moving smoothly and therefore cause damage to the organ. For instance, the death of

Chinese marshal Chen Yi from liver cancer in 1971 is widely believed to have a lot to do with the anger pent-up in his body due to the humiliations he suffered during the Cultural Revolution. As I can remember, the cases of liver diseases in China significantly increased during the Cultural Revolution.[2]

In the famous *Historical Annals* written more than 2,000 years ago, Sima Qian, a great Chinese historian, observed that Fan Zen, then premier to the King of Chu, died of a sudden occurrence of cancer shortly after he handed in his resignation because of his anger at the premier's neglect of his advice.

Anger can also lead to coughing up blood and even death, resulting from complete blockage of qi flow due to excess anger. The Chinese have known several people coughing up blood due to excess, sudden outbursts of anger. A well-known case is found in Chiang Kai-shek who, during his losing battles with the Communists, was well known to have twice coughed up blood.

Without a doubt, anger and stress can do a great deal of harm to our health. Indeed, they are diseases in themselves. If not effectively checked and managed, the body will feed on its energy reserves and fatigue will result. Worse still, the body's immune system will be damaged, opening up the body to attack from all kinds of diseases.

This direct relationship between emotions and health is clearly stated in terms of qi in *The Yellow Emperor's Classics of Internal Medicine* as follows:

Fury pushes qi up, joy calms qi down, grief dissipates qi, fear lowers qi, surprise scatters qi, fatigue wastes qi, thinking concentrates qi. Fury damages the liver, ecstasy damages the heart, worry damages the spleen, grief damages lungs, and fear damages kidneys.

Here, qi is seen as the key link between our mental health and physical health. Obviously, our emotions are directly connected with our health. Since the ideal status of qi is a state of peaceful balance, any excessive emotional activity directly impacts on our physical health, weakening our immune system and prolonging the healing process. For this reason, the ancient Chinese advised that effective emotional management is vital to holistic health and the healing process. This relationship between emotion and health is also described in "Su Wen" (a chapter in *The Yellow Emperor's Classics of Internal Medicine*) as follows:

If you cannot pacify your spirit, and if you let your mind be complicated with desires and worries, your disease will not be cured. To be healthy, you must avoid anger and worry, but keep your mind happy, your heart easy, and your desires at low levels. Only then can your qi energy flow smoothly and uninterrupted inside your body to promote health and cure diseases.

As if the discussion of emotional life is too abstract by itself, Su Wen tries to relate man's emotions with the changes of the seasons:

Spring is the season of birth. Everything comes into life during this time, so also should our emotional life be extending and happy. This is the rule of regimen dictated by the natural qi development in spring. . . . Summer is the season in which everything grows and ripens, and the heaven and the earth come into harmony with each other. . . . During this season, one must avoid anger. This is the rule of regimen dictated by the natural qi development in summer. . . . Autumn is the season in which qi in the nature is harsh. Therefore, one must keep his mind calm and easy. This is the rule of regimen dictated by the natural qi development in autumn. . . . Winter is the season of conservation and closing up. During this season, one must avoid emotional upheavals as if to hide such activities. . . . This is the rule of regimen dictated by the natural qi development in winter. . . . Thus, wise people take good care of their health by acting in accordance with the four seasons, taking life easily and managing their emotions, combining and regulating yin and yang. Hence, disease will not come to them, and they can enjoy long life with sharp eyesight.

This ancient Chinese belief of the inseparable link between the mind and body is beginning to dawn on the West. Scientists recently discovered that changes in emotional states change the biochemistry of the body. More and more scientific research indicates that emotional states have both an immediate and long-term impact on our health and well-being. Dr. Eugene P. Pendergrass, president of the American Cancer Society, is one of the first Western scientists who recognized the intimate relationship between the mind and body. He said: "There is solid evidence that the course of the disease in general is affected by emotional distress. . . . Thus, we as doctors may begin to emphasize treatment of the patient as a whole as well as the disease from which the patient is suffering."[3] Dr. Pendergrass realized that there is "the distinct possibility that within one's mind is a power capable of exerting forces which can either enhance or inhibit the progress of this disease (referring to cancer)."

Another Western pioneer in this field is Elmer Green of the Menninger Clinic in Topeka, Kansas.[4] Dr. Green believes that "every change in the physiological state is accompanied by an appropriate change in the mental emotional state, conscious or unconscious, and conversely, every change in the mental emotional state, conscious or unconscious, is accompanied by an appropriate change in the physiological state." That is to say, the body and mind are an integral system in which they affect each other.

Nowadays, it is widely acknowledged that there are psychosomatic factors in heart attacks, ulcers, insomnia, and hypertension. It has also been shown that the heart rate, blood pressure, brain-wave activity, and muscle activity can be brought under mental control. George Solomon, for instance, showed in the late 1960s that stress could suppress the immune response of animals while a healthy and positive mental state could enhance their immunity.[5]

Similar research has found the same rule applies to human beings. Scientists point out that a negative outlook can generate certain kinds of venomous compounds in our bodies, which weaken our immune systems. This can cause a number of ailments including liver disease and cancer, and even mental diseases. Dr. Pendergrass observed that "there is solid evidence that the course of the disease (cancer) in general is affected by emotional distress." He sincerely hoped that "we can widen the quest to include the distinct possibility that within one's mind is a power capable of exerting forces which can either enhance or inhibit the progress of this disease (cancer)."[6] In other words, not only can mental and emotional conditions cause or aggravate diseases, they can also contribute to healing.

In a study at the Harvard School of Public Health, 34,000 men were surveyed for common phobias such as fear of closed spaces, illness, heights, and crowds. Their health was monitored for two years. At the end of this period, researchers determined that the risk of fatal heart disease was 250 percent greater for those who scored highest on a phobia test than it was for those who were not so anxious. In actuality, panic and high anxiety can cause hypertension, heart spasms, and hyperventilation, which may trigger heart attacks.[7]

Several decades ago, George E. Vaillant, a doctor at Cambridge Hospital, in Massachussets, started an interesting study on the relationship between mental health and physical wellness. He kept track of the lives of 188 Harvard graduates for a period of thirty-two years, keeping records of their physical and mental health until they reached their early fifties in 1975. He found an insightful link between the two. Those whose lives had been emotionally stable reported less than half the physical illnesses than did those whose lives had been emotionally rocky.[8] The lesson of this study is clear: life is easier to live when you take it easy, because every cell in your body will reflect the status of your body and perform accordingly.

I remember my mother telling me that one of her best friends had died of a "broken heart"—she had never been really sick until her son was killed. Dying of a broken heart is equivalent to saying that chronic depression or an outburst of emotions can kill people. We read in history of people dying of extreme surprise or fear, or shortly after an outburst of anger. A fierce outburst of fury, for instance, often leads to coughing up of blood and sudden death. For instance, Chiang Kai-shek, a late President of the Republic of China, had been known to cough up blood at least twice during his losing battles with the Chinese Communists in the late 1940s. Liu Shaoqi is another example. This late President of Communist China also died of a broken—or angry—heart during the Cultural Revolution in the late sixties after being purged and persecuted by Mao Tse-tung, his boss and comrade-in-arms. In modern society, people with serious stress and depression often kill themselves. In fact, suicide is the ninth leading cause of death in the U.S.[9]

One reason why emotional outbursts can suppress our immune system is because such emotional changes consume a lot of qi energy, which is the material basis of our natural defense system. This ancient Chinese understanding is confirmed by modern science. Dr. Thomas H. Holmes of the University of Washington School of Medicine tells us that "we have only so much energy, no more. If it takes too much effort with the environment, we have less to spare for preventing disease. When life is too hectic, and when coping attempts fail, illness is the unhappy result."[10]

Neuropeptides are one more evidence of the unity between the body and mind. Neuropeptides are chemicals that regulate our moods. As a result, the mind-body connection is maintained. These chemicals also control the movements of monocytes—key cells of the immune system and essential materials for healing physical wounds. Monocytes also clean the body tissues of bacteria and help the immune system fight against diseases. In other words, the same neuropeptides that lead to emotional health also trigger bodily reactions that affect physical health. Moreover, the same chemicals that regulate the emotions also enhance the brain cells related to memory.

Another proof of the intimate body-mind association was provided by a five-year study of more than 8,000 subjects. The study found that the quality of a man's marriage can influence his risk of getting an ulcer. Researchers in this study said that men who felt they got love and support from their wives had only half the chance of developing ulcers as those who felt they received no support from their wives.

Networks of nerve fibers have been found that connect to the thymus gland, spleen, lymph nodes, and bone marrow. Thus, the brain may directly influence the immune system and therefore our physical health by sending messages down the nerve cells. Moreover, it is shown that immune functions can be altered by actions that destroy specific brain areas.[11]

Also proven is the fact that the word "feeling" has two meanings: one related to an emotional experience and the other related to a physical sensation. At a higher stage of sensation, the body and mind converge in a brain area known as the limbic system. Obviously, emotions are not just a matter of the mind; they have a clear physical connection, too. For instance, stress is not just a mental or psychological phenomenon. It is a physical state as well, and it leaves scars and hurts the body throughout. Dr. James S. McLester, former President of the American Medical Association, said: "The greatest tragedy that comes to man is the emotional depression, the dulling of the intellect, and the loss of initiative."

Stress is also a "killer" of sexuality. When stress levels rise, erections may "fall," both because of the psychological effects of anxiety and because of the physical effects of constricting capillaries. You may have noticed that while you are under stress, saliva flows less freely in the mouth, making your mouth and throat dry. Over time, this reduces natural bacteria control and causes dental problems. In addition, stress causes increased perspiration under the arms, and extra sweating robs the body of the minerals it needs, leading to muscle cramps. As mentioned before, stress is not just a psychological problem. It directly affects our physical health as well.

Stress, especially chronic, unrelieved stress, is probably the most common and neglected threat to our immune system. Along with worry, anxiety, anger, and depression, stress can trigger unfavorable chemical changes, releasing hormones in the body that cause the thymus gland to shrink, thus weakening the entire immune system. It is also known that stress constricts blood vessels in our arms and legs, increasing our heart rate. Affected by stress, the heart works harder, blood pressure rises, breathing becomes short and rapid, the flow of qi energy becomes blocked, and digestion slows down.

In a word, every function of the body is degraded as a result of mental stress and depression. This causes various forms of health problems to occur, such as colds, flu, diarrhea, insomnia, cramps, and heartburn. For instance, studies have shown that people who experienced a high level of anger and stress were four times more likely to develop a cold or flu than those who had a peaceful mind and a positive outlook.

Since our immune system is the body's first line of defense against disease, stress reduction is vital in maintaining health and preventing disease. While nobody wants to fall victim to stress, nobody can avoid it altogether. This is equally true for princes and paupers, the noble and the humble, the successful and the failing.

Indeed, worry and stress are a part of life, all the more so for modern humans. Life today inflicts all-around stresses upon us, internally and externally, with ever increasing intensity. There are bound to be days when you feel "buried in the blues," no matter who you are. It comes with all of life's daily hassles such as traffic jams, long lines, petty arguments, heavy workloads, job insecurity, financial strains, family dysfunction, unrequited love, sexual inability, and so on. Some of us feel down in the dumps, others are bored to tears, and yet others are stuck in a rut. Everyone gets his or her share occasionally, no matter who they are.

Actually, there is evidence showing that the more ambitious or successful you are, the more stress you will have. The fact that heart attack rates are much higher among successful people is just one example of this. When you are under stress, your body releases hormones called catecholamines, which increase the demand on the heart. If the heart is unable to meet this demand, it uses up oxygen faster than it can be supplied, and thus starts to kill heart muscle tissue—a heart attack.

A limited degree of stress can be a good thing. It makes us feel challenged and gives a sense of purpose to our lives. However, a high degree of stress as well as depression that occurs for a long time is decidedly harmful to our health and well being. The ancient Chinese warn us that chronic, unrelieved stress can pose a severe threat to our vital qi energy. It lowers the level of qi reserve, making the body tired and vulnerable to the invasion of disease. Modern research has confirmed this ancient theory by reporting that stress, together with depression, grief, and anxiety, can trigger chemical changes in our bodies, stimulating the release of neuropeptides, which negatively affect the immune system.

Living with continual stress means a constant exposure to glucocorticoid hormones. This can cause steroid poisoning, which is harmful to the body's immune system, causing the thymus gland, spleen, and lymph nodes to atrophy. Whenever we find ourselves in a stressful situation that we can't resolve, or get out of easily, our body generates a tiny dose of steroid poisoning. The accumulation and constant presence of this poison can lead to a number of health problems such as indigestion, insomnia, constipation, hypertension, mental disturbances, diabetes, heart disease, and often cancer. It is a direct result of the excessive production of corticoids associated with stress.

Another significant scientific discovery in this field is this: in responding to a stressful situation, virtually every bodily organ, gland, and cell is involved and plays its respective role. As we know, the human body thrives on a peaceful mind and orderliness of hormonal production. But the ultimate responsibility of restoring peace and reestablishing order rests with each and every cell in the body. Blood vessels, nerves, and the brain are all affected by stress. We can see how much of our precious energy is wasted due to stress, which in normal situations would be used for productive purposes, such as fighting diseases, helping digestion, boosting sexual vitality, and enhancing work efficiency.

Our immediate physical reactions to stress include:

- Trembling, teeth grinding, and nervous behavior.

- Increased heart rate (to move blood to the muscles and brain).

- Increased blood pressure.

- Shortness of breath.

- Increased perspiration.

- Slow digestion or loss of appetite.

- Dry mouth and throat.

- Insomnia and/or nightmares.

- Premenstrual tension or missed periods.

It is found that stress is linked to and/or causative in a variety of illnesses today. Christine A. Leatz, author of *Career Success/ Personal Stress*, cites the following diseases as stress-related: insomnia, fatigue, depression, upper respiratory infection, flu, chest pain, headaches, hypertension, jaw problems, lower gastrointestinal tract problems, menstrual irregularities, muscle soreness/pain, backache, repetitive stress injuries, dermatitis, eczema, acne, sores in or on the mouth, indigestion, gastritis, heartburn, gastroesophageal reflux, peptic ulcers, panic attacks, hyperventilation, mitral valve prolapse syndrome, drug use, alcoholism, tobacco use, sexual dysfunction including impotence, orgasmic dysfunction, diabetes, arthritis, asthma, and premenstrual syndrome.[12]

Prolonged or intensified stress causes a biochemical imbalance in the body, which in turn, weakens the immune system, thus opening the door to infection and disease. This triggers a vicious cycle with an even higher degree of stress. It is found that during times of stress, hormones (in particular, the previously mentioned glucocorticoids, actually) are released in the body that cause the thymus gland to shrink, lowering immunity. The longer and more intense the stress, the greater the risk of viral infection. Already, stress has been linked to insomnia, headaches, fatigue, aging, ulcers, hypertension, asthma, stomach ailments, heart attack, and cancer. It is significant to note that most heart attacks occur on Monday mornings, the time when we start to face a stressful situation at work after a weekend's relaxation.

Another significant experiment shows the cancer-inducing effect of stress. Researchers at the University of Pennsylvania injected mice with tumor cells, and then gave them electric shocks. The mice were divided into two groups: one that was allowed to escape the shocks and another that was not. The group of mice that was not allowed to escape developed cancer at a greater rate than those that were allowed to escape.[13] This shows that stress triggers malign pathological changes in animal cells (no similar studies have been done on humans though). Not surprisingly, as we are the most intelligent and sensitive of all animals, we are most susceptible to the negative effects of stress.

As already mentioned, anger is the greatest enemy of health. It is a bad, harmful emotion. Some people are more liable to anger than others. They are easily annoyed and angry when faced with life's frustrations. Researchers point out that anger and hostility are associated with heart disease. This is because anger causes the body to release adrenaline and other poisonous hormones into the bloodstream. As a consequence, muscle tension, blood pressure, and heart rate increase, digestion slows down, and arteries constrict and dilate. It also causes the liver to put cholesterol and triglycerides into the blood, and increases the testosterone level. Over a period of time, this causes wear and tear on the heart and blood vessels. This explains the link between repeated anger and the increased rates of heart disease and strokes as well as coughing up of blood.

Next to the heart, the digestive tract is considered the part of the body most vulnerable to mental stress. Scientists have found that although stress increases blood flow to the muscles and brain, it decreases blood flow to the digestive tract. During, and for a while, after meals, the digestive tract requires a heavy blood supply to fully accomplish the task of digestion. What happens is this. The stomach responds to stress by producing hydrochloric acid. Then the pancreas tries to balance this excess acid by releasing alkaline enzymes. Over time this can lead to low stomach acid and weakens the function of the pancreas, resulting in indigestion, nutrition deficiency and ulcers.

The ancient Chinese were aware of another source of stress and depression. This is wishful sex-oriented thinking. Thinking about sex is natural to anyone who has reached puberty. However, such thinking in excess can harm our health, leading to depression and loss of kidney qi energy. That is why it was regarded by the ancient Chinese as a thief of vital essence from our bodies.

The deeper you are drawn into such wishful thinking, the greater is your loss of vital sexual essence. This, as you will see later, affects not only your sexual vitality, but also your overall health and longevity. The nasty thing about sex-related thinking is that most of the harm it does to us goes unnoticed. That is one reason why many people find it easy to become addicted. However, the biological process triggered by this activity manifests itself in a variety of ways. These include loss of appetite, insomnia, chronic fatigue, low spirit level, lack of concentration, premature aging, and increased vulnerability to diseases. Normally, there is a lock on the tank of sexual essence reserve kept in

the "Gate of Life" for everybody. The Gate of Life refers to the right kidney in traditional Chinese medicine, which is the place where vital kidney qi energy is stored. This gate is opened up when one is sexually excited, such as when making love or lost in sexual or pornographic thinking.

According to the Chinese natural health care system, energy drainage through pornographic thinking and masturbation is even more harmful to our health than physical ejaculation as a result of intercourse. Actual intercourse gives you temporary satisfaction and more importantly, compensates you in many other ways as you will see later. However, one-sided sexual thinking goes totally unrewarded. All it entails is a meaningless waste of sexual essence, which we are supposed to conserve as much as possible for the sake of overall health and longevity. The earlier we become aware of this powerful truth, the longer and healthier we will live.

Whatever the cause, stress is an inescapable product of life, and threatens to become a way of life for modern people. In this modern hubbub world where stress is at an all-time high, mental discipline based on a healthy outlook on life has gained special significance. Just as stress and depression can negatively impact our immune system and our overall health, so can an easy heart and a happy and optimistic outlook strengthen our immunity and promote health. Recent studies show that this may not be entirely psychological, but have a neurological basis as well. It is, therefore, of special importance in terms of mental peace that we stay happy and keep stress at bay.

The ancient Chinese held that a healthy mind is a peaceful and serene mind. They refer to such a mental state as the smooth, windless surface of a lake, or a mirror. They believe that such a mental state is in itself a potent medicine and an effective defense against disease. To them, a healthy mind is reflected in a merry spirit that always hopes for the best, even when confronted with difficulties. A healthy mind is also an easily contented mind which refuses to compare itself with others.

Of course, such a mentality is not easy to achieve. The reality of life ensures that we are bound to have stress and worry. "Sorrows and anxieties are part of life," observed Confucius. "Those who do not have worries about the future will have sorrow near at hand." While clearly conscious of the sad side of life, Confucius was not pessimistic at all. In fact, he was a highly optimistic person. He believed that how one looks at life goes a long way in determining whether he will be healthy and happy or not. After all, everything in the universe is relative and changeable. It is largely our own attitude toward life that makes the difference between misery and happiness, health and illness. Confucius advised us to imitate the universe: do your best and leave the rest to heaven.

It may sound as if we are touching the border of cultural background and philosophy. There is no denying the fact that cultural patterns exert a significant influence on our health. After all, cultural patterns are largely responsible for creating vastly different sets of values and philosophies of life, which in turn give birth to feelings, emotions, beliefs, and the way people react to stress. Thus, the intensity of stress posed by the same situation can be quite different for different individuals, depending on their attitudes and philosophy toward life in general.

In a culture that emphasizes wealth, encourages hard work and competition, and bases self-esteem on productivity and monetary success, feelings are often suppressed and emotions held in the body. These pent-up feelings and emotions sometimes find an outlet in violence. In civilized societies, they more often result in chronic stress.

Obviously, stress has to be controlled and reduced in order for our body and mind to function in a healthy way. The ancient Chinese were the first to recognize that stress can weaken the body's natural defenses made up of qi energy, making one susceptible to the most severe and mortal diseases.

However, effectively managing stress is not an easy task. Many of us just do not know how to, and many others have failed in their efforts. I see this as partly a cultural and a social problem. In a society where capitalism and money are the primary drivers and determinants of activities and status in life, and where social inequality and injustice run rampant, it can be very difficult for the underprivileged to handle stress effectively and in a timely manner. Even if money is not a problem, stress can make its presence felt in many other ways, including sour relations and frustrated ambitions. Therefore, we need to learn some effective methods of stress control. Fortunately, the ancient Chinese left us some extremely important advice on this subject.

· Do not seek perfection in life.

· Keep life simple.

· Know various dimensions of happiness.

· Look forward rather than backward.

· Try to think of yourself as the happiest person in the world.

· Learn to forgive yourself and others.

· Know your own fate from a qualified reader.

· Learn to forget unhappy things.

· Learn some methods of active diversion.

· Exercise regularly.

· Practice qigong everyday.

· Learn to appreciate light music.

· Become involved in some religious or spiritual group.

· Eat a well-balanced, natural, and nutritious diet.

There is simply no such thing as perfection in the universe. One can even argue that the beauty of the world and of life lies in its imperfection, which ensures room for continual creation and progress. This idea of universal imperfection is well illustrated in the famous Chinese classic I-Ching, or the Book of Change, which significantly begins with the discussion of "Universe" and ends with the topic of "Unfinished."

Typically, people start their lives with many ambitions. As they reach the end of their life, they find that most of these objectives have not been realized. After all, the world is not created for you. All you can do is your best and leave the outcome to God. Otherwise, you are asking for worry and trouble. Think in these terms, and you will find the pressure of life greatly reduced. This means, among other things, checking your ambitions and taking life as it comes.

In a Chinese study that lasted for twenty-two years, psychologists found that people with strong personal ambitions and the desire to control and lead others experienced a 60 percent higher death rate than other people. They died from all kinds of diseases, especially those of the heart. The main reason, according to the study, is that ambitious and power-oriented people tend to release a much greater amount of adrenaline than ordinary people. Excess adrenaline reaches the blood vessels and adds pressure to them, leading to heart disease and strokes. This is all the more true for men. Ambitious men tend to work toward their goal on their own, and not solicit help from others.

Keeping life simple is not only the highest wisdom of life, it is also one of the most powerful weapons against stress and depression. In our modern society, numerous people have been driven to desperation by commercialism and credit cards which advocate a fancy, "comfortable" lifestyle in exchange for endless stress and depression. Many people are buried in debt trying to keep pace with our modern lifestyle. They may be driving fancy cars and living in luxurious houses, but their hearts are hardly at ease. The net result: lack of comfort. Keeping life simple gives you the wisdom to say no to many kinds of temptations in modern society, thus saving you endless trouble. The fact of life remains: the less you desire, the easier it is to be satisfied, and the happier you will be.

In order to minimize our level of stress and avoid depression, we also need the courage and wisdom to say no to our desires, greediness, and selfishness. You will find life much less demanding, and much more enjoyable. As the Greek philosopher Epicurus said over 2,000 years ago, "It is impossible to live pleasurably without also living wisely." To Chinese sages, a wise life is a simple life in terms of diet, dress, home, rest, recreation, and transportation. Such a lifestyle draws you closer to nature and gives you better health and greater happiness over the long run.

Living in this modern age, we need to repeatedly remind ourselves of three important facts about happiness. First, while money can produce happiness if wisely used, money itself is not tantamount to happiness. You cannot carry it to the tomb with you when you die. Neither will it ensure happiness for your beloved survivors. Indeed, it cannot even buy love and happiness for yourself. True happiness, as well as genuine love, is beyond the purchasing power of money. Of course, money is important to our existence in many ways. However, one should know the limits and when to stop.

Second, for all its beauty and convenience, wealth is not something that can be achieved by everyone. In fact, there is a limit to how much you are going to receive in this lifetime. Confucius, while far from being a fatalist, knew this very well. He acknowledged: "I am ready to be a driver for anybody if this can earn me a fortune." The greatest Chinese sage would like to drive for others if in so doing he could become rich! Obviously, he is saying that wealth is not won by diligence or cleverness. It is predetermined.

What Confucius meant to say is this: "I will do whatever dirty work if such work can ensure me wealth." In other words, success is largely determined by fate, not by personal choice of career or hard work. There is another popular Chinese saying which is more specific: "Small fortune can be won with one's diligence, but big fortune is predetermined by fate."

Happiness is primarily a matter of our own feeling about ourselves—our self esteem. This understanding takes us to the significant conclusion that the surest way to find happiness is to look inward, rather than outward, as most people blindly do. You do not need to compare yourself with others. Comparison is odious. When you yourself feel enough, it is enough. When you feel happy, you are happy, regardless of what others may think of you.

It is also important to look forward rather than backward. What has happened, happened. There is no use living the past. What we can plan for and do something about is tomorrow. Tomorrow is in our hands, and we must firmly grasp it. Look forward, keep your eyes looking ahead. It seems that this is dictated by the laws of nature. Otherwise why not have eyes in the backs of our heads?

Even more important than looking toward the future is firmly grasping the present. Today is the most tangible part of life and time. The most we can do about life is today, which is the link between the past and the future. Used wisely, today can help shape our future. The message is, therefore, to focus on the here and now. The secret of focusing yourself on the present is through meditation, which I am going to discuss in detail later in the book (see the appendices). The magic of meditation is in cleansing our minds and allowing us to concentrate on ourselves for a period of time, be it ten minutes, twenty minutes, or several hours.

Try to think of yourself as the happiest person in the world. This may sound like self-deception, but it is a useful way of managing stress and distress in life. Robert Louis Stevenson used to say: "The world is so full of a number of things, I'm sure we should all be as happy as kings."

I still remember a poem written by the great American philosopher Ralph Waldo Emerson, in which he depicts an argument between a mountain and a squirrel. The mountain laughs at the insignificance of the squirrel and boasts of its own strength to carry the entire forest on its back. The squirrel, knowledgeable and confident, ends the whole argument with this reply: "If I cannot carry forests on my back, neither can you crack a coconut."

It is no coincidence that the same philosopher made a bold statement to the world that health is the greatest wealth over the long run. Indeed, there is no need to compare yourself to others. Resisting the temptation to compare yourself is the first step to becoming happy and to stay happy. Just as stress and depression can adversely affect all aspects of your health, a happy and contented mind will strengthen your immune system. Thus, resistance to comparison can mean resistance to disease. What an interesting phenomenon!

Stop trying to be on top of everything, or to be in control of others. In the final analysis, the only person you can control and change is yourself. Nobody is perfect; even Homer agrees. It is only human to err. This basic understanding is a good beginning. But it is, or should be, human to forgive. The ability to forgive is not the monopolistic character of God. We human beings are capable of it. This is the teaching of Buddhism, and I think it goes into the foundation of all religions. Forgive not only other's mistakes, but also those of our own.

How do you know what is and what is not predetermined for you? Trying to achieve things beyond what is permitted by your own fate is to invite disappointment and depression. This is where genuine fortunetellers can offer valuable help. Knowing one's own fate presumes that for all the statements and good will on the part of statesmen and human rights leaders, men simply are not born equal in physical and mental abilities, and least of all in wealth and family happiness. This guarantees that competition will not be carried out on an equal footing, and that success will vary widely for different people who possess similar intelligence and work equally hard. The undeniable fact is that not every diligent person can realize the American dream.

In other words, material and marital success does not vary in direct proportion to the efforts you put into it. It is the popular Chinese belief that the kind of marriage you have is something predetermined. More specifically, what kind of spouse you will have is a matter of fate, not a function of hard work. Still, you have to work to make marriage happen, even though it is a bad marriage. When you know your own strengths and weakness, you are less tempted to try things that are impossible for you. You are also more able to laugh at difficulties and stressful situations when they come into your life. By knowing your own fate, you can resist the natural temptation to compare yourself with others.

Being able to forget unhappy or frustrating events can be as important to mental health as the ability to forgive. While a strong memory can be the envy of many, it can sometimes be a great disadvantage to our health.

Learning to forget things was advice given by the ancient Chinese as a means to achieving greater happiness. One of the famous artistic geniuses in China's history, Zhen Banqiao, said: "It is a rare thing to be foolish, and it is a blessing to be taken advantage of. Thus, pretending to be deaf and dumb is a effective way to prolong your life." This attitude of non-competition is emphasized again and again in the doctrines of Buddhism and Taoism, both as a means of promoting health and as a way of self-cultivation.

Find some activity or cultivate a hobby which you can fall back on in times of stress. Many people have discovered that as soon as they take their mind off the pain and engage in activities they enjoy, the pain disappears. This can be simply doing something you like, such as watching a movie, listening to music, or going fishing—there are untold ways that allow you to temporarily forget your worries. Often the best solution to stress is to stop thinking about it.

Exercise is one kind of mental diversion, and the best one at that. Indeed, exercises allow you to kill two birds with one stone—improve your health and eliminate stress. Regular exercise can boost your mental power and creativity, thus dissipating stress. This is largely due to the fact that exercise increases oxygen flow to the brain, and enhances your morale and self-confidence. The more inactive you are, the longer the depressive or painful mood will stay with you, which may lead to more serious or long-term effects (i.e., nervous breakdown).

Qigong is a comprehensive mind-body regulator that goes directly to the roots of stress response by releasing the triggers of stress. Meditation is at once a pacifier and an exercise for the mind. It can effectively cool down a mind heated up by emotional outbursts. It can clarify the mind for a more insightful view of life, making it oblivious to potentially difficult situations and more resilient to stress. Clinical observations conducted in China found that those who had been practicing qigong for years have much lower levels of cortical and adrenaline hormones. Consequently, their ability to cope with stress peacefully without disturbing the normal hormonal functioning of the body is much stronger. Meanwhile, practitioners of qigong have been found to be less anxious and expressed less anger, hostility, and irritability than nonpractitioners. (For more information on how to perform qigong, refer to appendix 1.)

In China, music has been used as a healing method for a long time. Confucius listed musical education as one of the compulsory courses in his curriculum. He advised his disciples to turn to music for the healing of physical as well as mental pain. He also advocated it for insomnia and relaxation. His disciples learned that pleasant melodies could bring about delicate changes in the body and mind, boosting spirits and immunity, and speeding the healing process. Listening to light and melodious music can transport you to an enlightened world where you can forget the stressful situation for a while. Apart from its magical ability to relieve stress and depression, music has been found to possess many other therapeutic effects. For instance, it can help relieve hypertension, insomnia, asthma, ulcers, and a range of physical disabilities and muscle pains. This is because music can promote endorphins—the body's own painkiller. It has been scientifically shown that certain styles of music can reduce psychological components of pain such as stress, depression, anxiety, and fear.[14]

A recent study conducted at the Women's Hospital in Baton Rouge involved two groups of premature infants. One group was exposed to slow tempo lullabies, while the other was not. The infants who listened to the music experienced higher levels of oxygen in their blood and more normal heart rates compared to the premature infants who did not.

Of course, musical melodies do not have to be those produced by musical instruments or the human voice. Nature itself offers us an abundance of choice in this regard if we pay attention to it. The sound made by the flowing of water, rustling of leaves, and birds—all these are natural healers that cost nothing but help enormously.

Religions have been widely regarded as food for the mind. Now that we know the interconnection and interdependence of body and mind, it is easier for us to understand the importance of feeding our mind with proper diets. Religion is one such healthy diet. A recent medical study conducted in Connecticut showed that nonreligious people have twice the mortality rate of people with a strong faith. It is safe to say that a strong religious belief can be a mental haven in time of stress, which is the time when one is more prone to diseases. In addition, researchers have found that people who regularly draw comfort and faith from religion have lower blood pressure, less heart disease, higher survival rates after major surgery, and distinctively lower suicide rates.

It is no wonder that the latest statistics show that about one-third of patients in the U.S. today ask their doctors to pray with or for them as part of the healing process.

The healing power of religion comes largely from its teaching of the existence of life beyond death. This can make the pressures and misery of the current life more endurable than would otherwise be the case. When the soul is lightened and nourished by the prospect of the next life, the current life becomes easier to manage.

The choice of religion is a minor issue from the viewpoint of mental health. As I see it, all major religions are basically the same. The differences are much more a matter of manner than matter. They all contain basically the same teachings and are all forces for good. They provide us a spiritual exit from the daily pressures of life. It is in this sense that we regard religions as healthy diets for the mind. As such, they are equally effective no matter if you believe in Christianity,

Catholicism, Buddhism, Taoism, Islam, or anything else. Speak with the believers of these different religions and they will give you convincing proof.

Eating a well-balanced diet is necessary not only for our physical health, but also for our mental health. The quality of food we eat inevitably affects our mental health and activities. It is a common observation that if we eat well, we are more mentally active and energetic, capable of working longer hours without sleep. The more energetic we are mentally, the less likely we will be drawn into stress and depression.

To complete this picture of a human being, we must say that as much as the mind affects the body, so also can the body affect the mind. The relationship between the two is one of close interdependence and interaction. Neither can survive without the other.

Endnotes

1. Hans Selye, *The Stress of Life* (New York: McGraw-Hill, 1956).

2. The Great Proletariat Cultural Revolution, 1966 to 1976, was a nationwide political campaign personally launched by Mao Tse-tung with the major purpose of purging his political rivals. It caused tremendous social and economic damage to the nation, and physical and mental damage to the Chinese people. It formally ended with Mao's death.

3. E. Pendergrass, "Host Resistance and Other Intangibles in the Treatment of Cancer," *American Journal of Roentgenology* 85 (1961): 891–96.

4. E. Green and A. Green, *Beyond Biofeedback* (New York, NY: Delacorte, 1977).

5. George F. Solomon and A. Amkrant, "Emotions, Stress, and Immunity," *Frontier of Radiation Therapy and Oncology* 7 (1972): 84–96.

6. Pendergrass, *American Journal of Roentgenology*, 891–96.

7. *Men's Health,* December 1994, 104.

8. George E. Vaillant, *New England Journal of Medicine* (December 6, 1979).

9. Allan R. Cook, *Men's Health Concerns Sourcebook* (Detroit, MI: Omnigraphics, Inc., 1998), 328.

10. T. H. Holmes and M. Masuda, "Life Change and Illness Susceptibility." Paper presented as part of the Symposium on Separation and Depression (Clinical and Research Aspects, Chicago, December 1970).

11. Allan R. Cook, *Immune System Disorders Sourcebook* (Detroit, MI: Omnigraphics, Inc., 1997).

12. Christine A. Leatz, *Career Success/Personal Stress* (McGraw-Hill, Inc., 1993), 207–289.

13. *Men's Health*, May 1997, 78.

14. *Journal of Music Therapy* XXIII (1986).

Chapter 7

Natural Health Secrets of Exercise

Exercise is one of the major tools for improving our health and treating diseases in the Chinese natural health care system. Thousands of years ago, the ancient Chinese discovered the truth that activity is life; inactivity is disease. In the I-Ching, the earliest book written in China and the most importance classic of Chinese civilization, it is stated: "The Universe evolves all the time, so a gentleman should also be active throughout his life."

Ever since their civilization began, the Chinese have been paying attention to physical exercise as a way of maintaining health. As has been mentioned before, daoyin, a set of Chinese exercises specially designed to improve health and treat diseases, has been in existence for 3,000 years. Hua Tuo, a famous Chinese doctor and one of the fathers of the Chinese natural health care system, liked to compare the human body with a door and water. In introducing his five-animal play series of exercises to the world, he argued convincingly that running water never gets stale because it keeps on moving. Likewise, a door pivot will not get wormed because it is often used. (In ancient China, doors and door pivots were made of wood, which were susceptible to attack by worms.) In exactly the same way, a human body that is exercised regularly will not get sick. On the other hand, lack of exercise is one of the major causes of disease.

This is even truer for people living today. Many of us are confined to electronic offices and computer terminals during our waking hours. We are subject to a greater degree of stress than our ancestors, and have replaced healthy walking with cars. The high-tension and sedentary lifestyle characteristic of modern life has been linked to everything from cardiovascular diseases to cancer. This seems to be the price humans pay for the convenience and productivity of modern life.

No wonder so many people complain about how the all-too-fast aging process is working on them. Many people experience thinning hair, wrinkles, ringing in the ears, blurring eyesight, memory loss, lack of sexual desire, and other phenomena, while still only middle-aged. This is largely the result of their sedentary lifestyles.

Since lifestyle is a personal choice, premature aging is not inevitable. If we are willing to modify or change our lifestyle to make it more active, we can reverse the aging process that has already set in. Exercise works its rejuvenating magic by making us breathe deeper. Scientists call the process that regular exercise brings about "maximal oxygen uptake." What this does, on a molecular level, is to infuse the cells of our body with oxygen.

Studies have proven that after the age of about twenty, when many of us start to get lazy, we process about one percent less oxygen every year. The consequence of this oxygen cutback is a commensurate decline in cellular activity. In other words, our bodies begin to suffocate. This is what I believe aging is about—that more fresh oxygen is good for health and will help delay the aging process. Experts now agree that most of the physical decline that older people suffer from stems, not from aging itself, but from simple disuse. Exercise can prevent bones, muscles, and internal organs from disintegrating and even revive the aging parts of the body.

A ready, natural, and free solution for this dilemma is regular exercise. Exercise can solve the contradiction between modernization and natural health. Exercise can prevent many forms of degenerative diseases from happening by keeping the heart and lungs strong enough to supply the amount of oxygen our bodies grew up with. The fact is that our bodies respond to physical stress by adapting and growing stronger. This response is what evolution is all about. Exercise also benefits our hearts and lungs. It has been shown that runners have cardiovascular systems that have twice the capacity and efficiency as those of people of the same age who are less active. We should not forget that the heart itself is a muscle and needs to be exercised regularly. Studies show that people who remain active as they grow older—especially those who remain very active—can maintain breathing capacities equal to those of people thirty years younger. (Here, active people refer to those who exercise for an average of one hour per day, and very active people refer to those who exercise for an average of at least two hours per day.)

Perhaps the most amazing fact is that regular exercise can even change our eating habits. One survey shows that regular exercisers are more likely to quit smoking, 40 percent more likely to eat less red meat, 30 percent more likely to cut down on caffeine, 250 percent more likely to eat low calorie foods, and 200 percent more likely to lose weight, than non-exercisers.[1]

Here are some of the benefits of regular exercise:

- Boosts the immune system.

- Lowers blood pressure.

- Increases good cholesterol (HDL) while lowering bad cholesterol (LDL).

- Increases the metabolic rate, speeding up the burning of excess fat.

- Sets the body's thermostat higher throughout the day.

- Improves respiration, and cleanses the lungs.

- Lowers the risk of breast cancer.

- Improves sleep and relieves insomnia.

- Increases blood and oxygen circulation to all parts of the body, thus improving our memory and immunity.

- Strengthens the heart muscle, protecting it, reducing the blood's tendency to form clots, and making it a more powerful and efficient pumping machine.

- Strengthens the bones by improving bone density and toning the muscles, thus preventing osteoporosis.

- Keeps us strong and trim; increases muscle mass and decreases fat.

- Enhances our mood and spirit.

- Accelerates bowel movements, speeding food through the colon, thus preventing constipation and colon cancer.

- Promotes the cleaning of our body through sweating and bowel movements.

- Encourages the growth of calorie-consuming enzymes and increases the power of the muscle cells to use glucose.

- Controls weight, helps prevent diabetes, obesity, and hypertension.

- Increases sexual vitality and helps cure impotence and loss of sexual desire.

- Relieves physical tension and mental stress.

- Enhances our ability to cope with crises.

- Stimulates morale and boosts energy.

- Smoothes and nourishes skin.

- Speeds recovery from the common cold by boosting the immune system.

- Slows the aging process.

Many people today are worried about wrinkles on their faces. Fundamentally, the best way to "iron out" these wrinkles is to keep fit. Actually, what makes the face red and sanguine—oxygen—also makes it rugged and wrinkled. The skin of athletes is more elastic than that of their sedentary peers. Scientists believe that our skin reflects an adaptation to habitual endurance training by increasing its mass and strengthening its structure. That helps explain why athletes look—and of course act—younger than their less active peers.

In addition, the oxygen that is pumped into our bodies during exercise is also pumped into our heads. The more fresh oxygen that gets to the brain, the more clear, active, sharp, and healthy the brain becomes. Exercise can, therefore, strengthen nerve tissue in much the same way as it does muscles. The increased oxygen supply, enzyme activity, and blood flow created by exercise safeguards the overall health of the central nervous system, which in turn favorably impacts on the physical well-being of the exerciser. There is a popular belief that exercise makes people become excited and overheated. In fact, exercise has a magic tranquilizing power over the body. Even moderate exercise can raise the temperature of muscles, making them less tense and therefore more comfortable.

Does exercise have anything to do with sexual ability? Of course it does. If you are attentive enough, you will notice that most sexually active people are physically active.

Modern scientists have confirmed this fact with the finding that exercise increases the flow of hormones that play key roles in the chemistry of arousal for both sexes. This agrees with the findings of James White, an expert on physical fitness and sex, and professor emeritus at the University of California at San Diego. He found that men who exercise moderately regularly report increased libidos, more satisfying sex, and fewer erection problems.

The *Journal of the American Medical Association* carried an article concluding that moderate exercise once a week can reduce the death rates of all female diseases by 24 percent.[2] Even better, moderate exercise four times a week can reduce the death rate of all diseases by 30 percent, especially heart and respiratory diseases. According to the study, regular exercise, even at a very moderate level, can prevent and cure many female-specific health problems such as menstrual dysfunction, because exercise can save female hormones.

The following statistics from various studies done in the U.S. clearly point to the benefits of regular exercises:

- Daily exercise speeds recovery from the common cold by boosting the immune system. Women who walked forty-five minutes a day recovered twice as fast— five days versus ten days—from colds than women who did not exercise.[3]

- Exercising five or more times a week can reduce the risk of type II diabetes by 42 percent.[4]

- Physically inactive people have, for one thing, a 35 to 52 percent greater risk of developing hypertension than those who exercise, independent of other risk factors for the disease.[5]

A recent fourteen-year long study on 25,000 women brings exciting news for women who are concerned about breast cancer. The study shows that regular exercise can reduce the risk of breast cancer by 47 percent for premenopausal women, and by 33 percent for postmenopausal women. This is because regular exercise decreases the production of estrogen, a female hormone that can lead to breast cancer.

Another study conducted for the Honolulu Heart Program found that among older people who practice exercise on regular basis, the incidence of stroke was only about one-third of that for inactive men.

Take the example one of the simplest forms of exercise—light walking. Walking has been shown to be one of the best exercises. It can prevent and relieve cardiovascular, respiratory and circulation disorders, aid digestion and sleep, control weight, and reduce stress and depression. A thirty-minute walk every day will lower the risk of developing or dying from some of the leading causes of illness and death in this country. It has been shown that regular walking can reduce your risk of dying prematurely from heart disease, colon cancer, and diabetes. It can lower your blood pressure, improve cholesterol levels, and reduce body fat. It can build and maintain muscles, bones, and joints, relieve arthri-

tis, and prevent hypertension. In addition, walking can make you sleep better, lowers your level of stress and depression, and boosts your energy.

The ancient Chinese recommended exercising twice a day on a regular basis, preferably once in the morning and once in the afternoon or evening. Ideally, exercise should be done on daily basis, rather than two or three times a week. After all, we must sleep each and every day, rather than just two or three times a week. Daily exercise is the most desirable because twenty-four hours represents nature's cycle. To maximize the health benefits of exercise, and indeed of most other things, it is important that we live in harmony with nature's rhythm. For people with special healing needs, the frequency of exercise can be increased and the duration of exercise reduced. The optimum length of exercise each time is somewhere around twenty to thirty minutes.

As far as the optimum times to exercise are concerned, the ancient Chinese provided us with important guidelines. According to traditional Chinese exercise physiology, the time between when you get up in the morning and breakfast is one of the best times for exercise. The earlier in the morning, the better and greater the healing effect. Typically, Chinese martial artists get up before 5 A.M. to start their daily exercises. For seventy years, my late teacher Dr. Wan Laisheng got up at 4 A.M. every day to practice qigong and martial arts. As he finished his training, the sun was just beginning to break with most people still in bed. He kept this schedule to the very end of his life.

There are many advantages to early morning exercise. First, it helps you get rid of the stale air that has accumulated inside your body during sleep (the Chinese ancestors considered night air as being yin in nature, which is not good for one's physical and mental health), and replaces it with fresh air (the ancient Chinese regard early morning air as highly nutritional and beneficial to overall health). Second, it clears your mind and boosts your spirit for a new day of work. This enhances your efficiency and productivity, making you more positive and confident, and better able to handle stress during the day. Third, it strengthens your digestion and boosts your appetite. Fourth, it increases your physical and mental adaptability to the environment, increasing your immunity to diseases.

My recommended schedule is to exercise at least twice a day, for about thirty minutes each time. I prefer to exercise once in the morning and again in the afternoon or evening. Weather conditions do not affect this regimen.

Exercise is best performed outdoors. This is because the air supply is ample and fresh. During exercise, your body needs more oxygen to keep up with the tempo of your heart rate and internal combustion. Fresh and abundant air supply thus becomes as essential as the exercise itself. As well, there is more to look at outside, which will enhance your interest in the exercise.

The ancient Chinese also warned us against exercising when we are tired, hungry, thirsty, or within half an hour of a meal. Exercise in times of fatigue drains our vital energy, making us weaker rather stronger as a result. That is something Chinese sages are very careful in avoiding. Exercise close to meal times takes the blood away from the stomach, causing indigestion and stomach ailments. It is also necessary to increase our water and nutrition intake in accordance with the amount of exercise. This is particularly the case during the summer months, which are considered to be the most consumptive time of the year. This means that we should drink more water and juice in the summer, and also eat more nutritious foods.

The ancient Chinese discourage "jumping into" vigorous exercise immediately after reading, resting, or sleeping. Neither should we rush into reading, resting, or sleeping immediately after vigorous exercise. The underlying moral is that the human body needs some transitional time to adjust itself from one state of activity to another, which may have a dramatically different heart rate. Therefore, it is essential that you give yourself a short period of transition from physical activity to mental activity. This is best accomplished in the form of a light walk before and after any vigorous exercise. My teacher Dr. Wan Laisheng used to tell me: "Neglecting to take a light walk before and after the practice of martial arts is a sure sign of stupidity." This is a golden rule to keep in mind. Violation of this principle will likely lead to heart problems, because a transitional period is needed for our heart to adjust to a different type of activity. In this sense, our body is somewhat similar to a car. For the sake of keeping our car working longer, it is recommended that after we start our car in the morning after a night's disuse, we wait for a period for the engine to warm up before actually driving it.

While appropriate and moderate exercise is necessary for health, too much exertion—for instance, heavy weightlifting, marathon running, and mountain climbing—can lower our immune systems and damage our health. While individuals vary in terms of strength and stamina, everyone should be able to tell when enough is enough. Here, as anywhere, too much is inevitably as bad as too little. According to David Nieman, professor at Appalachian State University in North Carolina, exercising near your maximum capacity for just forty-five minutes produces a six-hour "window" of vulnerability to disease afterwards. During that period of time, you are much more vulnerable to the invasion of disease because your immune system has been significantly weakened.[6]

It is also important that you never overstretch yourself during exercise. For this reason, I find traditional Chinese fitness exercises have distinctive advantages over more rigorous exercises. While all exercises share some common health benefits, there are some major differences between traditional Chinese exercises and conventional, popular ones in the West.

One of the major differences is that all Chinese fitness exercises are designed with the sole purpose of improving health, as contrasted with many forms of modern exercises which are designed mainly for competition, for example, taich'i, qigong, and Dharma's morning exercises. By contrast, soccer, basketball, running, and many other forms of exercise have competition as one of its purposes. This difference is highly significant from a medical standpoint. It not only leads to other major differences but also explains why Chinese fitness exercises are more suitable for the purposes of natural health and healing. Besides, Chinese fitness exercises are designed with the sole purpose of promoting health and curing disease. As such, there is no room for competition in them. This enables all their practitioners to play with a light heart, further enhancing the therapeutic effects of the exercise.

Just watching people practicing taich'i together in almost any park in China, you can see the marvelous rhythm of people moving in perfect harmony with each other. All of them share the sincere enjoyment of the exercise as well as each other's companionship. Here you sense the dominant spirit of peaceful co-existence characteristic of Chinese culture. This is only possible when competition is out of the picture. In an absolute sense, this is mutually beneficial. For one thing, if your neighbors are healthy, you have a greater chance of being healthy, too, if only because there is less infectious bacteria around you.

Another major difference lies in the very "softness" of Chinese fitness exercises, as contrasted with the muscle and toughness of Western sports. In exercise as well as in diet, the Chinese choose to take it easy and go slowly. They tend to think of life as well as health in the long term. They purposely regulate both the speed and the amount of exercise, exactly as they do with food. The Chinese know that while moderate exercise is necessary for health and the nourishment of vital qi, too much physical exertion can damage the vital qi and cause health problems.

Modern studies have confirmed this ancient Chinese wisdom. According to Dr. Thomas Brunoski, a physician in Westport, Connecticut, exercise at an extremely high intensity promotes the formation of free radicals for a brief period. These are substances that promote oxidation in the body and lead to premature aging and heart disease. Because traditional Chinese fitness exercises are soft and are performed in a leisurely manner, they make you feel doubly relaxed, a fact that can be greatly conducive to your mental as well as physical health. Thanks to their soft nature, they are suitable for virtually everyone. People of different ages, sex, and physical status can all benefit from doing these exercises as they have no adverse side effects. You can do them at any time and in any place. They are available to everybody because most of them require no equipment or facilities to practice.

The third major difference lies in the fact that Chinese fitness exercises emphasize the delicate coordination of body and mind. They require you to be completely focused on what you are doing, using your mind to guide your bodily movements. This is another direct application of the systematic philosophy that the Chinese hold with regard to the universe where the result is improved mental and physical health at the same time.

The fourth major difference is a very important one, and its importance can hardly be overestimated. It is the requirement of coordinating one's breathing with the physical movement. Due to the essential role breathing plays in our life and our health, the combination of regulated breathing and soft bodily movement greatly enhances the therapeutic effect of these exercises.

Here are a few points to keep in mind concerning exercise:

• Get prepared/warm up. Exercise should be preceded by a short period of warming up. Before engaging in any exercise you should perform some mental and physical preparations, and warm your body up for a few minutes. This warming-up preparation can be a light walk or some stretching exercises to improve the flexibility of the joints and muscles. The heat that is generated by this preliminary exercising will help boost blood flow to the muscles, increasing their oxygen supply. In addition, the increase in muscle temperature helps increase elasticity and joint mobility, thereby helping to prevent injury during the course of the exercises.

- Cool down. Take time to cool down after exercise, both mentally and physically. This means having a period of relaxation and gradual tapering off after exercise, rigorous exercise in particular. Cooling down after exercising is vital to avoid harmful side effects. This buffer period between exercise and work or sleep helps to gradually eliminate heat and prevent shock to the body system. In fact, if you suddenly stop exercising, muscle spasms and cramps may occur. Again, the best easiest way to cool down is to take a slow walk for a few minutes until your heart rate falls below 100 beats per minute. My teacher used to tell me: "It must be a fool who does not take a walk before and after practicing martial arts." In fact, this rule applies to all kinds of exercises, including the seemingly motionless breathing exercise.

- Go slowly. Begin your exercise routine, slowly build up momentum so that your heart, muscles, and lungs can adapt to the new demands exercise places on them. Sudden increases in duration, intensity, or frequency of a workout can lead to injury.

- Do not urinate immediately after vigorous exercising. Your heart is beating faster than usual, and your kidneys are in a state of strain. Like the heart, it takes a while for the kidneys to cool down. Urination at this time will cause damage to the kidneys and lead to the leakage of vital energy stored there. It is the belief of Chinese fathers that urinating immediately after exercise—intense exercise in particular—will cause subtle damage to the kidneys and possibly a fainting spell.

- Drink a cup of warm water and have a bowel movement before starting your morning exercise. This is because exercise makes you sweat. As a result, the body absorbs some of the water from the colon to keep balance. This may cause difficulties when having a movement later. Your body may also absorb some of the poisonous substances already dissolved in the waste to be excreted. This could damage your health. As drinking water and having a motion takes time, it makes good sense to get up early if you are serious about morning exercise.

- Do not exercise right after meal. This is because after each meal, a large amount of blood concentrates in the stomach to ensure that the food gets digested properly. The fuller your stomach, the more blood that is needed for this purpose. The digestion process take about an hour. Consequently, it is advisable to avoid vigorous exercise for at least an hour, if not longer, after a meal. However, a light walk is okay and even recommended after a meal.

- Wear loose-fitting clothes and light exercise shoes. No hat and no glasses, if at all possible. This is meant to give you greater relaxation, enhance your concentration of mind on the exercise itself, and promote the smooth circulation of blood and qi inside the body.

Please see the appendices, where I have outlined the characteristics, therapeutic effects, and instructions for five of the most effective forms of Chinese natural health and healing exercises.

Endnotes

1. "Look who's getting it all together," *American Health* 4, no. 2, 42–47.

2. "Physical Activity and Mortality in Postmenopausal Women," *Journal of the American Medical Association* (April 23/30, 1997): 1287–92.

3. Study by David Nieman, exercise physiologist, Appalachian State University, Boone, North Carolina, reported in "Physical Activity and Immune Function in Elderly Women," *The Walking Magazine* 25, no. 7 (July 1993): 823–31.

4. *Healing Unlimited* (New York, NY: Boardroom Inc., 1995), 116–117.

5. *Consumer Issues in Health Care Sourcebook* (Detroit, MI: Omnigraphics, Inc., 1995), 391.

6. David Nieman, *Fitness and Your Health* (Palo Alto, CA: Bull Publishing Co., 1993).

Chapter 8

Natural Health Secrets of Regulated Sex

Food and sleep are fundamental biological needs. So is sex. Sexual activities are the natural result of the production and secretion of sexual hormones. It is essential for the continuation of species. This is God's idea of creating two genders in all species to nurture each other and to ensure that the species continue. Indeed, man and woman are supposed to live together in harmony for mutual health benefits. Harmonious sex is highly desirable for overall health and happiness; therefore, lack of a normal sex life is not in the best interests of our health.

This idea of a male-female combination as a realization of universal Tao is clearly illustrated in the I-Ching, the classical Chinese Book of Changes that was written almost 3,000 years ago. In fact, one of the recurring themes it states is that yin alone will not reproduce, yang alone will not grow, and Tao is realized in the combination of yin and yang. It is this combination of yin and yang that gives birth to everything. Based on their understanding of the universal law of yin-yang, the ancient Chinese believed

115

that for the benefit of our health, we need to promote a harmonious sexual life so that both partners can complement and nourish each other. This is known as *qu-yin-bu-yang* (take the female yin to nurture the male yang) and *qu-yang-bu-yin* (take the male yang to nurture the female yin).

To derive the greatest benefit from sex, we need to know the law of yin and yang. For one thing, sex is a double-edged sword. It can work for the benefit of your health, but it can destroy your health as well. Exactly as yin and yang are two sides of the same picture, qu-yin-bu-yang and qu-yang-bu-yin are two processes occurring simultaneously during intercourse.

From a health point of view, the mutual benefits derived from sexual intercourse are manifold. Modern studies prove that sex stimulates the body's immune system and promotes the production of white cells. It accelerates blood flow and the metabolic process. In women, sex raises the level of estrogen in the blood, protecting calcium loss in the bones. In addition, sex releases a flood of endorphins, nature's own painkiller, thus providing hours of pain relief from arthritis and other aches. Moreover, sex is a great stress reducer, and can enable people to forget their worries and anxieties for a while.

Indeed, nothing relieves and soothes better than an orgasm. According to Ms. Sadoughi, Director of the Sex Dysfunction Clinic at Cook County Hospital in Chicago, sex is one of the best pain—and stress—relievers. "It could be any number of things,"

Ms. Sadoughi says, "something biochemical or hormonal. The emotional aspect is obviously important. Sex is a wonderful source of self-esteem, a great reliever of stress, and pretty fair exercise, to boot." Indeed, harmonious sex is not just a bliss of life; it is a potent health promoter and natural healer. In practice, sex has been used to relieve arthritis, allergies, and nocturnal emission. Researchers find that arthritis patients who go ahead and have sex despite the pain in their joints often report that their joints are free of pain for more than six hours afterwards. It is documented that heart surgeon Christiaan Barnard suffered from arthritis for years before he married a young woman named Barbara. He told people later that he virtually ceased to be an arthritis patient for several years after the wedding. To him, falling in love was the best arthritis medicine of all.

Researchers believe that sexual arousal touches off a chain of blissful hormonal changes, boosting the production of corticosteroid, a hormone that reduces pain and inflammation in the joints, as well as endorphins, the body's natural opiates. San Francisco allergist Alan Scott Levin is quoted as saying: "When I was really sick and nothing else helped, I can always count on sex." According to Dr. Levin, other patients also reported disappearance of allergic symptoms during and after sexual intercourse. It is also suggested that sex can be a preventer of prostate cancer.[1] As for the therapeutic effect of sex on nocturnal emissions, several of my friends have told me that their symptoms disappeared almost miraculously right after their wedding.

Again, while sex can improve your health, it can be a detriment as well. The difference lies in whether or not you know the Tao of yin and yang, i.e., whether or not sexual activities are regulated. Here, the vital thing is sexual essence, which means sperm. It is vital to health, as the Chinese fathers see it, and has been repeatedly verified by human experience. Indulgence in sex without mastering the Tao of yin and yang is bound to lead to a series of health problems. In other words, if the loss of sexual essence as a result of ejaculation can be more than compensated by sexual intercourse itself, it is regulated sex and will therefore benefit one's health. However, if the loss of sexual essence from ejaculation cannot be fully compensated by the sexual experience itself, it is unregulated sex, and will therefore damage one's health. It has been scientifically proven that ejaculation means a loss of zinc and other essential body nutrients. Zinc is a vital source of life energy, and it takes time and other forms of energy to replenish it. When zinc is not replenished, one's physical and mental health will suffer as a result. That is exactly why those who give themselves foolishly and willingly to sexual indulgences are eventually afflicted with chronic fatigue, low spirits, weak immunity, insomnia, ringing ears, sexual dysfunction, impotence, kidney diseases, neurasthenia, and other health problems.[2]

Obviously, regulated sex is mainly a male issue, as long as there is only one sexual relationship between the same couple for a long time, i.e., monogamy. This is because man is yang in nature, and yang energy is extroverted and outgoing. As such, yang energy is much more vulnerable to loss and drainage than yin energy, which is introverted and hidden inside the female body. Thus, regulated sex boils down to the issue of ejaculation control, of how frequently a man should ejaculate as he advances in age. As a general principle, ejaculation should be kept to the minimum. The less frequently you ejaculate, the greater will be the health benefits of sex. Waste of sexual essence means a lowered immunity and greater risk of all kinds of diseases. According to Dr. Wan Laisheng, "In the final analysis, the root cause of all male diseases can be boiled down to loss of sperm as a result of sexual indulgence or wishful sexual thinking."

Regulating ejaculation does not mean avoiding sex. It is not the frequency of intercourse, but the frequency of ejaculation that is to be regulated. Avoidance of sex is not a solution, because it is not the law of nature and, therefore, not in the best interest of health. For one thing, a chronic inability of a man to answer the sexual urge of nature will create a yearning for the female, a one-sided wishful thinking of sex. This will disturb the energy balance in the body, leading to unwanted leakage of sexual essence in the form of uncontrollable nocturnal emissions. Semen and vital energy lost in this way are far more harmful to one's health than conscious ejaculation during intercourse. Worse still, you get nothing back in compensation for your loss of semen and energy by engaging in wishful sexual thinking.

Normal, harmonious sex is good for your health for exactly the same reasons that avoidance of sex is bad for your health. A clinical experiment demonstrated that many single men who suffered from nocturnal emissions and neurasthenia were mysteriously healed of these diseases shortly after marriage, without needing doctors or medication. Their sleep improved, bedwetting suddenly stopped, and their energy levels and spirits grew. What happened? The harmonious sexual life of the newly married couples brought about the unexpected healing. Thus, we see that sex is a healer in itself, and a potent one at that, if you know the secret of regulated sex. It is the combination of frequent intercourse with regulated ejaculation that is in the best interest of our health.

Why should sexual intercourse be frequent but ejaculation infrequent? The answer lies in three parts. First, sexual intercourse represents the communion between yin and yang, the two basic energy types in the universe, and the harmony between earth and heaven. In the absence of this harmony and communion, nothing will come into being, nor will anything last for long. Yin and yang are supposed to coexist in harmony. This is the law of nature. Frequent sexual intercourse balances the yin and yang energies in the body, and creates a physical and mental state that is highly desirable for overall health.

Second, semen is a limited, precious substance of life. It is the prime source of male sexual vitality and the foundation of his immune power. Modern research finds that semen is rich in zinc and 20 percent of it is made of cerebralspinal fluid.[3] It is no wonder why those who squander away their semen freely and frequently are, without exception, afflicted with various degenerative diseases such as insomnia, headaches, poor memory, premature aging, and ear-ringing.

Worse still, the body's production of this precious substance is usually low, much lower than most people—especially younger people—would like to think. Therefore, if you willingly let your semen reserves fall below their desired level for a period of time, you are likely to cause trouble for yourself. The minimum level—I call it "strategic reserve level"—of semen in the body is determined by the biological nature of the individual. Usually each individual can feel his own strategic need, but unfortunately this is only possible in hindsight, and is often too late.

What remains to be answered is the question of how can a man benefit from a woman through intercourse and vice versa. This is qu-yin-bu-yang (take the yin energy to nourish the yang energy). It occupies the central place in the art of regulated sex. This rarely known fact is that the best of a woman's yin energy will not come out until she has reached orgasm. It takes both time and physical collusion for this to take place. Obviously, the man needs stamina. If he ejaculates prematurely, he cannot stay active long enough for his sexual partner to reach an orgasm, spoiling a good part of the game. The consequence is a loss for both parties. Premature ejaculation does nothing to enhance a man's self-image and self-confidence, nor does it allow him to receive the necessary yin energy to nourish his yang energy. Naturally, his partner will also feel dissatisfied and disappointed. He lost his precious semen without gaining any energy compensation from his partner in return. This is like adding humiliation to insult.

If a man does not know the art of regulated sex, the chances are high that intercourse will be a lose-lose situation for both partners. However, if he masters the art of regulated sex, he can turn intercourse into a win-win situation to the advantage and satisfaction of both partners. The net result is improved overall health and a better relationship between the partners.

Indeed, there is a lot to be gained by practicing regulated sex. It is said that Dr. Ma Yinchu, the late principal of Beijing University, made it a point to have sex each and every night. Despite all his ordeals during Communist rule, he died a healthy man at the age of 105! I do not have the slightest doubt that he must be a great master of the Tao of yin and yang, and benefited greatly from regulated sex.

According to the theory of the Chinese natural health care system, there are two essential rules governing the frequency of ejaculation. First, ejaculation has a lot to do with the person's age. As a rule, the younger you are, the greater your productivity of semen and therefore your sexuality, and vice versa. It takes five days for a normal male in his teens to replenish the semen lost in one ejaculation. However, it takes seven days for a normal man in his twenties to accomplish the same task, ten days for a man in his thirties, fourteen days for a man in his forties, one month for a man in his fifties, and three months for a man in his sixties to get the same job done. Moreover, it is a principle of Chinese natural health that ejaculation should be completely avoided after the age of sixty-four, the square of eight, at which a male has completed a full cycle of his biological evolution and is therefore ready for sexual retirement (meaning no ejaculation at all).

Second, ejaculation should be in harmony with the four seasons. Based on their understanding of the law of nature, the ancient Chinese held that summer is the season of evaporation, while winter is the season of conservation. Waste in the various forms of evaporation of body energy, such as sweating, can be tiring during the summer season. In this season, our Gate of Life is especially loose compared to other times of the year, making ejaculation all the more uncontrollable. When men ejaculate at this time of year, it is like a dam burst, as a large amount of semen is released. That is why men have to be cautious in controlling themselves and regulate their ejaculations in this season.

For opposite reasons, winter is not a good season for ejaculation, either. This is because the law of nature dictates that we preserve our semen during the winter season, as do snakes and bears as they enter their long winter hibernation. At this time, conservation of semen is the call of nature for the sake of combating the coldness in the environment. The mere task of combating the environmental coldness takes a great deal of energy. Strategic energy reserves should be used for this purpose first.

One should be doubly careful in regulating ejaculation during these two seasons. This is especially true for the two thirty-day periods in a year—one with the summer solstice as its midpoint, and the other with the winter solstice as its midpoint. Chinese regimen is opposed to ejaculation during these periods, no matter how young and healthy you are. Violation of this rule invites severe penalties, including an immediate lowering of immunity.

As well as this, the ancient Chinese were vehemently against ejaculation while under the influence of alcohol, with an empty or full belly, or shortly after recovery from illness. We should avoid ejaculation at these times. Ignoring this rule can be damaging to our health. Semen lost in these situations is considered to be one hundred times more harmful to our health than under normal conditions. Invariably, violators of this advice find themselves ill again, either with their original disease, some new disease, or in a dizzy mind shortly after the carnal pleasure. Under those situations mentioned above, a rule of thumb to follow is to avoid

sex altogether until you are well again.

As you can see, regulated sex is a highly involved art in the Chinese natural health care system. It has qu-yin-bu-yang (take the yin energy to nourish the yang energy) as its ultimate goal and *wo-gu-bu-xie* (intercourse without ejaculation) as its primary means.

We will come back to these interesting topics later in the book, in the chapter on "Secrets of Sexual Vitality." For the time being, remember that regulated sex is a powerful promoter of overall health and improved sexual relations. By striking a yin-yang balance between male and female partners through regulating ejaculation, our physical and mental health will improve, and we become able to heal our ailments in a pleasant way.

Endnotes

1. Stefan Bechtel, *The Practical Encyclopedia of Sex and Health* (Rodale Press, 1993), 19, 27 and 261.

2. This has been repeatedly proven in clinical observations in China. Modern science has found that zinc is a component of many enzymes and thus is involved in most metabolic processes. It plays an important role in the formation of protein in the body and thus assists in blood formation and general growth and maintenance of all tissues. Karen Bellenir, *Diet and Nutrition* (Detroit, MI: Omnigraphics, Inc., 1999), 22-23.

3. There are different conclusions about the content of semen. Saying that it has nothing to do with cerebrospinal fluid is against human experience. Almost all people who are sexually indulgent have experienced different degrees of headaches, insomnia, loss of memory, and ear-ringing.

Chapter 9

Natural Health Secrets of Environmental Hygiene

We are living in a world where environmental pollution has become part of life. Civilized humans today must live in cramped urban areas, drink contaminated water, take in polluted air, eat contaminated foods, and endure loud, disturbing noises. Global warming, acid rain, holes in the ozone layer, deafening city noise, and contaminated water, food, and air have all degraded the quality of life and caused many health problems. The grave environmental situation we face today is created entirely by humans. People today seem to be selfish, materialistic, and money-oriented, constantly undervaluing and ignoring the importance of our environment.

True, air costs us nothing and water is also cheap. There seems to be no limit of supply for these natural resources. This simplistic and selfish mentality has resulted in the serious environmental pollution around us. According to estimated statistics, each year we pour tons of pesticide into the air we breathe and vegetables and fruits we eat. The average person is exposed to over 700 chemicals in city drinking water and over 500 chemicals in the home environment, not to mention what we encounter at work and when travelling.[1]

This cannot help but have a great impact on our health. In fact, a number of diseases today can be directly associated with environmental pollution. For instance, polluted water and food are blamed for cases of diarrhea, stomach ulcers, and food poisoning. The noise pollution of modern cities often causes headaches, insomnia, deafness, stress, and mental disturbances, such as violence and suicide. The thinning of the ozone layer is thought to be the major cause of skin cancer, which is increasing rapidly. Allergic reactions and hypersensitivity ailments, for instance, are among the most common and costly of U.S. health problems, afflicting at least 35 million Americans at an annual medical cost of $1 billion.[2]

Three major reasons can be cited for the worsening situation of the environment we are experiencing today. One is the rapid growth rate of world population. Another is the expansion of industrialization. Yet another reason is a greedy drive for short-term profits and comforts, ignoring the well-being of the population and future generations, reminding people of the old saying: "After me, the deluge"—I don't care what will happen after me.

Population growth adds heavy pressure on water resources and solid waste treatment. In many parts of the world, waste-water and solid waste are barely treated before they are put into nearby rivers and oceans. This seriously affects the quality of the water we drink and the environment in which we live.

More people means more noise, more contamination in the air, and more destruction of natural resources to serve the needs of the whole population. Thus, we witness excess cutting of forests, arbitrary changing of water routes, and the leveling off of mountains and farmland to build houses and highways. We also witness the enormous amount of carbon dioxide from automobiles, industrial exhaust, and household sources released into the sky each day, polluting the air and causing severe damage to the ozone layer.

The greater the population, the fiercer the competition, and the more urgent the need to increase productivity. Here lies the second major cause of environmental pollution. This means, among other things, the excessive use of chemicals and hormones to boost the production of food and other necessities to meet the needs of humankind. Higher productivity means greater profits. While industrialization can enhance the quality of people's lives, at the same time it can cause harm. For example, oil leakage from ocean tankers puts millions of tons of crude oil into the water each year, poisoning and killing fish and sea birds and mammals. The excessive cutting down of forests has greatly weakened Mother Nature's power to neutralize the negative impact of industrialization in our environment, and is largely responsible for ever worsening flooding in China, year after year. Today, environmental problems are running in a vicious cycle. A growing population puts more pressure on the society's need to industrialize, while industrialization releases more wastes into our environment. To break this cycle will take enormous investment, education of the public, reduction of population growth, and restrictions on the greed of people around the world.

Environmental concern is not a recent issue. The ancient Chinese were keenly aware of the importance of environmental hygiene. They knew clearly that fresh air and clean water were essential to overall health and longevity. They also knew that the quality of air and water was better in mountainous areas than in crowded cities. Many of them traded the conveniences and comforts of city life for the fresh air, clean water, and quiet surroundings of the mountains. Typically, these were Taoist and Buddhist recluses, who chose to spend most of their enlightened lives in secluded mountainous areas in search of physical health and mental enlightenment. It is little wonder that most of the oldest living Chinese are enlightened people. Similar examples of longevity are found in Norway, Japan, Russia, and other countries, where the most long-lived people are found living in mountainous areas.

Ancient people did not eat much, nor did they have the comforts and conveniences provided by modern medical technology, but they enjoyed better health than modern people do. Indeed, most of the diseases that kill Americans today were simply unheard of at that time. How could they eat so little and yet be so energetic and healthy? The secret lies in the fact that they drew a lot of vital energy from Mother Nature. They drank clean water, breathed pure air, bathed in the mild sunlight, and ate raw fruits and vegetables that were nourished naturally by a healthy environment. These are unlimited sources of energy provided by nature. However, they are beneficial to us only when they are clean and protected from man-made pollution.

The following discusses several areas in the environment that can cause significant risks to your health. These are chemicals and other man-made pollutants, radiation (ultraviolet rays), air pollution, noise pollution, and water pollution.

Chemicals

There is abundant evidence in animal biology to show how pollutants destroy an animal's ability to reproduce and reduce its immunity to disease. One of the first modern clues that pollutants might affect the hormonal lives of animals came in 1977. A bird toxicologist studying sea gulls on Santa Barbara Island off the Los Angeles coast noticed a strange phenomenon: the balance between male and female sea gulls in one area was grossly disturbed—with a ratio of one male to nineteen females. Fry knew that for over two decades, 4 million pounds of DDT (a pesticide) had been pumped into the ocean from a nearby chemical plant. Obviously, he believed man-made pollutants were the root cause. Since then, wildlife experts worldwide have filed similar findings, reporting declining births, lowered sperm counts or testicular deformities in fish, panthers, alligators, and other animals in polluted areas.

Coincidentally, similar phenomena have been reported in humans. According to a 1992 Danish study, sperm counts in men around the world are only about half of what they were before World War II. Scientists believe that pollutants in the air, water, and food have a lot to do with this. Our food is thus filled with compounds that have estrogenic effects, such as in some red meat and some fish. Scientists have known for decades that DDT and similar chemicals are stored in human fat and accumulate there. It would be the height of scientific naiveté to conclude that what has caused health problems in animals would have no effect on humans.

Toxic organic chemicals are synthetic compounds that contain carbon, such as the pesticide DDT. Many of these compounds cause cancer in people and birth defects in other predators near the top of the food chain, such as birds and fish. A study in the *Journal of the National Cancer Institute* showed that women with high blood levels of DDE, a chemical from the pesticide DDT, had an increased risk of breast cancer.[3] This report adds to a growing body of research that raises concern about the potential risk of breast cancer from exposure to fat-seeking halogenated chemicals such as the now-banned DDT.[4]

Devra Lee Davis, formerly a policy advisor in the Department of Health and Human Services, and now a researcher at the World Resources Institute in Washington, D.C., argues that environmental pollutants are causing an increase in some cancers which may be preventable. She believes that foreign estrogen in the form of man-made chemicals can behave in the human body like hormones, mimicking estrogen or blocking testosterone. Said Davis: "We used to believe that only a woman's natural estrogen could turn the key on these receptors and cause breast cancer. It is now clear that many chemicals in plastics and pesticides can turn the key as well."[5] It is well known that pesticide residues leach into groundwater. Exposure to pesticides used on crops and lawns as well as certain cosmetics and plastic bottles may be partially responsible for an increase in hormone-related breast, testicular, and prostate cancers as well as infertility.[6]

Davis' argument is confirmed by Mary Wolff, a specialist in environmental medicine at the Mount Sinai School of Medicine. She looked at more than 200 New York women, and found that those with blood showing the highest levels of DDE—a breakdown product of DDT—were four times more likely to have breast cancer than those with the lowest levels of DDE in their blood.[7]

The widespread use of pesticides and agricultural chemicals has significantly polluted the soil we live on and the foods we grow. One devastating effect that agricultural chemicals and pesticides may have on humanity is the steadily declining amount of sperm in men worldwide. Recently, scientists in America, Scotland, France, and Denmark conducted independent studies on sperm levels from men in more than twenty countries. Their discovery is alarming: in the past fifty years, the average sperm count has decreased by 50 percent, with an annual decline rate of about 2 percent. Also, the quality of semen has gone down. While these findings have been disputed by other researchers, they do show that the reproductive capability of human beings is at risk. In the 1960s, only 8 percent of all males in the world had reproduction problems. Today, this percentage has increased to 40 percent. If we allow this tendency to continue, human beings may, in the not too distant future, lose the ability to reproduce and continue the species effectively.

Radiation

According to recent estimation by scientists, a high proportion of cancer is linked to factors in the environment, which include all nonhereditary influences such as air, water, tobacco use, and so on. For instance, due clearly to excessive exposure to ultraviolet sunrays, skin cancers are increasing at epidemic rates in the U.S. and around the world.

The earth's atmosphere shields the earth and its inhabitants from high doses of ultraviolet rays and other solar radiation. We are disturbing this atmospheric blanket with air pollutants. Among the cancer-inducing stimuli of our environment is the very energy source upon which life itself depends—the sun. This is because every day an enormous amount of carbon dioxide from automobiles, industrial wastes, and household products is being released into the sky, polluting the air and causing severe damage to the ozone layer. As a result, too much ultraviolet radiation invades our environment and our bodies, causing skin cancer, especially among people who work long hours outdoors. Scientific studies show convincingly that skin cancer, especially *squamous epitheliomas*, is induced by ultraviolet radiation. It is estimated that the cases of skin cancer will rapidly increase in years to come.

The negative effects of ultraviolet rays (UVR) impact not only our skin; it also affects our eyes and immune system. UVR negatively affect our immune system because they are biologically active. As such, they will cause the DNA in our body to undergo a variety of changes upon absorbing them.[8]

Air Pollution

The importance of air is self-evident. In the absence of it, nobody can last more than ten minutes without suffering permanent brain damage and death. We must breathe air all the time. We breathe about twelve times every minute, inhaling and exhaling a pint of air with each respiration. When the air we breathe contains impurities, the lungs have ways of getting rid of them. This is done by coughing, or by more complicated processes within the lining of the bronchial tubes or of the lung tissue. An excessive intake of impurities from the air, however, brings about changes in the bronchial linings and the lungs, which eventually result in disability and illness, including cancer and poisoning.

Since air is so crucial to life, the quality of life itself depends, to a large extent, upon the quality of air we breathe. Thus, a simple yet universally true equation of life reads: The cleaner and ampler the air supply, the healthier and longer will be your life, and vice versa. An ample supply of fresh air is essential to a sound blood circulation system, which, in its turn, directly affects the health and the efficiency of the mind. Moreover, fresh air is a cure for many kinds of diseases. It has a tonic effect on us. This explains why people who are exposed to fresh air for a good portion of their lives are found to have stronger lungs, with fewer incidences of asthma and other respiratory problems than those who are not.

According to scientific estimation, an inhabitant of an industrial city stands a better than average chance of contracting a deadly lung disease or suffering from heart trouble, just by breathing polluted air. Meanwhile, a research report presented by Birmingham University in the United Kingdom states that those born in areas within a three miles radius of a railway or highway have a high death rate from cancer. An even higher death

rate from cancer is reported for those born within a three-mile radius of a refinery, chemical factory, or high-temperature furnace. Children born in such places have a 20 percent higher chance of dying of cancer before they reach adulthood than children who are not born in such areas. This report also points out that the environmental conditions of our birthplace have a greater impact on our health than any later place of residence. This shows that the environment of our birthplace is a lasting factor in our health throughout life.

Air pollution alone is a serious environmental concern in many parts of the world. Millions of tons of harmful gases and particles are released into the air each year. Almost every major city in America is polluted. The polluted air we breathe everyday is at least partly responsible for the incidence and aggravation of coughing, sinusitis, bronchitis, heart disease, and lung cancer. Air pollution hurts the body both by directly inflaming and destroying the lung tissue and by weakening the lung's defenses against contamination.

Polluted air can contribute to the premature death of people with heart and lung diseases. It may pose an even greater threat to children in urban areas. Children are more vulnerable to air pollution in part because their lungs continue to develop throughout childhood. Damage from air pollution can impede lung development and may lead to chronic lung disease later in life.

It is well documented that in London, a "killer fog" in 1952, polluted with sulfur and particles, is estimated to have killed 3,500 Londoners. A Harvard study estimated that nearly 5 percent of deaths in the typical American city each year are linked to acidic particles in the air.[9] Another study estimates that 60,000 premature deaths each year can be attributed to air pollution. Occupational mortality studies from the United States, England, and Scandinavia reveal higher respiratory disease mortality rates among farmers than the general population, because farmers are more directly and frequently affected by the particles of agrochemicals floating in the air.[10]

We all know how bad smoking cigarettes is, but passive smoking or exposure to environmental tobacco smoke (ETS) can be just as toxic, or even more so, because it is not filtered. This is because when one smokes a filtered cigarette, the bulk of the nicotine contained in the cigarette is not inhaled by the smoker, but released into the environment. As it is not filtered, passive smokers take in even more tar and cancer-causing chemicals than the smokers themselves. Passive smoke can do a lot of damage to nonsmokers, causing eye and throat ailments, sinusitis, respiratory and circulatory illness, and lung impairment. A study involving 521 patients who experienced their first-ever acute stroke concluded that passive smoking leads to a significantly increased risk of stroke in men and in women.[11]

Another project studying female residents of five towns in Massachusetts between 1983 and 1986 concluded that passive-only smokers had twice as much the risk of breast cancer as people who had never smoked or been exposed to passive smoke.[12] Another population-based study was conducted in Beijing to explore the etiology of lung cancer in passive-smoking women. The study found a statistically significant risk of lung cancer, as their passive-smoking years accumulated to more than 200 cigarettes per year.[13]

Noise Pollution

Today, we live in an age where industry is all around us producing noises such as traffic and industrial noises, which disturb our biological balance and mental tranquillity. It becomes a burden that weighs on us, bringing to the surface submerged tensions and stress. It is estimated that 20 million Americans are exposed daily to noise that is permanently damaging to their hearing.[14]

Noise can interfere with sleep, aggravate medical cases, and delay recovery from disease. Traditional Chinese medicine maintains that a quiet environment is conducive to a good sleep, faster recovery from disease, and a peaceful mind. This theory is backed up by modern medicine. For instance, Dr. Samuel Rosen of Mt. Sinai Hospital in New York City warns us: "We now have millions with heart diseases, high blood pressure, and emotional illness who need protection from the additional stress of noise." Also, a growing number of evidence strongly suggests a link between exposure to noise and the development and aggravation of a number of heart disease problems. The reason is because noise causes stress and the body reacts with increased adrenaline, change in heart rate, and elevated blood pressure.[15]

A comparative study performed many years ago in China on 100 sufferers of heart disease and hypertension divided them into two groups and placed them in different locations. The first group went to a hospital located in the midst of noisy city center, while the others went to a hospital located in a quiet suburban area. Exactly the same medications and treatments were given to both groups. Six months later the group hospitalized in the suburban area showed a 30 percent higher rate of recovery than the group situated in the city center. The Chinese have taken this lesson seriously and have built all of their rehabilitation and recovery centers for patients of chronic diseases in suburban or mountainous areas. This allows the patients to take advantage of the powerful natural healers present in such areas: fresh air, clean spring water, and quiet and beautiful surroundings. The results have been very encouraging and convincing.

Unfortunately, many people do not have much choice in deciding where to live and work. It is highly advisable that these people get out of the office and into the open air as often as they can during the day. This en-

ables them to take in fresh air and rid themselves of the stale and polluted office air. By doing this, they will find themselves refreshed and invigorated, and their work efficiency increased.

Another kind of noise pollution is vibration pollution. Those who were born or live in areas close to railways and highways are among the worst impacted by this special kind of pollution. Several years ago, an entire line of trees planted alongside a busy highway in the U.S. suddenly withered without apparent reason. This aroused the curiosity of scientists who, after a lengthy examination, found that the constant, strong vibration caused by passing automobiles had killed the trees.

If trees can be affected by vibration in this way, we humans may be even more vulnerable to it. This is because the human body is equipped with many vibration "devices," which cause us to react in different ways to external vibrations with different frequencies. A scientific experiment performed several years ago had a man sitting on a chair receive different degrees of vibration through the chair, varying from low to high frequencies. It was shown that when the vibration was at a frequency of 1 hertz, he felt the vibration in his head, accompanied by muscle pains and other minor uncomfortable feelings. When he was given 2 hertzs, he felt sleepy, dizzy, and out of balance. As the vibration frequency exceeded 5 hertzs, it became totally unbearable for him. As a result, his breathing and speech were affected. The greatest human reaction to external vibration happens when the vibration falls between 4 to 8 hertzs. In other words, vibrations within this frequency range can cause the greatest harm to our health.

Water Pollution

Water stands next only to air in terms of priority for survival of life. Nobody can survive without water for more than a week. Water is listed as the first of the Five Elements that underlie the medical as well as philosophical thinking in traditional China. The importance of water can be seen from another angle. Nearly 70 percent of the weight of the human body is water. We need to maintain that bodily proportion in order to be fit and healthy. When the percentage of water in the body drops below that level, it is known as dehydration. Dehydration will lead to various health problems and even death.

Drinking plenty of clean water every day is an excellent way of ridding the body of impurities. Unfortunately, not only does air fill our body with pollutants, but also some water is so dirty that we have to use powerful chemicals to make it drinkable. The water is "purified" with chemicals such as chlorine, alum, and other inorganic minerals. Our bodies can only absorb organic minerals such as from vegetables, fruits, and meat. Inorganic minerals have to be eliminated from the body by use of vital qi, otherwise they can cause health problems. Consumption of city water "purified" with chloride has been asso-

ciated with rectal cancer in some studies and possibly with breast cancer, too.

What You Can Do

Here are some of the simple measures you can take to combat environmental pollution:

• Change the air in your house every day—your bedroom in particular—by opening the windows for at least two hours after getting up in the morning. Make sure that the places where you live and work are well ventilated and have plenty of fresh air.

• Walk or exercise in the open air at least twice a day, preferably by a waterfront or in a park.

• Make sure that the water you drink and use to prepare foods is clean. Boil it if necessary before using or use bottled water.

• Drink the juice of a carrot and a potato on a regular basis. This will cleanse your lungs of the pollutants you breathe in.

• Steam pig or chicken blood until it becomes solid. Cut the blood cake, fry or bake it together with some vegetables, and eat it as a meal. Regularly eating this once or twice a week can keep your lungs and intestines clean and healthy. The ancient Chinese tell us that pork and chicken blood can carry away pollutants in the lungs and intestines.

- Make your house, especially your bedroom, as soundproof as possible to eliminate outside noises. If this cannot be achieved and you are disturbed by noise, play some light music to neutralize the disquieting effects of noise.

- Keep a respectful distance from active cigarette smokers. Try to work in a non-smoking environment. If this is not realistic, leave the office temporarily when a smoker lights a cigarette.

- Avoid radiation from electric blankets, computer and TV screens, as well as digital alarm clocks. Do not place these electronic devices near your pillow in the bedroom.

- Wear protective clothing or sunscreen to protect you from ultraviolet rays.

- Wash all fresh fruits and vegetables to remove any pesticide residue.

Endnotes

1. David and Anne Frahm, *Reclaim your Health* (Colorado: Pinon Press, 1995).

2. Allan R. Cook, *Environmentally Induced Disorders Sourcebook* (Detroit, MI: Omnigraphics, Inc., 1997), 6, 7, and 36.

3. *Journal of the National Cancer Institute* (April 21, 1993).

4. Cook, *Environmentally Induced Disorders Sourcebook*, 125, 391.

5. B. Roberson, "Conferences Point to Growing Concern about Possible Links between Breast Cancer and Environment," *CMAJ* 154, no. 8 (April 15, 1996): 1253–5.

6. Amanda Spake, "Is the modern world giving us cancer?" *Health*, October 1995, 52–56.

7. Ibid.

8. Cook, *Environmentally Induced Disorders Sourcebook*, 581.

9. Allan R. Cook, *Environmentally Induced Disorders Sourcebook* (Detroit, MI: Omnigraphics, Inc., 1997).

10. Cook, *Environmentally Induced Disorders Sourcebook,* 75, 76, 79, 333, 567

11. R. Bonita et al., "Passive Smoking as well as Active Smoking Increases the Risk of Acute Stroke," *Tobacco Control* 8, no. 2 (Summer 1999): 156–60.

12. T. L. Lash et al., "Active and Passive Cigarette Smoking and the Occurrence of Breast Cancer," *American Journal of Epidemiology* 149, no. 1 (January 1, 1999): 5–12.

13. S. Zheng et al., "Studies on Relationship between Passive Smoking and Lung Cancer in Non-smoking Women," *Chung Hua Yu Fang I Hsueh Tsa Chih* (*Journal of Chinese Preventive Medicine*) 31, no. 3 (May 31, 1997): 163–5.

14. Cook, *Environmentally Induced Disorders Sourcebook*, 431.

15. Cook, *Environmentally Induced Disorders Sourcebook,* 432.

Chapter 10

Nature's Potent Healers

As we have already mentioned, the Chinese natural health care system was developed on the observation and understanding of the laws of nature. An essential part of this system is testing and documenting the therapeutic effects of natural products, especially foods. In China, remedies for diseases are handed down by word of mouth from generation to generation in an unbroken chain. These remedies are often ordinary foods, from the kitchen or garden, which can be used in their raw forms.

Nature has provided us with countless potent healers, which cost us very little and have no side effects. It is a long-held Chinese belief that dietary therapy is superior to herbal therapy, and that dietary nourishment is superior to herbal nourishment. This is because most pharmaceutical herbs are not naturally compatible with the biochemistry of the human body, even though they are natural products. As such, they cause side effects unless used with considerable care. Although herbs have fewer side effects than drugs, they can be toxic, too. One common side effect of almost all herbs is the negative impact they have on the function of the spleen, which is considered the general manager of postnatal life energy. According to the ancient Chinese, using an herb on a regular basis will significantly weaken the user's spleen. This neutralizes the value of the herb while causing digestion problems. Another common side effect of herbs is the damage they do to the qi energy in the body, leading to fatigue and lowered immunity. Sometimes, the use of herbs will cure one disease but cause another.

Most natural foods, however, are free from such side effects. Listed below are some of the common healers (not inclusive) in alphabetic order. Most are readily available and easy to use by anyone with an open and willing mind. Others may be harder to obtain, available only in Chinese grocery stores or restaurants or by special order. To obtain their medical benefits, these healing foods should be taken once a day for seven consecutive days, or until the symptoms disappear. This is the Chinese practice.

Ants

In some parts of China, ants have been used as both food and medicine. Ants can help our body resist rheumatism, arthritis, cancer and allergies, reduce swelling, and remove toxins, as well as relieve asthma, pain caused by arthritis and swelling, malaria, and cerebral thrombus. Modern science shows that ants contain more than fifty nutrients needed by the human body, twenty-eight amino acids and various minerals and chemical compounds that are good for our health. One kilogram of ants contains 120 milligrams of zinc. Of course, not all ants are edible. Only those living in nonpolluted fields can be used as food and medicine. In China, they come in a pill or powdered form.

Apple

The age-old saying "An apple a day keeps the doctor away" is still true. Clinical experiments have shown that apples—particularly in juice form—can relieve headaches, insomnia, fatigue, indigestion, constipation, cancer, toothaches, the common cold, and night blindness. The cancer-fighting properties of apples are largely derived from the elegiac acid and fiber they contain. Because they contain rich potassium and boron, apples can maintain healthy bones and prevent osteoporosis.

What gives apple the dual power to fight both diarrhea and constipation is a substance called pectin found in apple. In the case of diarrhea, pectin swells to form a thick mass that produces stools to stop diarrhea. In the case of constipation, pectin lubricates the bowels to facilitate the motion. An antibacterial substance called phloretin is found in apple. This substance is effective against a wide range of pathogens.[1]

Banana

Bananas are rich in potassium, tryptophan, sodium, magnesium, protein, glucose, starch, and L-tryptophan. Potassium is a mineral that relaxes arteries and reduces blood volume. Taking 2,300 milligrams of potassium a day can lower blood pressure 50 percent, as effectively as blood pressure drugs, but without the expense or side effects.[2] (A banana contains about 400 milligrams of potassium.) An eight-year study of 44,000 men in the health care field found that foods rich in potassium might help reduce the risk of stroke, especially in people with high blood pressure.[3] L-tryptophan is a natural chemical that can help induce sleep and relieve insomnia. Bananas have also been found capable of relieving constipation, diarrhea, indigestion, prostate ailments, impotence, heart disease, and stroke.

Bladderwrack

This is a tough, thick, and inexpensive sea plant that grows abundantly in high-tide zones. It is also known as sea kelp. Bladderwrack is a jelly-like substance that is easily visible on the water surface, and often drifts to shore by the tide. Nowadays, it is commercially grown in huge quantities and made into various food forms. Sea kelp pills are available at health food stores, and fresh and dried sea kelp are available in Chinese grocery stores or food markets. Dr. Sun Simiao in ancient China first discovered that this sea vegetable was very effective in treating sore or swollen throats, lumbago, and rheumatism. It is also rich in protein, vitamin C, and iodine. Modern studies show that bladderwrack can prevent blood clotting and therefore heart disease. It can also reduce plasma cholesterol and blood pressure, and relieve indigestion and food poisoning.

NOTE: Too much iodine can stunt your thyroid, so be careful how much you take.

Broccoli

This vegetable contains valuable anticancer properties. It is highly recommended that you include it in your regular diet for the sake of preventing and fighting various cancers. The active nutrients in broccoli that have cancer-fighting properties are sulforaphane, beta-carotene, and indolecarbinol. Since many of the nutrients in vegetables are either in, or just beneath, the skin where ice, light, and heat can destroy them, broccoli and other vegetables are best stored in a cool (not cold) and dark place. They should be washed in water, rather than soaked, and should not be cut until ready to be cooked. Keep the leftover cooking water and use it for soup.

Carrots

This vegetable is rich in vitamins A, B_1, B_2, and C, organic acid, beta-carotene, phosphorus, potassium, calcium, and iron. Beta-carotene helps protect your cardiovascular system, inhibiting LDL cholesterol from oxidizing in your body, thus lowering your risk of heart attack or stroke. Carrots can also help prevent and treat heart disease, stomach disorders, headaches, common colds, insomnia, eyestrain, diarrhea, night blindness, sinusitis, indigestion, urinary tract disorders as well as different cancers. They also enhance the immune system, protect the skin, and help treat skin diseases.

Regularly eating carrots can improve skin appearance and calcium absorption, thus preventing premature aging and osteoporosis, while also facilitating recovery from wounds, and promote the development of teeth and bones. However, carrot juice should be limited to no more than four cups a day since excessive intake of this juice can lead to yellowing of the skin, a condition known as xanthosis.[4]

Cherries

This fruit contains potent anti-inflammation and antiputrefaction properties. They stimulate the digestive and nervous systems. Cherries are a good "medicine" for indigestion, constipation, and premature aging. Most importantly, it ranks high as an anticancer food. Cherry juice is as effective as the cherry itself. For better medical effectiveness, cherries are best consumed raw.

Chestnuts

For centuries, the Chinese have been using chestnuts to relieve indigestion, diarrhea, frequent urination, sexual dysfunction, arthritis, rheumatism, and kidney disease. It is also one of the most recommended foods for people seeking immortality. Modern studies show that chestnuts are rich in protein, vitamins A, B_1, B_2, and C, and phosphorus, calcium, iron, and other nutrients. Chestnuts can be eaten raw or cooked.

Chinese Chives

This is a delicious, fragrant vegetable often found in Chinese kitchens. It is rich in protein, vitamin C, calcium, phosphorus, and potassium. As a dietary medicine, it can relieve asthma, diarrhea, constipation, hiccups, vomiting, frequent urination, sexual dysfunction, and impotence. You can either cook this vegetable alone, or slice it to mix with fried eggs, or fry together with shrimp.

Chinese Wolfberries

Medically known as *Lyceum chinese*, this wild fruit is held in high respect by the Chinese. For thousands of years, they have been using it to relieve sexual dysfunction, impotence, ear ringing, eyestrain, dizziness, liver disease, neurasthenia, and premature aging. It can also prevent and treat arteriosclerosis and help reduce cholesterol levels. Laboratory studies show that Chinese wolfberry contains carotene, vitamins B$_2$ and C, niacin, linoleic acid, calcium, phosphorus, and iron. There are several ways in which this fruit can be used. One is to cook them together with rice to make a porridge. Another is to stew them in water for half an hour and eat as a meal. You can also soak them in grape wine or rice wine for at least a week and drink a glass of this wine at bedtime. Wolfberries can be bought at most Chinese medical stores here in the States.

Chinese Yams

Chinese yams contains glycoside, choline, oxidized enzymes, multiple vitamins, folic acid, multiple amino acids, and other nutrients. They have traditionally been used in China as a treatment for diabetes, frequent urination, chronic fatigue, diarrhea, asthma, coughing, loss of appetite, nocturnal emission, and sexual dysfunction. You can cook them alone in water or with rice, steam them, or eat them raw. (See also "Yams.")

Crucian Carp

Carp is more than just a delicious food. Crucian carp is rich in protein, carbohydrates, vitamins A, B$_1$, and B$_{12}$, phosphorus, iron, and other nutrients. For instance, it can relieve kidney disease, lack of appetite, indigestion, chronic fatigue, lack of milk after childbirth, and prolapse (ptosis) of the stomach. Any carp has such medical benefits.

Danseng

Codonopsis pillosula is the medical name for this plant that is similar to ginseng both in form and function. Indeed, it is known as "small ginseng" in China, and is used to relieve asthma, hypertension, neurasthenia, diarrhea, loss of appetite, and premenstrual syndrome. Danseng can enhance the central nervous system, lower blood pressure, and boost the immune system. Danseng can be found in pill form in Chinese herbal stores, or you can cook it in water, or steam it together with chicken or fish to make a delicious dish.

Dates

Dates have been kept in both kitchens and pharmacies in China for centuries. Dates contain protein, vitamins A, B, and C, phosphorus, carotene, calcium, iron, and other nutrients. As a dietary medicine, dates can relieve loss of appetite, insomnia, diarrhea, premenstrual syndrome (PMS), anemia, sexual dysfunction, and neurasthenia. You can eat dates raw, cooked alone or together with rice, or used in baked goods.

Dong Quai

Chinese women have used this plant for centuries to relieve premenstrual syndrome (PMS), menopause symptoms, and infertility. In China, it is considered the most important female tonic and is used to treat menopausal symptoms and uterine cramping. Says Michael Sharon, author of *Nutrients A to Z*,

> *Dong quai has been used in China for centuries in the treatment of women's complaints, it has now been rediscovered by the West and found to have a balancing effect on estrogen activity and a tonic effect on the uterus. Dong quai is used to treat female conditions such as the hot flashes of menopause, pre-menstrual tension and vaginal dryness. It is also used to promote a healthy pregnancy and delivery.[5]*

In America, dong quai is becoming popular as an ingredient in women's supplements. It is rich in volatile oil, folic acid, and vitamin B_{12}. These stimulate the production of blood cells, nourish the blood, and promote blood circulation, all of which are vital to the health of women. It also is good for chills of the limbs, anemia, and general tiredness. It is the dried root of this herb that is used. It is available in standardized form, which can be purchased in almost any Chinese herb store and is taken in doses of 200 milligrams, three times a day.

Dove

Considered a messenger of peace in the West, dove is used as both a high-quality delicacy and an effective medicine in China. Modern studies show that dove contains protein, vitamins B and B_2, phosphorus, calcium, iron, and other nutrients. As a dietary medicine, dove can help cure diabetes, chronic fatigue, sexual dysfunction, impotence, weakness after serious illness, and food poisoning.

Duck

This is another favorite food in China. It has been used to effectively relieve kidney disease, edema, chronic fatigue, asthma, sexual dysfunction, and increase the strength of people recovering from illness. Basically, duck has the same nutritional content as chicken, but has different medical effects, mainly because a duck spends a lot of time in the water. Since water stands for kidney in Chinese medical medicine, Chinese fathers think that duck must be beneficial to kidney and sexual health. Also, since water has a cooling effect, ducks is therefore better than chicken when eaten in the summer, which is a hot season, serving to balance the heat in the nature.

Eggs

The reputation of eggs has suffered in the West where it is considered a contributing cause of heart disease due to its high cholesterol content. However, the Chinese seem never to tire of this delicious, nutrient-laden food. Actually, eggs have a quarter less cholesterol than most people believe. They are low in fat and calories but rich in vitamins A and B, and minerals such as iron, calcium, zinc, phosphorus, selenium, potassium, and sulfur. Egg yolk is rich in vitamins A, B_1, B_{12}, E, and K, all of which are vital in maintaining the sexual and reproductive function of humans. Therefore, eggs can boost sexual vitality, relieve infertility in both sexes, improve memory, and relieve chronic fatigue and dizziness. Egg yolk is also a rich source of amino acids, cysteine, and methionine, which enhance immunity against disease. Egg white contains lysozyme and vitamins. Lysozyme can enhance one's immunity against many kinds of bacteria.

True, egg yolks contain 275 milligrams of cholesterol but this is balanced by an abundance of lecithin (1,700 milligrams), which emulsifies cholesterol. The only people who should avoid eggs are those with the condition known as hyperlipoproteinemia, who should avoid all foods containing cholesterol.[6] Recently, eggs have been taken off the forbidden list except for those with the most serious cholesterol problems, simply because eggs are not high in saturated fat.[7]

Fish Glue

This is the white, slippery part of fish that is found in the intestines. The Chinese discovered that this part of the fish has high therapeutic values as well as culinary values. For a long time, the Chinese have used it to treat hemorrhages, premature aging, chronic fatigue, nocturnal emission, heart disease, and sexual dysfunction. Recently, clinical experiments found that fish glue can also be used to treat cancer. Modern studies show that fish glue is rich in protein, omega-3, calcium, phosphorus, iron, and other nutrients. You can get fish glue from Chinese herb stores or Chinese grocery stores. (Or you could also just buy a fish and eat it.) You can cook it together with the fish. If it is from an herb store, it must be dried already, therefore, you have to soak it in water for several hours, and then steam or fry it before eating.

Fish Oil

Fish oil is a primary source for the omega-3 fatty acid, which is the healthy, unsaturated fat for our heart and overall health. It can significantly reduce the risk of heart attack by warding off blood clots, lowering blood pressure, and bringing down high triglycerides. Therefore, fish oil provides economical "insurance" against heart disease. An Italian study involving 11,000 patients with heart disease found that taking omega-3 fish-oil pills on a daily basis cut the risk of further heart problems by 10 to 15 percent.[8]

According to Dr. D. Q. Bao, regular consumption of dietary fish rich in omega-3 fatty acids can lower blood pressure levels and reduce cardiovascular risk.[9] It is also reported that a diet rich in fish oil has shown to modulate the course of several experimental models of renal disease.[10]

Garlic

Garlic can be found in almost every Chinese kitchen, where it has been a folk remedy for thousands of years. Garlic is a strong antitumor, antibacterial, and antiviral vegetable, with marked antibiotic effects. Among other qualities, garlic aids in digestion, relieves and cures dysentery and typhoid, kills bacteria and other parasites inside the body, helps prevent and cure the common cold and flu, treats stomach ulcers and diarrhea, cleanses the blood vessels and the stomach, prevents and cures pneumonia and tuberculosis, eliminates toxic wastes in the body, lowers blood pressure and cholesterol levels, prevents and relieves heart disease, cures sinusitis, boosts sexual vitality, relieves sexually transmitted diseases, promotes antibody production and circulation, help prevent fatal blood clots and cancers of the stomach and colon, and even looks promising as a treatment for AIDS. Indeed, it is hard to believe that this multitude of magic medical effects are all contained in one homely food—garlic!

Most of the medicinal power of garlic comes from its drug-like compounds, such as allicin, ajoene, allyl sulfide, and polyphenols. Polyphenols can protect your heart. Allicin, the major component in garlic, is a potent antibiotic, fungicide, and cancerfighter. Researchers at Memorial Sloan-Kettering Cancer Center showed in 1997 that substance in garlic can significantly slow the development of prostate cancer cells. Commercial garlic extract has also slowed the growth of breast, skin, and colon cancers in mice.[11]

Recently, scientists have discovered that garlic is a strong antimicrobial and antiviral vegetable. Allicin has been proven to be more effective than penicillin in suppressing certain types of viruses. Austrian scientists also discovered that the use of garlic produces three kinds of chemicals—allyl ethyl sulfide, diethyl sulfide, and acetone. All of these are powerful in breaking up cholesterol in the blood. A recent study shows that even a small amount of this pungent vegetable can go a long way in lowering cholesterol and triglyceride levels, reducing the clotting ability of blood. In a 1995 study, volunteers with high cholesterol who took an aged-garlic extract saw their total cholesterol fall by 7 percent and their artery-clogging LDL cholesterol fall by 10 percent.[12]

It is best to eat garlic raw. This is because allicin, the essential enzyme in garlic, is destroyed by heat. One or two cloves taken of garlic at mealtime will be medically beneficial. However, you need to chew it raw to get the most benefit, because its nutritional contents will be better released and absorbed by the human body after chewing.

Ginger

The Chinese have used ginger as both a seasoning and as a medicine for many years. When they have digestion problems, such as diarrhea and indigestion, or the common cold and flu and their related problems, this plant naturally comes to mind. Generations of experience tell them that ginger can help relieve these ailments and, moreover, raise the body's metabolism, promote circulation, eliminate cell toxins and products of infection, as well as enhance the immune system.

Like garlic, ginger is a strong antiviral and antibiotic product. Its phlegm- and mucus-loosing properties make it a great expectorant. Modern studies have shown ginger capable of lowering cholesterol levels and reducing blood clotting.[13]

To incorporate ginger into your daily diet, you can slice it and eat it raw, or cook it together with other foods. Some Chinese have added ginger juice to their bath water to treat a cold, allergic skin, and sore feet.

Ginkgo

A highly recommended food for seekers of immortality, ginkgo is known in China as the "elixir of youth." Its leaves were recently found to contain substances capable of protecting the membranes of brain cells and reversing the aging of the brain. Since ginkgo appears to increase both the blood supply and oxygen supply to the brain, it can delay the aging process, strengthen memory, im-

prove circulation, and benefit the sufferers of degenerative diseases such as dementia in the elderly.[14] Numerous well-controlled studies show that ginkgo improves blood flow to the brain and the extremities, and alleviates vertigo and ringing in the ears. It can also help recover lost memory. Recently, ginkgo has been clinically used to treat Alzheimer's disease as well as ischemia, hypoxia, and head injuries. Clinical experiments show that it is effective in treating Raynaud's disease and dizziness associated with inner-ear disorders.[15] You can steam, cook, or fry it.

Ginseng

This plant has become famous around the world, although as the name implies, the Chinese were the first to use it. The Chinese have used ginseng for thousands of years, and have found it to be a powerful booster for vital qi energy and sexual vitality. It is effective in relieving chronic fatigue resulting from qi deficiency or as an aftermath of a serious disease. It can also be used to treat sexual dysfunction, nourish the brain system, delay the aging process, and strengthen the body's immune system.

The best way of consuming ginseng is to chew it thoroughly before swallowing. Alternatively, it can be stewed in water to make a soup. It should be eaten on an empty stomach, but not too close to mealtime. You should not drink water for a while afterward, to allow the ginseng to be absorbed by the body.

Gooseberries

Closely related to currants, gooseberries are very tart fruits that change from pale green to amber as they ripen. They are as big as a cherry, and taste a bit sour, but ripened ones are sweet. This wild fruit is rich in vitamins C and E. It can calm an upset stomach, treat a loss of appetite, food poisoning, and fever, and even prevent the development of certain cancers. A 1995 study at the University of Illinois shows that extracts of wild berries inhibited the activity of an enzyme that can lead to cancer.[16] Most gooseberries are used for pies, though a bright yellow type is sweet enough for eating raw.

Grapes

This common fruit is among the most potent of all natural food medicines. Grapes are rich in multiple vitamins, calcium, phosphorus, iron, and other nutrients. The sugar they contain—mostly pure glucose plus some fructose and levulose—is exactly what is needed for cellular metabolism. The Chinese have a long history of using grapes to treat many kinds of diseases such as the common cold, flu, constipation, arthritis, gastritis, indigestion, insomnia, anemia, chronic fatigue, liver disease, sexual dysfunction, incontinence, and impotence. They are also helpful to pregnant women and new mothers because of the iron they contain. Recent scientific studies show that grapes contain rich procyanidolic oligomers (PCOs), which possess much stronger antioxidant power than those of the vitamins C and E. Because their chemical structures are incorporated within the cell membranes, PCOs are excellent cellular bodyguards. In addition, PCOs can strengthen veins and capillaries, and inhibit the destruction of collagen, consequently preventing heart disease and delaying the aging process. Most important, grapes are a rich source of unusually potent antioxidants called flavonoids, which help tiny blood vessels in the body to dilate. This may partly explain why regular grape eaters and wine drinkers are less likely to die of heart disease than those who don't eat grapes or drink wine. For medicinal purposes, the black or dark red variation of the grape family is considered the most potent of all.

Heshouwu (Fo-ti)

Heshouwu (pronounced "ho-sow-woo") literally means "turning any hair dark" in Chinese. *Fo-ti* is the Japanese name. It is used in China for preventing and treating a number of diseases, such as premature aging, declining memory, sexual dysfunction, and neurasthenia. The story goes that in the Tang dynasty, a poor scholar was so frustrated with his repeated failure in imperial examinations that his hair became completely gray when he was still in his forties. One day, he wandered into the mountains, and fell asleep. When he woke, he was extremely hungry. He could find no food but saw some vines spreading in front of him. He tracked them to their roots, which he cleaned and ate raw. His hunger disappeared, and he felt more energetic than ever before. He had accidentally found the heshouwu plant. He stayed in the mountains for several days, eating nothing but heshouwu. When he returned home again, his family and neighbors were surprised to find that his hair had turned dark again. He told them what he had been eating, and Heshouwu found a permanent place in the Chinese pharmacy.

The ancient Chinese believed that heshouwu could boost the kidney qi energy, nourish the spleen and liver, and enhance the body's overall immunity. Modern studies show that heshouwu has the ability to reduce artherosclerotic lesions and cholesterol deposits in the arteries, relieve high blood pressure and arteriosclerosis, and increase the superoxide dismutase (SOD) enzyme, which is closely associated with longevity. (From a traditional Chinese viewpoint, heshouwu can enhance the brain and kidney systems, which are the two pillars of longevity.) Today, it is also used in clinics for treating cancer and AIDS.

Heshouwu is available in any Chinese herbal store. It comes in different forms: raw, pill, or liquid. To consume it, soak it in water for a few hours together with peanuts, then steam for half an hour. Drink the soup and eat the peanuts. Do this once a day for seven days.

Honey

The Chinese hold that as bees collect honey from hundreds of different kinds of flowers, which are also considered medicines, honey therefore possesses multiple medicinal values. They believe that honey can nourish the liver, moisten the lungs, and reduce the heart rate and blood pressure. For centuries it has been widely used in China to treat various ailments such as anemia, insomnia, liver and heart diseases, stomach problems, asthma, constipation, eyestrain, neurasthenia, bronchitis, coughing, sexual dysfunction, hypertension, and food poisoning. Modern studies show that honey contains multiple sugars, protein, multiple enzymes, vitamins A, B_1, B_2, B_6, C, D, and K, as well as organic acids such as citric acid and folic acid. You can either eat it raw by itself, or use it with other foods such as on breads or in tea.

Lemons

This common fruit contains fruit acid and multiple vitamins. It can treat diabetes, hypertension, asthma, coughing, and indigestion. It can also boost the production of saliva, which is essential to immunity, and keep the skin smooth and soft. Usually, the juice alone is consumed. Oftentimes in China, people brew tea together with lemon slices. Rarely do people eat the whole fruit.

Lotus Root

This is both a delicious food and potent medicine in China. Wherever there is a lotus plant, there will be lotus root. The two are different parts of the same plant grown in water. As a medicine, it has been used to relieve vomiting, hiccups, diarrhea, jaded appetite, strokes, and food poisoning. In terms of nutrition, this food contains protein, starch, multiple vitamins, digestive enzymes, and minerals. It looks like a tree root, but has holes in it like a bee nest. You can eat it raw like vegetable, or slice it and fry it as a dish, or make it into a powder to make a meal. You can get it fresh, dried, or powdered from most Chinese grocery stores or Chinese herb stores.

Lotus Seeds

This is the seed from the lotus plant that grows in lakes or ponds. Lotus seeds look like peanuts. There are two kinds of lotus seeds: one black and one white. Both have the same medical and nutritional effects. For centuries lotus seed has been considered a highly respected food medicine in China. It is used to relieve sexual dysfunction, impotence, nocturnal emission, chronic diarrhea, jaded appetite, incontinence, frequent urination, neurasthenia, insomnia, leucorrhea,

heart disease, hypertension, and heat stroke. Its medical effects are derived from the rich protein, iron, calcium, phosphorus, and multiple vitamins it contains. To eat lotus seeds, you usually steam them in water for half an hour, add some sugar, and eat. Lotus seeds can also be cooked together with rice to make a porridge.

Mushrooms

Mushrooms are rich in potassium, phosphorus, copper, and iron. They are also a good source of vitamin B_1 and B_2. Clinical studies show that eating mushrooms on a regular basis can significantly lower blood pressure and cholesterol levels, prevent blood clotting and therefore heart problems, improve digestion, strengthen the immune system, relieve skin ailments, and prevent and fight many kinds of cancer. They also have antibiotic properties, and can boost immunity against disease by increasing white blood cell count.[17] Mushrooms are easily digested and can be cooked alone, together with other foods such as chicken or pork, or eaten raw. They are recommended for all who have digestive problems.

Oatmeal

Oatmeal is suitable for patients with heart, stomach, and skin diseases, as well as hypertension. It can also help prevent premature aging. Oat bran is known for its ability to lower bad cholesterol while maintaining the good cholesterol. Oatmeal contains protein, calcium, silica, iron, lipids, and vitamins B and E. It contains these nutrients in a well-balanced way, aiding digestion and easy absorption by the body. Oatmeal is also useful for conditions such as weakness, diabetes, hepatitis, indigestion, and bloating. Thanks to the rich calcium and silica oats contain, oatmeal can strengthen bones, and prevent and treat osteoporosis. Oat oil keeps the skin soft and supple, and relieves various skin problems.

Olives and Olive Oil

Olives are considered a "longevity fruit" in China. Therapeutically, they are used to relieve indigestion, hypertension, obesity, toothaches, jaded appetite, premature aging, constipation, kidney stones, and high cholesterol levels. Olive oil is the healthiest kind of all edible fats (besides omega-3). Olives and olive oil can help lower cholesterol and control blood pressure, two significant ways to help prevent diabetes and heart disease. Olive oil can also be used externally to treat burns, bruises, and sprains.[18]

Use olive oil for cooking or to season other foods. It is suggested that olives should be eaten at least once a week.

Onions

This spicy vegetable is a favorite seasoning in the Chinese kitchen. It is best known for its antibacterial power. Onions contain large quantities of potassium (a mineral easily lost through sweating), phytochemicals, allicin, mustard oils vitamins A, B_1, B_2, and C, sulforaphane, and allylic sulfides—a strong class of anticancer compounds. A clinical study in the Netherlands on more than 3,000 people found that consumption of at least half an onion a day can reduce the risk of stomach cancer by half.[19] The reason seems to be that allylic sulfides activate enzymes that neutralize cancer-causing substances. Thanks to flavonoids they contain, onions can reduce blood stickiness, preventing blood clots and heart attacks. Onion has been shown to lower high blood pressure and cholesterol levels. They conduce respiration in very much the same way as garlic does, and relieve colds, kill bacteria in the body, boost the appetite, relieve hypertension, and aid in digestion. They have also been used externally to treat sores, mosquito bites, and burns.

Oranges

As well as being a delicious fruit, the orange is highly respected for its therapeutic value in China. In fact, it is kept in both Chinese pharmacies and grocery stores. The medical value of an orange lies in its rich vitamins, especially vitamin C, potassium, and folic acid it contains. Vitamin C disables the free radicals that harm the linings of blood vessels. Oranges also prevent and relieve colds and flu, headaches, indigestion, asthma, coughing, eye diseases including cataracts and night blindness, teeth problems, and cancer. They also enhance the immune system and speed up the recovery from diseases and wounds. The major cancer-fighting property of oranges comes from bioflavonoids and vitamin C. Oranges are also rich in potassium, a mineral capable of controlling high blood pressure and therefore preventing stroke.[20] For pregnant women, folic acid from oranges can significantly reduce the risk of premature delivery and neurological birth defects. To take the maximum advantage of this common fruit, it should be consumed together with its rind.

Oysters

Oysters have always been a major aphrodisiac in Chinese dietary therapy. Ancient Chinese discovered that oysters could boost the production of semen, enlarge the penis, and greatly enhance one's sexual drive. As oysters are rich in zinc, a mineral vital to sperm production and sexual drive, consumption of oysters can nourish kidney qi energy, boost sexual vitality, and help treat various diseases resulting from a deficiency of kidney qi energy. These include impotence, premature ejaculation, impotence, incontinence, frequent urination, chronic fatigue, insomnia, lumbago, and strained lumbar muscles. Since oysters are considered a yin food that possesses a potent cooling effect, they make an excellent food during the summer season. They can also treat toothaches caused by overeating fried foods. To derive the maximum therapeutic effects, oysters should be consumed raw and fresh, or lightly cooked.

Peanuts

As another "fruit of longevity," peanuts have been a favorite food in China for centuries. They are widely used as dietary therapy for diseases such as asthma, coughing, pneumonia, indigestion, constipation, lung and kidney diseases, sexual dysfunction, and chronic fatigue. Peanuts lubricate the intestines and are useful for the alleviation of ulcers or digestive tract tumors. They are also known to increase milk flow in nursing mothers, improve hearing, and curb internal bleeding. Indeed, peanuts make an ideal dietary component for patients with almost any disease. Peanuts derive their medicinal effects from protein, amino acids, alkaloids, calcium, iron, phosphorus, vitamins A, B, B_2, B_6, and C. For medicinal purposes, do not eat fried peanuts. Eat them raw or cooked in water.

Pears

The Chinese use pears to relieve asthma, coughing, loss of voice, constipation, lung disease, hypertension, diabetes, urinary difficulties, indigestion, and heatstroke. Pears are considered a yin food able to counterbalance the effects of heat. Pears contain pectin, citric acid, calcium, iron, potassium, and vitamins B_1, B_2, and C. To consume pears, eat them raw or steam in water for a few minutes. In both cases, pears should be peeled first.

Peppers

Peppers of all colors are an excellent source of beta-carotene, vitamin C, calcium, phosphorus, sodium, and potassium. The Chinese believe that peppers can boost the appetite, promote digestion and circulation, stimulate one's sexual desire and ability, and reduce swelling. It is therefore very helpful in treating the common cold, flu, headaches, arthritis, and various forms of ailments caused by humidity and cold weather. Peppers can be used in cooking, or soaked in rice wine to receive its medicinal effects. However, hot peppers are usually not recommended for medical use except in very cold weather or cold areas such as in northern China. Another word of caution: peppers are an allergen to some people. For these people, either avoid peppers or use cooked peppers only. Cooked peppers are much less allergenic than raw ones.

Pilose Antler

This antler of a deer was considered a potent aphrodisiac by the ancient Chinese. It is used in China to boost the sexual vitality of both men and women, relieve impotence and sexual dysfunction, premenstrual symptoms, prostate ailments, frequent urination, incontinence, chronic fatigue, and ulcers. Scientists find that pilose antler contains male and female sex hormones, in addition to calcium, magnesium, and twenty-five kinds of amino acid. It is available in various forms. It is best consumed on an empty stomach.

Pineapples

Pineapples are grown in the southern part of China. The ancient Chinese discovered that this fruit has a healing effect on colds and sinusitis, because it opens the air passages in the nose, without any side effects. In China, it is also used for the treatment of burns, wounds, and invasive injuries to the skin.

Pineapple contains a substance called bromelain, which has shown distinct pharmacological promise. Its properties include interference with the growth of malignant cells, inhibition of platelet aggregation, fibrinolytic activity, anti-inflammatory action, and skin debridement properties. These biological functions of bromelain, according to Dr. S. J. Taussig, have therapeutic values in interference with tumor growth, blood coagulation, inflammatory changes, debridement of third-degree burns, and enhancement of absorption of drugs.[21] It is also found that unripe pineapples contain a violent purgative. Therefore, such pineapples could be used to empty the stomach in cases of poisoning or drug overdose.[22]

Placenta

The Chinese believe that the placenta produced by a healthy mother can nourish the kidney qi energy of others, promote the development of breasts in prepubescent females, boost the appetite, enhance immunity, and relieve sexual dysfunction, impotence, chronic fatigue, asthma, breast cancer, and even AIDS. Modern scientific studies show that the placenta contains rich hormones and ovarian hormones, as well as choline, multiple acids, and protease. These nutrients are good for the immune system and qi energy. This substance is widely used in China, mostly in pills and fluid forms.

Pork Blood

Pork blood is a nourishing food for humans, especially for women and those afflicted with anemia. This is because pork blood contains a large amount of iron. This is organic iron, which is far superior to the inorganic iron that is sold in pharmacies. Regularly consumption—once a week or once in a month—of pork blood strengthens the body and relieves anemia and chronic fatigue. It was highly recommended by Dr. Sun Yat-sen, the father of the Chinese Republic, who was professionally trained as a doctor. While unusual to Americans, it is common in China. If you want to try, you can get fresh pork blood from a Chinese grocery store even here in the U.S. To eat, just steam it and add some salt and oil.

Potatoes

Potatoes can relieve arthritis, ulcers, heart disease, hypertension, and strokes. They are rich in potassium, a mineral that can regulate the heart rate and lower blood pressure. As a specific remedy for arthritis, Dr. Vogel recommends potato juice, from at least one potato daily, sipped slowly on an empty stomach in the morning.[23] Moreover, potatoes can also treat burns, diarrhea, stomachaches, bronchial asthma, and allergic skin reactions.[24]

You can eat potatoes in any cooked form. However, for medical applications, potato juice is the most effective and preferred form. For instance, to treat skin burns and allergic skin, apply the juice to the inflicted part of the body. To treat arthritis, diarrhea, stomachaches, bronchial asthma, or to regulate your heart rate, drink one cup of potato juice each day on an empty stomach.

Radishes

Known in China as the "small ginseng," radishes are rich in vitamins A, B, and C, carbohydrates, calcium, iron, sodium, phosphorus, potassium, sulphur, as well as digestive enzymes, and possess many therapeutic uses. Clinical research shows that radishes can improve digestion and urination, kill bacteria, diminish inflammation of the gums and stomach, reduce phlegm, and treat asthma. Radishes are also useful in treating coughing, laryngitis, sore throat, diarrhea, headaches, gallbladder problems, depression, kidney stone, and many kinds of cancer, especially stomach cancer. German scientists have discovered that a particularly strong decrease of stomach cancer was associated with consumption of radishes and onions.[25] The Chinese also use radish juice to treat the coughing up of blood, food or alcohol poisoning, chilblains, furuncles (boils), and blisters resulting from being scalded. Radishes are particularly effective in treating kidney stones. Half a cup of fresh radish juice each morning on an empty stomach usually dissolves even the most stubborn kidney stones, passing them out of the body in the urine.[26] To derive the maximum therapeutic effect, radishes are best consumed raw on an empty stomach. You should avoid other foods for half an hour.

Red Wine

Made from red grapes, this liquor contains important antioxidant flavonoids such as quercetin and tannins, which account for an amazing phenomenon known as French paradox. The fact is that although the French are among the highest consumers of red meat, their rate of heart disease is lower than in other industrialized nations. The major reason is believed to be that the French are also the biggest consumers of red wine. Red wine contains a rich content of procyanidolic oligomers (PCOs). PCOs are one of the most potent groups of antioxidants, and produce strong vascular protective actions helpful to deterring atherosclerosis. In addition, red wine contains rich polyphenols that have been found to reduce the accumulation of bad cholesterol and deter the formation of platelets in arteries, thus lowering the risk of heart disease and stroke. Researchers at Tripler Army Medical Center in Honolulu found that wine was more effective at killing the bacteria that cause diarrhea than bismuth salicylate, a popular medical cure.[27]

Reishi Mushroom

For thousands of years, the Reishi mushroom (*ganoderma* mushroom or *lucidum*) has been called the "flower of longevity" and the "herb for immortality" in China. Medically, it slows down the aging process, nourishes the heart, provides kidney and liver qi energy, improves eyesight, quiets the mind, relieves rheumatism, and lowers blood pressure. Clinical experiments in China, Korea, and America have shown that this mushroom can kill cancer cells, lower blood pressure, improve immunity, and suppress proliferation of peripheral blood mononuclear cells.[28] Naturally, it is being studied as a potential cure for AIDS. The Reishi mushroom contains proteins, amino acids, alkaloids, resinic acid, multiple vitamins, and enzymes, as well as polysaccharide. Polysaccharide gives it the ability to contain, and eventually kill, cancer cells. It is best to either grind them into a powder and make a tea, or stew them in water and drink as soup. The Reishi mushroom is best consumed on an empty stomach.

Salt

Despite the fact that salt is blamed for hypertension and other diseases, this popular seasoning is, if properly used, an effective and excellent medicine for many kinds of health problems. (For those who are told by their doctor to restrict their salt intake because of heart problems, they should only use salt externally instead of internally, as in the case of nasal and gum bleeding. They should rinse the salt away after using it.) For centuries, the Chinese have used salt to stop bleeding in the nose, gums, and stomach; bleeding caused by ulcers; and temporary relief of stool bleeding and urination bleeding. Salt also diminishes inflammation of the gums and skin; detoxifies the body of alcohol; sterilizes foods; neutralizes chemicals on the skin; and relieves sore throats, toothaches, constipation, and bad breath. Apply salt externally when treating nasal and gum bleeding as well as skin inflammation, but drink a cup of slightly salted water in the morning when treating ulcer, stool, and urination bleeding.

Sesame Seeds and Oil

Sesame is popular in China as it can help prevent premature aging, keeping people looking youthful. It can also relieve chronic fatigue, constipation, asthma, sexual dysfunction, food poisoning, stiff joints, weak knees, nervous spasms, as well as lack of milk after childbirth. Sesame contains rich oleic acid, lecithin, vitamin A and E, calcium, protein, unsaturated fatty acids, magnesium, and other nutrients. It is usually used in the form of an oil or porridge. A mixture of sesame and rice makes an excellent porridge.

Shrimp

Shrimp is an excellent source of protein with low fat and low cholesterol. In China, it is considered both a delicious food and a potent healer for sexual dysfunction, chronic fatigue, infertility, and lack of milk after childbirth.

Snake

This reptile is a potent medicine in China and is used to help relieve food poisoning, eye diseases such as eye inflammation, red eyes, and general eye pain, arthritis, rheumatism, coughing, bronchitis, and cancer. There is a famous saying in China: "Use poison as an antidote for poison." Snake fulfills this perfectly and is one of the most famous antidotes for these ailments. It can be cooked for eating, or soaked in wine to make snake wine. Only those snakes that can be found in Chinese restaurants should be eaten.

NOTE: Consult a Chinese doctor before taking snake for medical use because of possible allergic reactions.

Soybeans

Soybean and soy products such as tofu, soymilk, and soy powder are becoming widely known for their beneficial qualities. They have been a favorite food in China for thousands of years. Dr. Sun Yat-sen, the father of the Chinese Republic, highly recommended tofu as "the meat for the vegetarians, which contains the nutrition of animal meat but is free from the poison of animal meat." Soy food contains protein, plentiful fiber, vitamins B_1, B_2, B_6, B_{12}, folic acid, choline, calcium, phosphorus, plant estrogen, and nonatherogenic oil. The genistein that is abundant in soybeans functions like estrogen. It can lower cholesterol, check the growth of breast cancer cells, and maintain bone density in women, while easing the hot flashes and night sweats of menopause. Medical researchers find that Chinese and Japanese women have a considerably lower rate of breast cancer and hot flashes than their American and European counterparts. One major reason is that Oriental women consume much more soy products. Recently, it was found that soybeans contain rich phytochemicals called isoflavonoids, which seem to possess powerful disease-fighting properties. For instance, the isoflavonoids in soy can prevent breast cancer by preventing the estrogen from changing normal cells into cancer cells. Other phytonutrients in soy include soy fiber, saponnins, phytosterols, lecithin, and phenolics, which all help boost the immune system.

Soy foods can also prevent and relieve osteoporosis because soy can increase the bone density and drives out the humidity in the body. Soy milk is used in China to relieve asthma, urination problems, and food poisoning. A common product of soybeans is tofu, which was invented by Liu An, King of Huai Nan in the Han Dynasty. According to Peter Jaret, dozens of studies—including an overview featured in the summer of 1995 in *The New England Journal of Medicine*—have shown that soy protein can dramatically lower cholesterol.[29] There is also evidence that the phytoestrogen found in soybeans can relieve some side effects of menopause and even slow down osteoporosis. In countries like China and Japan where soybean is served at almost every meal, rates of heart disease and many forms of cancer are unusually low. In Shanghai, the average cholesterol level hovers around 165 as compared to 200 in the U.S. Based on animal tests, scientists suspect that the isoflavones in soybeans bear so close a resemblance to the hormones in a woman's body that they may be able to be used as a replacement when her own levels start to fall. Also, according to Mark Messina, a former program director at the National Cancer Institute, who organized the first international symposium on soy foods and health, isoflavones can alleviate hot flashes and night sweats in menopausal women. He is optimistic: "I'd bet good money soy protein will become a widely accepted alternative to estrogen replacement therapy within the next few years."

Sparrow

Like the dove, this bird is both a delicacy and a dietary medicine in treating sexual dysfunction, chronic fatigue, incontinence, and frequent urination.

Spinach

This is a favorite vegetable of the Chinese, and everyone from emperors to the common people enjoy it. The famous emperor Qianlong of the late Qing dynasty had a special love of spinach. He nicknamed it the "green parrot with a red mouth." As a dietary medicine, spinach can be used to relieve diabetes, anemia, constipation, liver disease, cataracts, eyestrain, night blindness, hypertension, cancer, tooth and nasal bleeding, as well as facilitate the healing of wounds. Dr. Brown L. and Chasan-Taber L. reported that both spinach and broccoli were most consistently associated with a lower risk of cataracts.[30] Spinach is also a good preventative of strokes, thanks to the rich potassium it contains. An eight-year study of nearly 44,000 men in the health care field concluded that foods rich in potassium such as spinach, bananas, tomatoes, and oranges may help reduce the risk of stroke, especially in people with high blood pressure.[31] Spinach may also prevent cancer because of the glutathione it contains. Glutathione is a tripeptide that is widely distributed in animal and plant tissues, and it functions in various redox reactions: in the destruction of peroxides and free radicals; as a cofactor of enzymes; and in the detoxification of harmful compounds. In addition, spinach contains other beneficial nutrients such as carotene, riboflavin, sodium, potassium, vitamins B_1, B_2, and C, as well as formic acid, phosphorus, calcium, and iron.

Sugar Cane

Sugar cane contains glucose, protein, calcium, phosphorus, iron, and vitamins. Sugar cane can be taken to treat vomiting, constipation, food poisoning, and premature aging. Many people in China who enjoy longevity report that they were in a habit of drinking a cup of sugar cane juice every day. Sugar cane is also being used to treat cancer in China. To consume, drink the juice once a day, or suck the juice directly from the cane.

Tea

For thousands of years, Chinese families have enjoyed their daily cup of tea. Only at the turn of the century was it introduced into the Western world. It is both a pleasant, tasteful drink and a potent medicine. Tea, especially green tea, is regarded in China almost as a cure-all. If someone has indigestion or stomach discomfort, they drink tea. If someone has a headache or cold, they think of tea. When they are intoxicated, have food poisoning, feel low-spirited, or have a hangover, they drink tea. It is the perfect remedy. Tea can also help treat the common cold, liver disease, heart disease, high cholesterol, hypertension, obesity, diarrhea, diabetes, stomach ailments, and various kinds of cancer.

In China and Japan, many epidemiological studies have found that people who drink a few cups of tea a day have a lower-than-normal incidence of cancer.[32] In the past decade, global cancer studies have supported this conclusion. W. H. Chow of National Cancer institute in Bethesda, Maryland, reported a significant reduction of stomach cancer in women as a result of daily tea drinking.[33] More and more American scientists are increasingly vocal about

drinking green tea because it may help prevent or control a host of ailments.[34]

What gives tea this magic, therapeutic power? The answer lies in the polyphenols and catechin it contains. Polyphenol—a kind of chemical compound made of carbolic acids—gives tea its taste and medical power. Over 10 percent of green tea is made up of polyphenols, as compared to 5 percent in black tea. Modern studies show that green tea, because of the high percentage of polyphenols it contains, can speed up the free radical scavenging in our blood by nearly 50 percent. This benefits many organs in the body. For instance, the liver's detoxification system is enhanced by the ability of tea to eliminate free radicals that would otherwise weaken the liver.

The heart also benefits. Tea lowers the cholesterol in our body by speeding up the rate at which our body burns fat. It interferes with the accumulation of plaque on the arteries, and dissolves blood clots. In addition, tea can lower the risk of cancer in many areas: lung, breast, stomach, colon, prostate, and pancreas. Tea can also help stop leukocytes and liver tumor cells from duplicating themselves.[35] Dr. S. Gupta and other scientists in Case Western Reverse University of Ohio concluded that many laboratory experiments conducted in cell culture systems have shown the usefulness of green tea against prostate cancer. According to them, the epidemiological basis for this possibility is two-fold: first, people who consume tea regularly have a lower risk of death from prostate cancer; second, the incidence of prostate cancer in China, a population that consumes green tea on a regular basis, is the lowest in the world.[36] Catechin—a crystalline astringent principle from catechu—and phenolic compounds found in green tea are given the credit for these findings. Also, tea contains fluoride that helps protect our teeth against decay.

Tea should be drunk two to three times a day, one cup each time, but not within a half an hour of bedtime, for fear that sleep will be disturbed. Any green tea is considered good.

Tomatoes

Rich in lycopene, vitamin C, and other nutrients, the tomato is a potent antioxidant. A regular, sufficient consumption of tomatoes has been linked to a lower rate of ulcers, prostate cancer, and stomach cancer. (A tomato a day is regular and sufficient.) The major cancer-fighting ability of tomatoes comes from lycopene—an antioxidant.

A Harvard study of 48,000 men showed that those who had two to four servings a week of tomato sauce had a 34 percent lower risk of prostate cancer. Dr. Omer Kucuk, an oncologist who led a very recent study in Detroit's Karmanos Cancer Institute aimed at finding exactly how tomatoes can help fight cancer, said: "We can conclude that lycopene caused regression of tumors and make them less aggressive."[37]

Trepang

Known as "sea ginseng" in China, this seafood is a highly nutritional food containing calcium, phosphorus, iron, sodium, organic acid, and protein. The Chinese use it to nourish the kidney qi energy, strengthen the urination function, and to relieve sexual dysfunction, incontinence, nocturnal emission, diabetes, kidney disease, and liver disease. Trepang looks like a big, long bean. It does not have much taste by itself; all depends on how you cook it and what seasonings you put into cooking it. You can just fry it with some sauce to make a delicious dish, or together with other foods such as pork, beef, chicken or shrimp. Eating it once in a week is recommended.

Vinegar

For centuries the Chinese have used vinegar to prevent and treat a variety of ailments such as the common cold, headaches, indigestion, diarrhea, urinary problems, food poisoning, drug overdose, skin ailments, sprained muscles, and joint strains. Scientists have discovered that organic vinegar is a natural storehouse of vitamins and minerals that can fight many of the things that make you sick.

For therapeutic purposes, vinegar can be used in three different ways. The first is to drink it, two to three spoonfuls at a time. This is good for indigestion, the common cold, flu, pneumonia, and diarrhea. Another way is to cook the vinegar and let it evaporate in the room. This kills bacteria and is a preventive measure against cold, flu, and pneumonia germs. Yet another way is to directly apply it to the wounded part of the body, as in the case of arthritis, sprained ankles, and other injuries. This is because vinegar can promote the blood circulation blood in the body. It is also believed that vinegar restores the acid balance of the skin and face, keeping it smooth and youthful looking.

Walnuts

Walnuts are rich in vegetable fat, carotene, multiple vitamins, calcium, protein, phosphorus, and iron. They nourish the brain, lungs, and skin, strengthening one's memory and lungs, and making the skin lustrous. Walnuts are long thought to be a brain food and is sometimes called a "fruit of longevity." Regular consumption of walnuts can nourish the brain, prevent Alzheimer's disease, and delay the aging process. They can be used to relieve ringing in the ears, insomnia, chronic fatigue, kidney stones, constipation, asthma, sexual dysfunction, and infertility.

Warmed walnut oil is a home remedy for inflammation of the ear. Walnuts can be eaten as often as you want. Also, they can be eaten by themselves or together with other foods. Walnut oil is used as a cooking oil, and is an excellent choice for salad dressings.

Water

Few people think of water as a medicine. In fact, water is both an essential dietary component and a potent healer in itself. Water is needed for transporting nutrients, lubricating joints, helping digestion, regulating body temperature, eliminating internal wastes, cleaning the body, and keeping the skin smooth and healthy. Even the smallest deficit of water can leave you sick with constipation, dizziness, headache, heatstroke, and so on. This is especially the case during the summer.

Drinking plenty of water can greatly relieve fevers, and prevent premature aging by moistening the skin and face. It can even prevent and relieve cancer by cleaning up the internal body. University of Washington researchers surveyed 462 men and found that those who drank more than four glasses of water each day had almost a one third lower risk of colon cancer. The ancient Chinese also believed that consuming plenty of clean water helps longevity. Drink six to eight glasses a day, at least.

Whole Wheat and Grains

As commonplace as these foods are, they are actually very potent and effective preventives and healers of many kinds of diseases. Nutritionally, whole wheat and grains are rich in multiple vitamins, minerals, starch, protein, and other nutrients. When refined, these foods are largely deprived of their valuable fiber and other nutrients. In combination with selenium, magnesium, and other minerals and vitamins, rich fiber contained in whole wheat and grain can effectively ward off diabetes, breast cancer, uterine cancer, colon cancer, and heart diseases. Scientists hold that whole wheat is a potent weapon against cancer. That is because wheat is an excellent source of the trace mineral selenium. Years of studies among Chinese peasants have produced encouraging results of the cancer fighting ability of whole wheat.[38] The reason why fiber can prevent diabetes is that it reduces the absorption rate of carbohydrates in the food.

A high-carbohydrate diet that is low in fiber can cause serious illness. For instance, researchers have found that people who eat white bread and white rice as their staple foods have two-and-a-half times the risk of diabetes and colon cancer than those whose diet is mostly whole wheat and grains, as well as vegetables and fruits. Foods like whole-grain breads, brown rice, wheat germ, and whole-wheat oatmeal are good choices.

Yams

This simple and delicious food has been a favorite staple for millions of Chinese for thousands of years. It is useful and effective in fighting hypertension, constipation, indigestion, high cholesterol, heart disease, and sexual dysfunction. Yams contain fiber, multiple vitamins and minerals, as well as carbohydrates and protein. It is also easily digested and absorbed by the body, and is therefore useful for people of any age and health condition. To eat, you can slice them and cook in water, or steam them or cook together with some rice as is often prepared in China. I know some people eat yams on daily basis, but others only once or twice a week. It really depends on your individual needs and tastes.

Endnotes

1. Thomas Squier, *Herbal Folk Medicine: An A to Z Guide* (New York, NY: Henry Holt and Company, Inc., 1997), 40.

2. *Health*, September 1997.

3. *Seattle Post-Intelligencer*, 2 September 1998: A3.

4. Michael Sharon, *Nutrients A to Z* (London U.K.: Prion Books Limited, 1998), 62.

5. Ibid, 86.

6. Ibid, 88.

7. Michael D. Lemonick, "Eat Your Heart Out," *Time*, 19 July 1999, 43.

8. Cynthia Drake, "Looking for heart-friendly food? Go fish," *Investors Business Daily*, 26 March 1999.

9. D. Q. Bao et al., "Effects of Dietary Fish and Weight Reduction on Ambulatory Blood Pressure in Overweight Hypertensives," *Hypertension* 32, no. 4 (October 1998): 710–7.

10. O. K. Eberhard et al., "Short- and Long-term Effects of Fish Oil on Protenuria, Morphology and Renal Hemodynamics in the Milan Normotensive Rate Model of Spontaneous Glomerulosclerosis," *Kidney Blood Press Resources* 22, no. 3 (1999): 128–34.

11. *Health*, March 1998, 90–91.

12. Ibid.

13. Squier, *Herbal Folk Medicine: An A to Z Guide*, 90-92.

14. Sharon, *Nutrients A to Z*, 112–3.

15. Squier, *Herbal Folk Medicine: An A to Z Guide*, 92–93.

16. *Health*, July/August 1998, 42.

17. Sharon, *Nutrients A to Z*, 167–8.

18. Ibid., 174.

19. *Men's Health*, May 1997, 78.

20. Squier, *Herbal Folk Medicine*, 40.

21. S. J. Taussig, "Bromelain, the Enzyme Complex of Pineapple and its Clinical Application. An Update," *Journal of Ethnopharmacol* 22, no. 2 (February/March 1998): 191–203.

22. Squier, *Herbal Folk Medicine: An A to Z Guide*,144–5.

23. H. C. A. Vogel, *The Nature Doctor* (Edinburgh: Mainstream Publishing, 1990).

24. Henry C. Lu, *Chinese System of Food Cures* (New York, NY: Sterling Publishing Co., Inc., 1986) 95–96.

25. H. Boeing et al., "Dietary Risk Factors in Intestinal and Diffuse Types of Stomach Cancer: A Multicenter Case-control Study in Poland," *Cancer Causes Control* 2, no. 4 (July 1991): 227–330.

26. Sharon, *Nutrients A to Z*, 203.

27. *Men's Health*, May 1997, 122.

28. J. Zhang et al., "Antitumor Active Protein-containing Glycans from the Chinese Mushroom Songshan Lingzhi, Ganoderma tsugae mycelium," *Bioscience Biotechnology Biochemistry* 58, no. 7 (July 1994): 1202–5. G. Wang et al., "Antitumor Active Polysaccharides from the Chinese Mushroom Songsan Lingzhi, the Fruiting Body of Ganoderma tsugae," *Bioscience Biotechnology Biochemistry* 57, no. 6 (June 1993): 894–900. S. C. Jong et al., "Medical Benefits of the Mushroom Ganoderma," *Advance in Applied Microbiology* 37 (1992): 101–34. R. S. Kim, "Suppressive Effects of Ganoderma lucidum on Proliferation of Peripheral Blood Mononuclear Cells," *Molecules and Cells* 7, no. 1 (February 28, 1997): 52–7.

29. *Health*, October 1995, 30.

30. *American Journal of Clinical Nutrition* 70, no. 4 (October 1999): 509–524.

31. Squier, *Herbal Folk Medicine*, 40.

32. S. Okabe, et al., "Mechanistic Aspects of Green Tea as a Cancer Preventive," *Japanese Journal of Cancer Research* 90, no. 7 (July 1999): 733–9. I. F. Benzie et al., "Consumption of Green Tea Causes Rapid Increase in Plasma Antioxidant Power in Humans," *Nutrition and Cancer* 34, no. 1 (1999): 83–7.

33. W. H. Chow et al., "Risk of Stomach Cancer in Relation to Consumption of Cigarettes, Alcohol, Tea and Coffee in Warsaw, Poland," *International Journal of Cancer* 81, no. 6 (June 11, 1999): 871–6.

34. Glenn Garelik, "Call Green Tea the Cure-all of Cure-alls," *Investor's Business Daily*, 28 September 1998.

35. R. Haufbauer et al., "The Green Tea Extract Epigallocatechin Gallate Is Able to Reduce Neutrophil Transmigration through Monolayers of Endothelial Cells," *Wien Klin Wochenschr* 111, no. 7 (April 9, 1999): 278–82. For the medical effects of green tea on liver disease, see H. Tsuchiya, "Effects of Green Tea Catechins on Membrane Fluidity," *Pharmacology* 59, no. 1 (July 1999): 34–44.

36. S. Gupta et al., "Prostate Cancer Chemoprevention by Green Tea," *Seminars in Urologic Oncology* 17, no. 2 (May 1999): 70–6.

37. James Peter Rubin, "A Tomato a Day May Keep Doctors Qway," *Investor's Business Daily*, 21 April 1999.

38. *Health*, April 1997, 16.

Chapter 11

Secrets of
Sexual Vitality

I t is stated in the I-Ching that "Yin alone cannot reproduce, nor can yang alone develop. Tao lies in harmony
and balance between yin and yang." The message contained in this statement is clear: the law of nature requires
that man and woman live in balanced harmony so that
both can enjoy good health and longevity, and the human
species can continue. Since yin-yang balance is the basic
law of nature, the Chinese natural health care system believes that our health can be significantly improved and
our life prolonged, if we can maintain such a balance between men and women.

Mencius (370–290 B.C.), a great Confucian sage, obviously agreed when he wrote: "Love of food and sex are
among human nature, wherein lie the two greatest desires
of mankind." Today, this view of Mencius has been universally accepted, largely thanks to the monumental work
performed by Sigmund Freud in this century. One would
assume that Mencius himself was a great lover of food
and women. This is not an insulting assumption, for he

once admitted that a man of great talents must also have great desires. Indeed, the intensity and scope of one's desires vary in direct proportion to one's talent. The history of humankind has repeatedly confirmed this truth—China's Mao Tse-tung and Chiang Kai-shek, Franklin D. Roosevelt, and John F. Kennedy are famous examples—placing Mencius in the top rank of all psychologists who have ever lived. One can even say that there is no escape from Mencius.

From both biological and sociological points of view, a harmonious sexual relationship is vital to the happiness of both parties. In fact, it is one of the most significant cornerstones of human happiness. Biologically, from puberty onwards, we humans spend most of our lives in sexual awareness, if not in sexual relations. The power of the libido is overwhelming, omnipresent, and irresistible. As a matter of course, sex and sexual vitality have a significant impact on our happiness, even more so than money or power.

If we compare the number of people committing suicide due to broken relationships and those committing suicide due to the loss of power or money, we can readily appreciate the essential importance of sex to life. Louis XV of France, who openly preferred a beautiful woman to a kingdom, must have won much sympathy for his royal simplicity. A survey conducted by the Rev. Andrew M. Greeley, a sociology professor at the University of Chicago, offers convincing evidence of this point. His study showed that the happiest elderly people in the United States are married couples who have sex on a regular basis even after the age of sixty.

Contrary to general belief, sex remains a vital part of most people's lives into their seventies and even beyond. A survey of 4,246 American men and women aged between fifty and ninety-three found that 60 percent of married couples in their seventies still have regular intercourse, with an average frequency of three times a month; more than 75 percent of single men remain sexually active in their seventies; and that 50 percent of single women of that age are sexually active.[1]

This, of course, does not mean that all men are sexually vital. The grim fact is that about 30 million American men have chronic impotence problems.[2] Sad to say, the greatest threat to matrimonial happiness in modern American society is not infidelity, but sexual inability. Countless couples have ended their relationships because the husbands could not fulfill their sexual duties to their wives. Today, a growing number of American males are complaining about the shrinking of their penises, a premature decline in sexual vitality, declining sexual urges, premature ejaculation, and impotence. At least 10 million American men are impotent. This figure does not include those who are too shy to go to a hospital or clinic to seek help for their problem.

In a broad sense, sexuality impacts not only on our ability to have sex, but also on our basic needs for intimacy, affection, approval, and acceptance. Sexuality affects how we love, how we show affection, how we value ourselves, and how we bond with and befriend others. While the desirability and importance of sexual vitality is beyond any doubt, the answer is not simply "just go for it." Unlike food, which we can eat even in the absence of a biological need, intercourse cannot happen, or will not happen satisfactorily, without sexual vitality. This vitality depends on our health status. In fact, sexual vitality itself is a significant indicator of overall health. For one thing, the penis depends on a smooth and vigorous flow of blood for its sensitivity and duration of erection, something that cannot happen without good health. Therefore, a healthy man who has plenty of blood and smooth blood circulation tends to function better in bed than an ill man.

It must be pointed out that the sexual dysfunction prevailing in this country is not a natural part of aging. Conventional wisdom tells us that our sexual vitality starts to decrease after the age of forty. Let me tell you that this is simply not true. It is an age-old Chinese belief that a man who is still sexy after sixty bodes well for longevity. As has been mentioned before, the Yellow Emperor of China was still busy with his sexual affairs as well as national affairs when he was over one hundred years of age! China's Mao Tsetung was very proud of referring to himself as "an old man fond of seeking youthful pleasures" in his eighties. Do not let yourself or others say "no" to your sexuality.

Biologically, sexual vitality is primarily a function of sexual essence, which means

semen and male sexual hormones for a man, and ova and female sexual hormones for a woman. For a man, semen and androgens are the prime driver of his sexuality. These substances are produced in the testes. When called into action, semen (sperm) flows out of the testes through the coiled tube. Semen is not only the material basis of sexuality, it is one of the most precious substances of life. Semen builds up the immune system and life energy. Generally, the Chinese believe that people with high reserve levels of semen are energetic, healthy, sexually vital, and less vulnerable to diseases.

Actually, premature aging is diagnosed in Chinese medicine as a deficiency of kidney qi energy resulting primarily from sexual indulgence. Kidney qi energy is what keeps one youthful and energetic. The more of this energy one has, the longer he or she will live.

Since the male body's production of semen is generally limited, and the urge to "spend it" is always strong, there is an imbalance characterized by demand far exceeding the supply. Typically, the production of semen takes dietary nutrition, effective digestion, proper rest, and time. Economic theory tells us that the lower the supply, the higher the price. This is exactly what makes semen so precious. Also, as you age, it takes your body longer to reproduce the same amount of semen lost in one ejaculation.

Based on this understanding, the ancient Chinese laid down some golden rules regarding the frequency of ejaculation for different age groups. Thus, a man in his twenties should not ejaculate more than once a week; a man in his thirties should not ejaculate more than once in two weeks; a man in his forties should not ejaculate more than once a month; a man in his fifties should not ejaculate more than once in two months, and one should avoid ejaculation at all after the age of sixty-four.

Thus, conservation of semen constitutes the central theme in male sexuality, health, and longevity. Violation of this principle will lead to declining sexuality, premature aging, and death. In fact, one of the crucial reasons why husbands are usually survived by their wives and not the other way around is this: husbands give out the precious semen while wives receive it.

We know that women have a biological phenomenon called menopause. Equally true but less known is the fact that men also have a male menopause, which normally occurs at around the age of sixty-four, the square of eight, which is the typical male cycle. At this age, it is believed that the production of semen stops and that a man will experience great difficulty achieving an erection unless he knows how to preserve semen and improve sexuality early in life. This coincides with the progressive impairment of testosterone production after puberty, and especially after fifty. Male menopause, however, does not mean the loss of reproductive ability. In fact, male fertility can persist until an advanced age if one knows and practices the secret of sexual vitality. Many elderly men have been found to possess androgen

levels that can be considered normal for young men.

Normally, a woman will see the production of her hormones in the endocrine system declining after the age of thirty until it completely stops at around fifty. The key female hormone is DHEA, which is converted by the body into active sex hormones like estrogen, testosterone, progesterone, and corticosterone. Estrogen is the name for a class of female steroid hormone compounds of which there are about twenty members. It plays an important role in promoting the overall health of a woman. It helps in the development of female secondary sexual traits such as breasts and uterus development and fat deposits.

Progesterone also has a direct impact on female sexuality. The functions of progesterone include boosting one's libido, helping use fat as energy, normalizing blood sugar levels, maintaining secretory endometrium, ensuring that a fetus develops in a healthy way, and so on. The major difference between male and female menopause seems to be that women almost stop their ovary secretion completely after menopause, while men can still produce semen, although at a very low rate.[3]

The conventional response to declining sexuality is hormone injections. This can be a dangerous measure with some serious side effects. A recent breast cancer study published in *The New England Journal of Medicine* involved almost 70,000 nurses during an eighteen-year observation.[4] It found that artificial injections of estrogen can greatly increase the risk of breast cancer. Of those women who took progesterone with estrogen, there was a 54 percent greater risk of developing breast cancer compared with women who never took any synthetic hormones. As another side effect, hormone supplements, especially the use of artificial estrogen, which an estimated 11 million American women take, have been shown to increase the risk of heart attacks in women by a dramatic 40 to 50 percent. This challenges the long-held notion that hormones shield against heart disease.[5]

The ancient Chinese, on the other hand, offered a completely natural set of solutions toward the problem of declining sexuality, if only because they knew nothing about science. For males, they proposed the idea of regulating ejaculation through intercourse as the major solution. This is known as *wo-gu-bu-xie* (hold fast and not ejaculate) in the Chinese natural health care system. To borrow a military metaphor, this means being engaged with the enemy but not firing, or bending the bow but not shooting.

It is typical of the Chinese way of thinking to liken all serious activities bearing heavily on the choice between life and death to battle. Thus, a bedroom is referred to as a flowery battlefield. The principle is to be engaged but not to fire. Here lies the difference between regulated sex and unregulated sex. The latter seeks mere carnal pleasure from sexual intercourse, while the former uses sex to improve overall health including

sexual vitality. The key difference lies ultimately in whether or not to ejaculate. The reason why the ancient Chinese proposed intercourse without ejaculation is, so to speak, "to use poison to relieve poisoning," or to use sex to promote sexuality. In other words, it is ejaculation, not intercourse itself, that should be regulated.

Any man with sexual experience can you tell that regulating ejaculation during intercourse is no small task, a little short of "turning the tide." Indeed, the very idea of holding fast to one's semen during intercourse runs directly counter to the conventional premise of sex, which is the pleasure obtained by ejaculation. At issue here, however, is not only whether to ejaculate or not, but in the final analysis, to live or to die. Nu Dongbin, one of the famous Eight Great Immortals, underscores this relation in a poetic form:

> *Delicate are the waists of a young lady,*
> *Wherein hangs a sharp knife for the*
> *folly.*
> *While nobody gets beheaded,*
> *All will be marrowless and dead.*

According to Chinese philosophy, sexual intercourse represents the communion between yin (female) and yang (male), and suggests the image of fire (sexual desire) cooking water (sexual essence). The fire can burn up the limited water in a bottle in a hasty flame lasting a short while, or slowly warm the water without drying it out. The fiercely boiled water will evaporate quickly, while slowly warmed water will last for a long while, making both parties involved happy and healthy. Here lies the difference between stormy sexual ecstasy and lasting sexual pleasure and vitality. If you know how to control your ejaculation during intercourse, you can fight a hundred battles in the "flowery battlefield" and come out the winner.

Actually, the image of fighting a battle is not an accurate one. For in military battles, one either wins or loses. But in sexual intercourse, or flowery battle, the outcome can be, and should be, a win-win situation, with both parties feeling satisfied, happy, and healthy. It goes without saying that the male is largely responsible for creating such a situation, for he is the giver, the prime driving force in the entire process, on whose sexuality and duration depends the outcome of intercourse. A win-win situation is characterized by the female's orgasm, which makes her enchanted and enlightened, but requires the penis to remain erect inside the vagina for a long while.

This ability of a male to stay for a length of time inside the female gives him considerable sexual nourishment and enhanced sexuality. As a result, his energy and immunity are enhanced. In the Chinese natural health care system, this phenomenon is known as *qu-yin-bu-yang* (take the female yin energy to nourish the male yang energy). Indeed, the nourishing and therapeutic effect of regulated sex is a two-way street—it simultaneously benefits both the male and the female

involved. Thus, such intercourse can cure a woman of many diseases, especially those related to menstrual dysfunction. (A position with the woman lying on her back is strongly recommended during intercourse.)

Why is it so important for a male to control his ejaculation during intercourse? There are several reasons for this. First, ejaculation means loss of semen, a precious substance with very limited supply for all of us. Second, being able to control ejaculation means longer intercourse, a factor directly contributing to female orgasm. Third, according to the Chinese fathers, the semen thus conserved will travel directly upward to the brain, nourishing the brain and the spirit while promoting sexual vitality.

Regulating ejaculation is the highest secret of male sexuality and the bedroom arts. In his classic *Precious Prescriptions*, Dr. Sun Simiao tells us:

> *Actually, the bedroom art is very simple, but most people are ignorant of it. How can I intercourse with ten women in a night without feeling tired? I just hold fast to my semen and do not let it go. This is the climax of bedroom art.*

While it is solely a man's responsibility to control his ejaculation, a woman can do a lot to help her partner in realizing this goal. Her role is to passively and harmoniously cooperate, avoiding sudden and overzealous body movements. Obviously, a man must go through more demanding training to do his job. Most important, he has to learn the art of coordinating his mind, breathing, and physical movements during intercourse.

Sexual urges start with the mind as a result of visual or audio stimulation, physical contact, or mere imagination. Sexual excitement speeds up the heart rate and shortens the breathing cycle, which in turn pries open the Gate of Life and lets out the precious semen. Thus, we see ejaculation as a trilogy composed of mental stimulation, respiratory acceleration, and physical stimulation. The more sexually excited you are, the faster your heart will beat and the harder it will be to control ejaculation. Since the mind is the primary trigger of ejaculation, it stands to reason that regulation of ejaculation must begin with the regulation of the mind.

The ancient Chinese advise us that the right way to approach a woman is to keep the mind as calm as possible, like the water in a windless lake. This should be done from the very beginning of intercourse, not at the brink of ejaculation. When you feel like ejaculating, the Gate of Life may already be open and ejaculation may be inevitable. It takes little imagination to know that such a mental state is impossible if the purpose of intercourse is to merely seek carnal pleasure. Only when you realize the vital value of semen and make it a point to use intercourse as a chance to promote your health and sexuality, can you maintain a serene mind throughout the act.

For all its necessity, mental preparation alone is not enough to perform the job of regulated sex. Learning proper breathing exercises is also helpful. Deep, regulated breathing is a powerful tool in reducing mental excitement and keeping sexual urges under control. A calm mind is reflected in deep, rhythmic breathing. Thus, regulating breathing and regulating the mind must go hand in hand to achieve the desired goal of ejaculation regulation. The better trained you are in Chinese breathing exercises, the greater will be your chance of success for regulated sex. That is why masters of regulated sex in China are invariably masters of qigong, the Chinese breathing exercise. Moreover, by practicing qigong during intercourse, you greatly facilitate the transforming of conserved essence into vital qi energy and be able to nourish the brain. As a result, many kinds of diseases related to the brain and memory can be relieved. Little wonder practitioners of regulated sex are never found to be inflicted with Parkinson's or Alzheimer's diseases. Their memory is very good, and their mind functions like that of a young person.

To further aid in the task of regulating ejaculation, the ancient Chinese recommended that body movements, particularly that of the penis, be synchronized with the tempo of regulated breathing during intercourse. Regulated breathing teaches the special skills of "nine shallows and one deep" and "eight shallows and two deeps." Here, "shallow" and "deep" symbolize the degrees of penetration into the vagina by the penis. In other words, if a man penetrates ten times, only one or two of such penetrations should be deep ones, the rest should be shallow ones. Of course, this is just a rule of thumb. Individual practitioners can develop their own "style." The whole idea behind this is to ensure that a man can "penetrate in a dead state but withdraw alive," with his penis still erect and strong before he ejaculates. This is the best way to naturally promote one's sexuality and "win one hundred flowery battles" without losing one.

The health benefits of this practice of alternating deep and shallow movements are summarized by Dr. Sun Simiao in his book *Cultivating Nature*:

The secret to make a sexual couple live long and healthy is to insert the penis deep into the vagina, and hang on there without moving for a few minutes. As the female feels warm in her face, the male should lose no time in kissing her and absorbing the breath in her mouth. Meanwhile, take deep breathing and imagine that there is a big red bean in the navel. Afterwards, gently move the penis inside the vagina for a few dozen times. Before you feel like ejaculating, resolutely withdraw your penis. Practice this every night and both partners will live longer and healthier.

Sooner or later, frequently or infrequently, one will ejaculate. There are several measures to minimize the loss or to recover at least part of the loss resulting from ejaculation. To Chinese sages, it is never too late to "mend the fence," but the sooner you take action, the less will be the loss and the better off you will be. One course of action is to cover the vagina with your left hand immediately after ejaculation, while breathing deeply and thinking of dantian, the lower abdomen. This will enable you to recover some of the vital qi lost in the ejaculation. Another course of action to minimize the loss is to promptly contract your anus muscle for a dozen times right after the ejaculation. This will allow you to close up the Gate of Life, and stop the further flow of semen. The third course of action is to press the perineum with your middle finger and hold it there for a few minutes. This will serve the same purpose. Whatever the course you take, take it promptly.

It is good to know that one's sexual vitality is related not only to one's own health, but to the health of one's descendants. A sexually vital father will give birth to healthy babies, while a father given to sexual indulgences will have descendants who are born with sexual dysfunction, impotence, infertility or other problems. Pu Yi, the last emperor of China, was a well-known example. He was born an impotent man because his father and grandfathers had been playboys and wasted too much of their sexual essence. This cannot but negatively affect the primordial and prenatal qi energy of their offspring. Thus, sexual vitality is not only a matter of personal health and happiness; it is also a eugenic consideration for humankind.

As well as all this, the Chinese art of regulated sex also involves a set of taboos with regard to the location and timing of intercourse. These taboos fall into three major categories: heavenly taboos, manly taboos, and earthly taboos. Thus, one should avoid sexual intercourse when the weather is extremely hot or cold, when there is a hurricane, a tempest or thunderstorm, or when there is a solar or lunar eclipse. These are called heavenly taboos. Similarly, one should avoid places such as temples, churches, cemeteries, and kitchens for intercourse. These are earthly taboos. Manly taboos refer to times when one is hungry, tired, intoxicated, or sick. Violating these rules lead to various diseases including sexual dysfunction for yourself and your children.

Besides bedroom arts, the Chinese natural health care system has many other ways to promote sexual vitality. This system runs the full spectrum from diet and sleep to clothing and exercise.

In terms of diet, the Chinese have the following potent yet natural aphrodisiacs to offer: deer antler, soft-shelled turtle, oysters, mussels, clams, shrimp, eggs, honey, animal kidney and penis, animal tails, sea horses, Chinese chives, peppers, onions, walnuts, chrysalis of the silk worm, garlic, ginseng, grapes and grape wine, pumpkin seeds, venison, and soy products (also see chapter 10 on potent healers). In Buddhism, vegetables such as garlic, chives, onions, and peppers are considered "meat dishes in vegetables" for their aphrodisiac ability, and are to be avoided for fear of sexual urges. For the promotion of female sexuality, soy products are especially helpful. Modern scientific studies show that soy contains rich phytochemicals called isoflavonoids, and are a natural source of estrogen, one of the major female sex hormones. Therefore, regular consumption of soy products can prevent breast cancer, promote sexual vitality, and delay the aging process. Another dietary recipe for female sexual problems is to stew dong quai together with chicken and eat it as a dish. Foods to avoid are those loaded with caffeine, sugar, or fat, which can dampen one's sexuality.

So far as clothing is concerned, Chinese fathers vote for loose underwear and against tight underwear, for fear that tight-fitting underwear will dampen a male's sexuality and fertility. This is because tight underwear hinders the smooth blood circulation to the area and the growth and development of the private parts. Modern medicine finds that tight-fitting underwear may raise testes temperature to a point where it interferes with sperm production, leading to sexual dysfunction and infertility.[6]

Another natural way to promote sexuality is to frequently accumulate and swallow saliva from time to time. Referred to as "the golden liquid" and "water of the flowery pond," saliva was held in high respect by the ancient Chinese for its ability to promote sexuality and immunity, and to delay the aging process. In addition to its important medical roles as teeth protector and digestive aid.[7] American and Japanese scientists recently discovered that certain hormones in saliva can delay the process of aging, prevent disease, and enhance sexual vitality. To maximize the therapeutic effects of saliva, the ancient Chinese tell us to gently swallow it once it fills the mouth, thinking of the lower abdomen—dantian—as it goes down. Since dantian is the "sea of qi energy" and the area where the Gate of Life is located, sending saliva directly to this area will double the therapeutic effects.

Yet another natural tool advocated by the ancient Chinese for promoting sexuality lies in regular, proper exercise. Modern studies show that exercise increases the flow of endorphins, androgen, and adrenaline, sexual hormones that play a key role in the arousal of both sexes. Also, exercise increases the capillary network throughout the body. This means there is plenty of blood to spare when the brain signals for an erection. People who exercise enjoy a better supply of blood and oxygen and complete nutrition, resulting in heightened sensations of pleasure, greater arousal, and stronger stamina—thus, enhanced sexuality.

In particular, stamina is essential for successful intercourse. When a female is close to orgasm, her vaginal muscles begin to contract, requiring more stamina and staying power on the part of the male to continue the thrusting motions of the penis. Lack of stamina is responsible for many a lover's failure in his romantic undertaking, when on the verge of success. Thus, people who exercise regularly have a much longer and stronger sexual life than those who do not.

However, not all exercises are good for sexuality. Actually, some can even stifle it. Bicycling, for instance, is one such exercise. A recent study conducted at the University of South Carolina School of Medicine found that male cyclists who ride one hundred miles per week may become temporarily impotent. Another study conducted in 1995 at Boston University reported that 250,000 Americans are impotent because of pelvic and perineal sports injuries. Repeated sitting pushes the groin against the seat, damaging the critical nerves and blocking the penile arteries.

Biologically, when you become sexually excited, two arteries in the penis stretch to about twice their normal size and pipe at least five times the usual amount of blood into two tubes of spongy tissue, which in turn become enlarged, resulting in an erection. If these arteries are blocked, erection becomes difficult. Besides, damage done to penile arteries can also lead to painful, persistent erections.

The best exercises use no mechanical equipment or cause exertion, which leaves Chinese fitness exercises the best options for our purpose, such as taich'i and qigong.

In addition to those popular Chinese fitness exercises, Dr. Wan Laisheng taught me the following skills designed to enhance sexual vitality. (Several of these are also described in appendix 5, "Dharma's Internal Exercises.")

Rub the Abdomen

The abdomen is where dantian is located, and dantian is the "sea of vital energy." As sexual vitality is a function of vital qi energy, it makes sense to keep this part of the body in good health by gently rubbing it.

Performance

Use your right hand to rub the entire abdomen in clockwise circles twenty times, then use your left hand to rub the abdomen in exactly the same manner, but counterclockwise. (See also page 446 in appendix 5.)

Rub the Waist

The waist is where the "Gate of Life" and the kidneys are located, on which depends our sexual vitality. In Chinese literature, impotent or sexually weak men are described as being weak in the kidneys. Frequently rubbing the waist can strengthen kidney qi energy, fasten the Gate of Life, and consequently enhance sexuality.

Performance

Use both hands to massage the waist, up and down thirty-six times. Keep the trunk as upright as you can. (See also page 446 in appendix 5.)

Shake the Heavenly Pillar

This exercise has a similar effect as rubbing the waist. Both massage and train the kidneys and the Gate of Life.

Performance

Put both hands in fists besides your waist, knuckles facing outward. First turn your upper body to the left, eyes looking backward as fast as possible. Then, reverse the position and turn to the right. (See also page 447 in appendix 5.)

Rub the Neck

The Chinese are the only people to have discovered the association between the neck and sexual vitality. They believe that frequently rubbing the neck can strengthen one's sexuality.

Performance

Rub both hands against each other first before applying them to the neck. Rub the neck rhythmically up and down thirty-six times. Adjust the strength to your comfort level. (See also page 445 in appendix 5.)

Clench the Teeth

This is another unique discovery by the ancient Chinese who held that both teeth and sexuality are measures of the strength of one's kidney qi energy. Teeth gradually decay as the kidney qi energy significantly weakens as one advances in age. Therefore, teeth and sexuality are connected in an indirect way. By strengthening the teeth, one enhances his or her sexuality, and vice versa.

Performance

Gently clench the teeth several times a day, just as if you were chewing food. (See also page 448 in appendix 5.)

Contract the Toes

What on earth do the toes have to do with sexuality? The ancient Chinese held that one's sexual nerves are linked to one's toes. By contracting the toes, you can boost the sexual nerves and therefore enhance your sexuality.

Performance

To perform, one just contract and let loose one's toes in alternation. Do this for thirty-six rounds each time, with one contraction and one loosing being defined as a round.

Contract the Anal Muscles

The anal and pubococcygeal muscles are the ones you need to contract in order to stop the urine flow or essence flow. The anal sphincter muscle is located at the base of the penis. Therefore, exercising these muscles can strengthen your control of the Gate of Life, giving you greater stamina and staying

power during intercourse. This can also relieve wet dreams and incontinence.

For women, there are three sets of pubococcygeal muscles: one is found at the entrance to the vagina; another is located deeper inside the vagina; and the third is found around the anus.

Performance

As you inhale, contract the muscles as if you were to stop the flow of urine. Hold for several seconds. Then, as you exhale, release the muscles. Repeat thirty-six times.

Massage the Soles

Rubbing both soles many times, especially right after taking a bath, is believed to have a positive impact on sexual vitality and overall health.

Performance

Rub your hands against each other until warm. Turn the left sole upwards and rub it with your right hand. Do this thirty-six times. Then repeat on your right sole. (See also page 448 in appendix 5.)

Pull the Ears

The ancient Chinese believed that ears, like teeth, are connected with one's sexual nerves in some delicate ways. Pulling on the ears will strengthen sexual vitality and improve one's sexual performance.

Performance

Use your index fingers to support the upper corners of the ears, while pulling down the earlobes with the thumbs and middle fingers. Do this many times a day.

Press Acupoints

The following acupoints are considered to be related to sexual vitality and functioning: Zusanli, Sanyinjiao, Chenfu, Earlobes, Fengmen, Guanyuan, Guanzhong, Juque, Mingmen, Qihai, Yaoyangguan, Yinlinquan, and Yongquan. (Refer to appendix 7 for instructions and illustrations of these exact locations.)

Gaze at the Morning Sun

The ancient Chinese believed that the first gentle rays of the morning sun are helpful to one's sexual energy and health. Therefore, they asked us to get up early in the morning and gaze into the sun for one minute as it first rises. While doing this, breathe deeply and think of dantian, the lower abdomen.

NOTE: Looking directly into the sun could be dangerous to some people with sensitive eyes. Remember that it must be the early morning sun, as it is just rising above the horizon, not when it's high in the sky.

Endnotes

1. Edward M. Brecher, *Love, Sex and Aging: A Consumer's Union Report* (Boston, MA: Little, Brown and Co., 1984).

2. E. Douglas Whitehead, *Management of Impotence and Infertility* (Philadelphia, PA: Lippincott-Raven Publishers, 1994).

3. Stefan Bechtel, *The Practical Encyclopedia of Sex and Health* (Emmaus, PA: Rodale Press, 1993).

4. *New England Journal of Medicine* (June 1995).

5. *The Seattle Times*, 19 August 1998: A1.

6. Allan R. Cook, *Men's Health Concerns Sourcebook* (Detroit, MI: Omnigraphics, Inc., 1998), 381.

7. Simeon Margolis. *The Johns Hopkins Medical Handbook* (New York, NY: Rebus, Inc., 1995), 202.

Chapter 12

Secrets of Rejuvenation and Longevity

I n traditional Chinese culture, longevity is considered to be as important a contributor to happiness as wealth and social position. It has always been something highly desired and jealously coveted. When the New Year comes, friends and dear ones are fond of saying: "I wish you have as much good luck as the water in the East China Sea, and as high a life expectancy as the Southern Mountains."

Long-lived historical figures in China's history have been a recurring literary theme. They are a constant inspiration to many Chinese who find consolation and pride in longevity itself, even though they may be poor. Such historical figures include Lao Tze, the author of *Tao Te Ching*, who left the world at the age of 180; Peng Tze who is said to have lived to an impressive 800 years of age; and Liu Jing, who is said to have died at the age of 305.

One modern story goes that in the early 1930s, John Fairbank was hired by Qinhua University in Peking as a professor of economics. He had heard a great deal about

Dr. Hu Shi, the famous intellectual leader and scholar in modern China, and arranged to call on him during his visit to Peking University. After arriving at Hu's residence, the American sinologist was shown immediately to a reception room by a handsome, baby-faced gentleman and offered a seat. After they finished exchanging greetings, the American professor asked: "I have come to interview your leader Dr. Hu Shi. May I see him now?" The man replied: "Surely, I am Hu Shi!" Mr. Fairbank had expected to meet a much older man and was surprised to find that the famous Chinese scholar was so youthful in appearance in his late forties.

I am sure Dr. Hu Shi can be an object of envy for many people who are haunted by the idea of premature aging. Today, too many Americans just "get old and tired and want to retire" while still in their forties. Their bodies don't move as they should, their eyes become blurred, their hearing gets weak, their memory fades, and their hair turns gray. Enormous sums of money and much research has been spent in an effort to find effective solutions to such signs of aging, but all to little avail. Apparently, the answer does not lie in money and technology. Is there something in nature and within ourselves that can offer a solution?

My students and American colleagues frequently ask: "How do you manage to look so young?" "Can you teach me some secrets about keeping young?" As can be expected, there is no simple answer to these questions. Nor is it an accident that Dr. Hu Shi and many other Chinese look younger than they actually are. The fact is that since time immemorial, the Chinese have systematically and constantly sought natural methods to help them achieve their dual goal of rejuvenation and longevity. One of the earliest researchers in this field was the famous Yellow Emperor of China, who lived to an agile age of 111. Until his death, he had the ability to personally handle state affairs and make love regularly. Not surprisingly, he must have had some secrets and precious lessons to offer in this regard. The following are some of the ageless conclusions found in *The Yellow Emperor's Classics of Internal Medicine*:

> *The way to longevity involves being moderate in eating and drinking, abstinent in ejaculation, regular in living habits, calm in heart and indifferent to fame and gains, and avoiding the bad influence of extreme weather. Following these rules and the genuine qi energy will permeate the body, and your spirit will be on high alert against any disease. How can you be sick this way? Therefore, it is desirable that we reduce our earthly desires, keep the mind easy and calm, free from fear and emotional outbursts, and keep the body active but not tired. . . . On the contrary, to drink wine like water and engage in sexual intercourse in a drunken state; to spend the precious sexual essence freely and lead an irregular way of life, ignorant of the vital importance of semen and energy*

conservation—these are sure ways to get old and die prematurely.

It is a significant phenomenon in the Chinese natural health care system that an intimate relationship is set up between sexual essence and aging and death. This should come as no surprise if we understand that the Chinese fathers always regard sexual essence as the primary driver in life. Again, let us turn to *The Yellow Emperor's Classics of Internal Medicine* for a detailed explanation:

For a female, her kidney qi energy (the equivalent of sexual essence) starts to develop at the age of seven, characterized by changes in teeth and hair. As she reaches 14 (2 x 7), her Ren channel opens up and menstruation starts. Thus, she is able to conceive and deliver a baby. As she reaches 21 (3 x 7), her kidney qi continues to grow and her teeth grow to their fullest. At 28 (4 x 7), her physique is at its strongest and her hair at its longest. At 35 (5 x 7), her kidney qi energy starts to decline. Consequently, her face begins to wither and her hair starts to fall. At 42 (6 x 7), her kidney qi energy becomes deficient. As she reaches 49 (7 x 7), her Ren channel becomes weak and menstruation stops as a result.

For a male, his kidney qi energy starts to grow at the age of eight, as is manifest in the growth of his teeth and hair. As he reaches 16 (2 x 8), his kidney qi becomes strong and he is able to intercourse and ejaculate. At 24 (3 x 8), his kidney qi continues to cumulate until he reaches 32 (4 x 8) when his kidney qi arrives at its apex and he is at the peak of his physical life. As he reaches 40 (5 x 8), his kidney qi energy starts to decline. At 48 (6 x 8), this decline in kidney qi accelerates. When he reaches 56 (7 x 8), his kidney qi becomes deficient. As a result, not only the function of kidneys, but also that of the liver and heart, are affected. At 64 (8 x 8), his kidney qi energy is almost exhausted and his teeth and hair fall out.

As we can tell from the above description, the ancient Chinese consider seven to be the cycle for a female and eight the cycle for a male. Thus, the squares of seven (forty-nine) and eight (sixty-four) are taken to be the full circles of the physical life of a female and male respectively. Moreover, the rotation of these cycles is closely associated with the rise and fall of kidney qi energy based on sexual essence. To delay and reverse the biological process of aging, it stands to reason that we need to accumulate and conserve our sexual essence. Therefore, the theory and practice of rejuvenation in China constantly focuses on the conservation of sexual essence.

As explained earlier, the ancient Chinese are keen observers and modest students of nature. Indeed, all the principles of Chinese regimens are based on such observations. In terms of rejuvenation and longevity, the ancient Chinese repeatedly asked themselves this question: "Why does the universe never get old?"

It seems that nature is in a never-ending process of rejuvenation. Thus, winter stifles all life in the field only to be rejuvenated by the coming of spring. Snow and ice freeze the field only to give way to refreshed beauty shortly afterwards. This cycle continues endlessly, year after year. What makes nature behave like that and remain forever young? The answer lies, as the ancient Chinese found, in that nature does not have emotion. In other words, unsentimental and unemotional is the way of nature in her never-ending work of evolution and rejuvenation.

Emotional upheavals and stresses are the major drivers of the human aging process. "To think of you makes me old" is a poetic expression of this understanding in China. If thinking alone can drive one old, how much more will it be if one is stressful and depressed? To delay aging and prolong life, therefore, the ancient Chinese tell us to minimize all kinds of emotion, be it joy or sorrow. Again, we find Dr. Sun Simiao an authoritative voice in this regard.

Those who are good at taking care of their health have less worry, less thinking, less desires, less speech, less laughing, less anger, less likes and dislikes than those who are not. This is the key to good health and longevity. For excess worry makes the heart timid, excess thinking makes the mind tired, excess desire makes the spirit dull, and excess speech makes the qi deficient. Similarly, excess laughing hurts the internal organs, *excess anger makes the pulse fluctuate, excess likes make us prejudiced, and excess dislikes make us depressed.*

Based on this understanding, Sun Simiao went on to lay down a list of "don'ts" and "lesses" as a guide for health and longevity.

The Seven Don'ts

1. Don't lift any weight beyond a comfortable level for you.

2. Don't worry too much.

3. Don't be angry.

4. Don't feel miserable.

5. Don't laugh too much.

6. Don't overwhelm yourself with joy.

7. Don't eat too much fat and delicious foods.

The Nine Lesses

1. Less thinking to keep your spirit clear.

2. Less worry to keep your mind concentrated.

3. Less desires to make you happy.

4. Less speech to save your saliva.

5. Less social life to keep yourself comfortable.

6. Less laughter to keep your spirit at home.

7. Less anger to protect your liver and lungs.

8. Less ejaculation to conserve your vital energy.

9. Less jealousy to keep your heart peaceful and in harmony with nature.

In the final analysis, according to Dr. Sun, the Tao of rejuvenation and longevity lies in balance and moderation. That is to say, excess is as harmful as deficiency. Therefore, reading for too long will hurt your essence, listening for too long will harm your spirit, lying in bed for too long will hurt your qi energy, sitting for too long will hurt your arteries and veins, standing for too long will hurt your kidneys, and walking a long way will hurt your bones. Likewise, excess anger will hurt your liver; excess worry will hurt your heart; excess sorrow will hurt your lungs; excess melancholy will hurt your spleen; excess fright will hurt your kidneys; excess eating will hurt your stomach, and so on.

Another important contributor to the youthfulness of the Chinese is that they enjoy a slower tempo of life than Westerners. In traditional Chinese society, there is less stress and competition than in the U.S., although there is a much larger population in that country. In the U.S., life is characterized by rushing here and there to meet demands of work and family, demands of a competitive business world, and stress from feelings of job insecurity and an uncertain financial future, if not about life itself. Stress alone can lead to premature aging. Modern studies show that stress can adversely affect the hormone-producing system of the body, mainly that of the thyroid and adrenals. Every time we are in a stressful situation, adrenal hormones are released in a biological effort to strike a balance, thus causing an increase in heart rate, respiration, and blood pressure. This is an involuntary waste of limited body energy simply to prepare the body for "imagined" threats or worries. By draining our body's vital energy reserve, stress cannot help but speed up the aging process and lower one's immunity.

Following regular living habits is yet another reason why the Chinese look relatively younger than their Western counterparts. For thousands of years, the Chinese have been advised to go to bed early and wake up early, following the rise and fall of the sun. As the Chinese see it, the rising sun is nature's call to work, and the setting sun is nature's call to retire. To live a healthy and long life, we must be in harmony with nature. There is a biological clock inside the body that regulates the activities of the central nervous system. For instance, our pulse, our blood pressure, our respiration, and our metabolism all have their own tempos and cycles. Thus, as the day breaks, we have a natural tendency to wake up. As the night falls, we feel low-spirited and ready for sleep. Keeping a regular, natural living habit promotes the functioning of our biological clock and therefore the functioning of our central nervous system, making us happy, healthy, and youthful. On the contrary, an irregular living habit confuses the biological clock, disrupts the functioning of the central nervous system and all the internal organs under its command, making us sick and age prematurely.

As is now clear by now, diet also has a lot to do with our aging process. It is universally acknowledged that the Chinese diet is a healthy one. One less known reason for the health of the Chinese diet is that most culinary principles in China are worked out by doctors and Taoist adepts rather than by cooks. Such a diet contains plenty of natural, organically grown fresh foods such as vegetables, fruits, and wholesome grains, and little caffeine. Fresh vegetables and fruits invigorate our systems and keep our skin smooth and youthful. Wholesome grains are rich in chromium, a nutrient which has been shown by chemists at Bemidji State University in Minnesota to be able to lengthen the life of rats by one third of their normal life span. By living close to nature and eating foods provided by nature in their original forms, the Chinese are able to get the best nourishment they need for a healthy and long life.

Born and bred in a cultural soil fertile in the teachings of Lao Tze, Confucius, and Buddha, the Chinese have developed mellow, flexible, and noncompetitive modes of thinking and living. We cannot say that they have no worries or stress, but most Chinese, rich or poor, have a profound sense of humor. Perhaps they can smile more easily and laugh more heartily than other people. When confronted with worries and tricky problems, they like to remind themselves of the ancient advice: "Why worry so much while in less than 100 years all of us will be buried in the ground?" It is this understanding of life that enables them to tell internal things from external things, and to laugh away worries in life. This is another reason why they have a relatively youthful appearance.

In the eyes of most people, hair is a measurement of age. Its color and thickness usually indicate the age of its possessor. Thus, black hair is associated with youth and middle-aged people, while gray hair and thinning hair usually mark the evening of life. This, however, can be misleading because these days many people in their forties and even thirties have gray hair. In traditional Chinese medicine, gray hair and balding are diagnosed to be a matter of deficiency in kidney qi energy. Normally, as one reaches fifty, one's kidney qi energy is significantly weakened, resulting in white hair and thinning. The fundamental means of rejuvenating the hair lies, therefore, in conserving and promoting kidney qi energy, or sexual essence. Another reason is that there are not as many commercial shampoos and bathing soaps in China as there are in the West. These chemicals have a dampening effect on the health of hair and the skin. Regular use of them cannot but rid the hair of its luster and the skin of its natural moisture, hastening the aging process.

Skin is another measurement of age. My teacher, Dr. Wan Laisheng, told me that his teacher Immortal Liu used to clean his body with a raw sponge of towel gourd, and rub his body with his own urine right before a bath. As a result, Liu's skin looked like that of a teenager even when he was more than 150 years of age!

Hu Shicong (1095–1183), who for more than four decades was doctor to Ghengis Khan's family of the Yuan dynasty, summarized his understanding of the secrets of rejuvenation and longevity in his book *Essentials of Diet*:

> In ancient times, people who understood Tao lived in harmony with Nature. They were careful in their diet, regular in their living, and moderate in work and exercise. Hence, they enjoyed long life. Nowadays, however, people behave in a quite different manner. They lead an irregular life, and are undiscriminating in diet. Moreover, they have too many desires, and are ignorant of the principle of moderation, conservation and abstinence. It is little wonder that many of them just get old before fifty.

The key to rejuvenation and longevity lies in constant maintenance, and the guiding principle of maintenance is moderation. Through moderation you avoid the mistake of both too much and too little. If we have excess desires, we will be sick. Therefore, it is the principle of regimen to avoid excesses and conserve vital energy. As such, one will have stronger immunity against negative external factors.

> What is regimen, after all? Regimen means simplifying your diet, saving yourself from excess thinking and worries, abstaining from excess desires, avoidance of anger and excessive labor, conservation of vital qi energy, limiting your speech, belittling material gains and losses, and pacifying your mind and spirit. If the mind is peaceful, how can ailment enter you?
>
> Thus, those good at regimen do not eat until they are hungry, and stop eating before they feel full. For they know that excess eating damages the stomach, just like hunger damages the qi energy. Besides, one should not go to bed right after a meal. Hence, do not eat a heavy dinner. The thing to be avoided each day is a heavy dinner. The thing to be avoided each month is excess drinking at the month's end. The thing to be avoided each year is long travel away from home at the year's end. The thing to be avoided in lifetime is to have sexual intercourse with light on.
>
> Nor should you take a shampoo right after a meal, otherwise you will suffer from wind diseases. While taking a bath, do not let the wind go directly through you. Otherwise, all kinds of external affections will invade you as your pores are wide open.
>
> Sleeping alone for a single night is superior to taking nourishing herbs for a hundred days. Do not sleep with lights on. Otherwise, your spirit will go woolgathering, and nightmares will visit you. Do not speak on bed or at dinner table, otherwise your qi energy will be hurt. Do not blow off the light with mouth, for fear that your qi will be wasted (although it is fashionable nowadays to

blow off candles on a birthday pudding with bare mouth).

Before going to bed at night, rub your face and eyes with warm hands. This will keep your face tender and youthful. Taking a warm bath of feet at bedtime can save you cold diseases and a lot of dreams.

Hu also went on to discuss healthy ways of life in accordance with the four seasons:

In spring, go to bed early and rise early in harmony with the sun. Meanwhile, as the weather starts to get warm, take more wheat products to slightly cool down the qi.

In summer, the heavenly qi and the earthly qi merge. It is important that you go to bed late in the evening but get up early in the morning. Do not feel tired of the long summer day, but keep a calm, happy mind. Meanwhile, eat plenty of foods that are cool in nature.

In autumn, the heavenly qi is moving fast and the earthly qi is clear. During this time of the year, you should go to bed early and get up early. Meanwhile, conserve your spirit and qi energy. Do not let it dissipate by chasing after various desires. Since autumn is a dry season, it is advisable to eat plenty of juicy foods.

In winter, the earth is frozen. This is a closing and saving season. During this time of the year, you should go to bed early in the evening but get up late in the morning after the sun is out. This is the way to conserve your energy and

avoid external affections. Meanwhile, eat more foods that are warm and hot in nature. This is the way to health and longevity.

Dr. Wan Laisheng has additional words to say concerning rejuvenation and longevity:

- Practice qigong regularly on daily basis. Qigong can promote the blood and qi circulation, and give you a smooth, sanguine complexion and a youthful face. Clinical studies in China show that those who regularly practice qigong have a lower heart rate and blood pressure, better vision and hearing, sounder sleep, and higher spirits than those who do not. Basically, their body is in a better and younger shape than people of the same age who do no qigong.

- Practice fitness exercises every day. Physical exercise greatly retards the aging process, especially Chinese fitness exercises that are leisurely and forbid exertion. Actually, most of the physical decline that older people suffer from stems not from age but from simple disuse of their minds and bodies. There is no longer any doubt that regular exercise is one of the best ways to prevent and treat almost all kinds of disease. Exercise can potentially charge up the immune system to stop the spread of viruses and diseased cells. With no requirement for exertion, soft Chinese exercises are the best form of exercise. They lack the side effects that some vigorous sports cause.

- Frequently accumulate saliva in the mouth and swallow it down to dantian. Saliva is a precious bodily fluid with magical therapeutic and rejuvenating powers. The Chinese have regarded it with the highest respect for thousands of years, although its value is just starting to "dawn on the West." Saliva can nourish the brain, aid in digestion, detoxify the body, increase flexibility, add luster and smoothness to the face and skin, enhance sexuality, and strengthen immunity—all functions that fight the effects of aging.

- Frequently think of dantian, the lower abdomen. Dantian is a unique discovery by the ancient Chinese, who regarded this portion of the body as the reservoir of vital qi energy, the converging point of viscera. Frequently thinking of it helps to promote and conserve the vital qi energy, thus delaying the aging process.

- Gently knock your head and ears. Your head is the headquarters of your life. Gently knocking it every day by performing Dharma's internal exercise, "Beat the Heavenly Drum," will promote the mental functioning, improve memory, prevent and relieve ringing in the ears, Parkinson's and Alzheimer's diseases—conditions that are more and more companions of old age these days. (See appendix 5 for instructions.)

- Frequently comb your hair with your fingers. Frequently combing the hair with bare fingers can promote the blood and qi circulation in the head, promote mental ability and memory, as well as keep the hair black or in its natural color.

- Gently clench your teeth several times a day. Teeth are another important marker of age. Loss of teeth is often associated with old age. To preserve them, the ancient Chinese tell us to gently bite our teeth against each other. This will not only strengthen the teeth, and prevent them from decaying prematurely, but will also promote sexuality and mental power. Teeth movements directly affect mental functioning and sexual performance. (See appendix 5 for instructions.)

- Rub the soles several times a day. A Chinese story goes that several generations of a family all lived to more than 100 years of age. When asked the secrets of longevity, the family members said they all would frequently rub their soles. The sole is where the starting point of the kidney meridian is located. This is the acupoint of Yongquan. Therefore, frequently rubbing your soles can strengthen kidney qi energy, and serve to commune the kidneys and heart, a process known in Chinese natural health classics as *shui-huo-ji-ji* (water and fire balancing each other). (See appendix 5 for instructions.)

- Frequently contract and release the anal muscles and toes. This is designed to promote sexuality, kidney qi energy, urinary function, and other functions often associated with age. If lowered sexual vitality and incontinence are symbols of premature aging, frequently contracting and releasing the anal muscles and toes in a rhythmic manner can delay the aging process by preventing such medical conditions from occurring. (See chapter 11 for more instructions.)

- Do not allow your stomach to become more than 70 to 80 percent full at any meal, even if your diet is healthy. This ancient Chinese wisdom is confirmed by a recent scientific experiment that shows that the best way to delay aging and prolong life in mice is to underfeed them, giving them just enough nourishment to stay alive. Mice who were regularly underfed not only lived 35 percent longer than those fed to fullness, but they were also far less likely to contract cancer and other diseases. Overeating damages the stomach, wastes energy, and makes you feel sluggish and tired. Therefore, for the sake of health, better to err on the less-than-enough side than on the more-than-enough side in terms of quantity.

- Drink three spoonfuls of soup at the start of each meal, and you will be saved a lot of trouble in old age. Ancient Chinese believe that this practice can enhance one's appetite and promote digestion, and therefore prevent diseases in the digestive system. Of course, "three" here is not a fixed number to stick to. What it tells us is just to drink a few mouthfuls of soup at the start of each meal.

- Drink plenty of clean water each day. Water is the first of the Five Elements, and plays a vital role in the proper functioning of our bodies. The fact that about 70 percent of our physical weight is made up of water speaks for itself. Water is needed to moisturize the skin, limber the joints, clean the body, aid in digestion and bowel movements, and many other vital biological functions. Even a slight deficit in water will make you feel tired and sick.

- Do not smoke. Cigarette smoking constricts blood vessels and impairs blood circulation which, in turn, leads to premature wrinkling. Just look at the faces of chronic smokers and you will see. As well, smoking disturbs the hormone function and depresses hormone production, negatively impacting the thyroid and the entire endocrine system, consequently speeding up the aging process.

- Make sure you have enough good quality sleep each and every day. Lack of sleep puts added pressure on the body, draining tour strategic reserves of energy, disturbing the qi and blood circulation, and weakening the mental and immune systems. Basically, it hastens the body's aging process. While sleeping, keep the bedroom well ventilated, but do not allow drafts or breezes to blow directly on you.

- Spend a considerable amount of time outdoors each day. Walk a mile after dinner. This is meant to give you enough fresh air and natural sunlight each day. Fresh air and sunlight are to life what oil is to a lamp, in the absence of which no life would have been possible. The ancient Chinese believed that fresh air and gentle sunlight contain alive qi energy which can nourish our lungs, heart, brain, and skin, making us energetic and youthful.

• Treasure your sexual essence. The aging process and one's life span depends directly on sexual essence. Actually, sexual indulgence is the major cause of premature aging and death in the whole course of human history. In modern times, people mature earlier than their ancestors did a century ago. This has a lot to do with pornographic materials that are widespread and serve to stimulate sexual urge and maturity on the part of teenagers. As a law of nature, the sooner one matures the sooner one will die. Specifically, the maximum life span of humans as well as animals is governed by the rule of seven, i.e., seven times the age of maturity. This makes the conservation of sexual essence all the more relevant.

• The following foods are conducive to rejuvenation and longevity if taken on regular basis—ginseng, pork or beef marrow, Lingzhi mushroom, peanuts, walnuts, pine nuts, soybeans and soy products, milk, sesame, tremella, red dates, raisins, coconut, turtle meat, pomegranates, and chrysanthemums.

Indeed, the Chinese do not believe that decrepitude is inevitable. They believe that we all have the natural tools needed to live to the age of ninety or more. In the animal world, the life span rule seems to be seven times that of the age of maturity. Thus, a horse reaches maturity at three years and generally has a life expectancy anywhere between twenty and twenty-five years. A dog can live to fifteen years because it normally matures at around the age of two. Rabbits have a life expectancy of seven years because they normally mature at one year old.

Applying the same rule to human beings, we can all reasonably expect to live more than ninety years ($14 \times 7 = 98$ years for women and $16 \times 7 = 112$ years for men). According to a report by the Chinese National Committee on Aging, there are more than 8,000 people in China today who are 100 years old or older, while the number above ninety years of age is climbing 5 percent per year. Indeed, it is up to us to explore this potential longevity that nature has endowed to every one of us. At least in this sense we can declare that all men are born equal.

Chapter 13

The Road
to Immortality

It may sound ridiculous to Westerners to insert a chapter on immortality into a book on health and longevity. This is not, however, the case to someone well trained in the traditional Chinese culture and its natural health care system. To such a mind, immortality is a natural extension of longevity. The Chinese culture is one of humanism, in which man occupies the central place and plays the central role in the trinity of heaven-man-earth. In such a culture, nothing is impossible to man so long as he is willing. The fact is that health and longevity are not the ultimate goals sought by many Chinese. They see health and longevity as a means to a supreme end—immortality. The relationship between good health and immortality is a close one. According to the ancient Chinese, good health is a necessary foundation and prerequisite of immortality, which is the supreme sublimation of a healthy, long life.

As the Chinese see it, life is a continual cycle that almost everybody has to go through over and over again, in the form of life and death. This process is known as reincarnation. Since life is full of pain and worry, it would be wonderful if one can transcend the process of reincarnation once and for all. To a willing mind, this is not an insurmountable task, although it is obviously an extremely difficult one. The cycle is broken by a process called xiutao, or "cultivating Tao," in Chinese culture. In plain English, this means seeking immortality through consistent effort guided by Taoist principles. In order to attain immortality, one has to cultivate it. Those who succeed in becoming immortals are said to have attained Tao. Remember that Tao is the Way of Nature. As such, to have attained Tao means to have merged into nature.

According to Dr. Wan Laisheng, there are three kinds of immortals, reflecting different levels of attainment. They are (in ascending order of attainment and lifespan): manly immortals, earthly immortals, and heavenly immortals. Manly immortals are made by seeking Tao with some special methods short of a comprehensive understanding of the Way of Nature. Earthly immortals are those who have attained the bulk of Tao through persistent effort under the guidance of other immortals. Heavenly immortals are the highest achievement with full understanding and complete attainment of Tao.

Manly immortals are not immortals in the absolute sense of the word, because they still have to go through incarnation, but the cycle of their incarnation has been extended to 500 years. In other words, they can live up to 500 years of age in a single lifetime. Earthly immortals can live to 1,000 to 2,000 years, thanks to their higher attainment of Tao. Heavenly immortals have no limits because they have completely transcended incarnation and totally merged into Nature. In other words, they can live as long as nature lasts. When they reveal their true feature, so to speak, heavenly immortals appear in purely golden form. For this reason, they are also known as Golden Immortals.

Although the immortals are different in their levels of attainment of Tao, there is a universally applicable, standardized procedure through which one has to go through in order to achieve immortality, be it manly, earthly, or heavenly. Essentially, this procedure is composed of four interrelated, ascending steps:

1. Refine foods into sexual essence.
2. Refine sexual essence into vital qi.
3. Refine vital qi into primordial spirit.
4. Merge primordial spirit into nature (immortality).

These steps lay down the three goals or milestones in seeking immortality. Thus, the journey in search of immortality starts with the effort to refine foods into sexual essence, and ends with the completion of merging one's refined spirit into nature.

The whole idea is to use fire (mind) to boil water (essence) into vapor (qi), and guide qi energy to circulate in the body. Spirit is generated in this circulation, until eventually the spirit becomes internal elixir and merges into nature.

The most important method to refine foods into essence is fitness exercises, which improve digestion power and enhance sexual vitality. Of course, healthy foods are needed for the production of essence. They do not have to be made of animal protein, but instead beans, whole wheat, plants, and vegetables. Fish is even preferable to red meat.

The aim is not to generate sexual essence for intercourse, but to produce as much essence as possible to be refined into qi energy. As can be readily verified, there is a direct relationship between the amount of essence one has and the level of qi energy one possesses. The more essence one has, the higher will be one's level of qi energy, and the stronger will be one's immunity and health. None of the later goals can be realized without the foundation of good health; in the absence of which, digestion will be poor, and the body will not be able to make the best use of the foods it consumes. This relationship between excellent health and immortality is well explored by the ancient Chinese who used the term "internal elixir" to describe refined spirit, and the term "external elixir" to describe robust health. In other words, before one can embark on the journey in search of immortality, (i.e., to refine the internal elixir) one must first refine one's external elixir, (i.e., have good health). Indeed, external elixir is an indispensable material to be used in the refinement of internal elixir.

Alternatively, the cultivation of internal elixir is referred to as xingong, or the "training of the spirit," aimed at refining qi into spirit, while the cultivation of external elixir is referred to as mingong, or the "training of the body aimed at refining essence into qi." The concept of xingong and mingong are of vital importance to the understanding of the immortality process. The fathers of Chinese civilization held that as a fetus, body and soul are in oneness. Later, when the baby comes to into the world, the two become separated, with xin residing in the heart and min residing in the kidneys. One of the basic tasks for cultivating immortality is to restore the primordial balance between xin and min, or body and spirit. Xin is the root of the heart, and spirit is the root of xin. Min is the root of kidney, and essence is the root of min. Xin symbolizes heaven and fire, while min symbolizes earth and water. While seemingly contradictory to each other, they are really two sides of the same coin. Just imagine a hot summer without water, or a cold winter without fire, and you will come to appreciate the interdependence of xin and min. The ideal status is one in which fire and water are in balance. This is known in the Chinese natural health care system as *sui-huo-ji-ji*, or "harmonious communion between heart and kidneys," or alternatively, "calling down the dragon to control the tiger." Here dragon stands for xin and tiger stands for min, an image specifically referring to the process of using one's mind to control one's sexual desire.

There is nothing strange about this interdependence between xin and min, internal elixir and external elixir, if we understand the requirements of cultivating immortality. For one thing, the search for immortality is a very arduous and long process, which requires that anyone serious about it have robust health and be able to sit cross-legged for hours on end in meditation without becoming tired.

For another thing, the cultivation of immortality takes a great deal of sexual essence as raw material to be refined into vital qi, so that much vital qi can then be refined into primordial spirit. It is common knowledge that only healthy people are sexually vital, and the production of sexual essence takes good digestion and circulation. Therefore, one has to have a strong external elixir in order to create an internal elixir. That is to say, one has to train his body first in order to possess excellent health as the springboard for the search of immortality. In this respect of training, all Chinese fitness exercises and the rules of diet, sleeping, regulated sex, and so on are meant to give you an excellent external elixir, enabling you to live healthier and longer. Whether you want to further pursue the goal of internal elixir is your own personal decision.

For all the intimate relations between min and xin, a healthy person will not automatically become an immortal, if only because most of us spend or waste most of our precious sexual essence during the course of life. In the end, there is little left to be refined into qi, even less to be refined into spirit. For a serious seeker of immortality, however, the challenge begins with conscious and timely conservation of sexual essence, and then refining most, if not all of it into qi energy. True, sexual essence will, in a sense, become qi energy naturally by itself, and vital qi will nourish the spirit as a natural process. But the difference between the results of conscious effort and natural biological process lies in both quantity and quality.

For most people, only a very small amount of sexual essence is actually transformed into vital qi. The bulk of it is wasted either through sexual indulgence, wishful sexual thinking, internal leakage without your notice, or physical and mental exhaustion for the sake of worldly gains, be they money, power, or glory. Even if sexual essence is biologically transformed into qi, it is not the pure form of vital qi needed for immortality. By contrast, seekers of immortality use the unpolluted essence (unpolluted by sexual thought and external temptations) to generate vital qi, making it superior both in quality and quantity. In fact, a key factor accounting for the difference among immortals in terms of attainment of Tao lies in whether their mind is completely devoid of sexual thought during the course of cultivating immortality.

The second stage of cultivating immortality aims at refining as much essence as possible into qi energy. Here, we are confronted with the technical aspect of xiutao. The primary tool for accomplishing this goal, and indeed the later goals, lies in qigong, the Chinese breathing exercise. Qigong has been widely practiced in China for thousands of years, although most people practice it merely to cure disease, promote health, and prolong life. Only a few do it for the sake of immortality.

Reasons may differ, but the tool remains roughly the same. By refining sexual essence into qi energy and eventually into primordial spirit, qigong causes essence to travel upward through the body, as contrasted with the typical situation of essence traveling downward in the form of ejaculation. Essence going downward in this way results in new lives, as new babies are born. Essence traveling upward leads to immortality. Chuang Tzu, the great Taoist sage who was second only to Lao Tzu, made a solemn statement more than 2,000 years ago: "Those who give birth to new lives will die; those who kill new lives will live." In other words, those who give birth to new lives are those who spend their essence in sexual intercourse, resulting in new babies. Those who "kill new lives" are those who refuse to spend sexual essence that way, i.e., remain celibate, resulting in no new life, which is tantamount to killing new lives. Instead, they constantly conserve and refine sexual essence into vital qi, a higher form of substance. This is the key difference between mortals and immortals.

Indeed, qigong can help one in the attainment of Tao in many ways. First, qigong helps purify and uplift the mind, mentally preparing it for the attainment of Tao. Second, it promotes physical health which is indispensable to the attainment of Tao. Third, it causes essence to travel upward. Third, it serves as the link between our physical existence and the spirit in the nature so that one can merge into the nature as time arrives.

It must be pointed out, however, that qigong alone is not sufficient for the training of xin, or internal elixir. Indeed, our heart in which xin resides must be purified before we can seriously consider seeking immortality. For most people, the strongest temptations in life are sex and money. These are the archenemies of immortality. It is hard to rid your heart of these temptations. It takes the right education and considerable first-hand experience for one to see through life and realize the vanity of worldly temptations, be they sex or money or fame.

In this regard, the ancient Chinese teach us that beautiful girls are boats sending you to the shore of death, worldly wealth is alien to life, and children are the debt of current life. You cannot take them with you when die, and they will give you lots of trouble while you live.

Therefore, learn to go gently with life. Do not compete with others, do not seek worldly wealth and pleasure, and do not envy others. Rather, be patient, simple in mind and life, and kind to people. This is the way to cultivate your heart, an essential step in the cultivation of Tao.

Of course, this is easier said than done. Only when you have gone through the due process of life including romance and marriage can you hope to see its true colors. Many young people embark on the pilgrimage for immortality with great enthusiasm without first living through life. Naturally, they fail because they were distracted by worldly desires.

A story goes that a group of monks came down from the deep mountains to a city center after living in the secluded area for many years. Some of them were still in their thirties with little sexual experience. During their tour of the city center, they came across many beautiful women. The head monk lost no time in telling his young colleagues that they (the beautiful women) were venomous snakes which would kill people. After a day's tour of the city center, including a luxurious shopping area, they retreated back into the deep mountains. When asked about the most impressive objects they had seen during their tour, all the young monks replied that they liked the snakes the best. Even if physically insulated from the polluted world, their heart was by no means dead to temptations. This is why all immortals started their pilgrimage toward immortality after forty or forty-five years of age, when they already had consid-

erable life experience and a genuine disillusion about mortal life and worldly affairs.

For the mere sake of promoting health and healing disease, natural breathing combined with meditation will carry you a long way. For the purpose of cultivating immortality, however, two additional challenging tasks must be accomplished. These tasks are the creation of the Minor Heavenly Cycle and the Major Heavenly Cycle, in that order. These two orbits are the ideal routes inside the body along which qi circulates. The route of the Minor Heavenly Cycle begins at the acupoint of Baihui (myriad confluence) located at the top of the head. It then goes down the Functioning channel along the middle line in the front of the body, passing through dantian (abdomen) until it reaches the acupoint of Huiyin, or the perineum, located between the legs at the midpoint between the genitals and anus. From there it starts its upward journey along the Governing channel running along the middle line of the back all the way to the apex of the head, thus completing a full cycle. The purpose of the Minor Heavenly Cycle is to completely connect the two vital channels in the upper body, (i.e., the Functioning channel and the Governing channel,) in order to better refine essence into qi.

The Major Heavenly Cycle, as the name implies, is a much longer route for qi circulation than the Minor Heavenly Cycle, and therefore harder to achieve. In addition to the full cycle of the Minor Heavenly Cycle, the Major Heavenly Cycle carries on to include the lower body. This is how the Major Heavenly Cycle runs: rather than ending at the perineum, it travels further downward in two parallel lines along the legs until it reaches the soles of the feet. Then, as you inhale, it starts its ascending journey, first retreating along the same parallel lines in both legs until the two branches converge at the perineum, and it then follows the Governing channel and continues its upward journey until it reaches Baihui, located at the very apex of the head, ending your exhalation and completing a full cycle of its own.

It must be pointed out that the Minor Heavenly Cycle is not a naturally complete cycle for ordinary people. There are two broken links in the chain. One happens in the mouth between the Functioning channel and the Governing channel, and the other is found in the diaphragm, separating the upper abdomen and the lower abdomen. In order to make the Minor Heavenly Cycle a full cycle, one has to make conscious, persistent efforts in the breathing exercise to mend, so to speak, the broken links.

There are some special skills passed down to us by the ancient Chinese to help accomplish this task. One of these vital skills is called "building a magpie bridge." What this means is to put your tongue slightly against the upper palate during qigong exercise, thus bridging the gap between the upper face and the lower face, mending one of the broken links in the Minor Heavenly Cycle. For most people not well trained in qigong, mending the broken link in the area of the diaphragm presents a gigantic hurdle in the creation of the Minor Heavenly Cycle. Typically, the air cannot descend directly to dantian because the diaphragm prevents it from passing through unchecked. Thus, the first major challenge confronting a seeker of immortality is to "remove" the diaphragm so that qi can go to dantian and the lower part of the body unchecked. This should be done in a natural way, and it takes considerable time.

The correct way to remove this hurdle is through natural, conscious guiding of qi with your mind to go down the body along the Functioning channel. Any attempt to get through this hurdle by force will be counter-productive and harmful to your health. In an absolute sense, haste makes waste. During each session of qigong, use your mind, not force, to guide the flow of air along the Functioning channel all the way down to dantian in your lower abdomen as you exhale. In practice, as you inhale, imagine that the air comes all the way up from the acupoint of Huiyin, or the perineum (located between the legs at the midpoint between the genitals and anus), along your spine until, at the end of the inhalation, it reaches the acupoint of Baihui at the apex of the head. Then as you exhale, imagine that you are sending the air down your body, from the very top of the head along your mouth and throat, all the way down the Functioning channel to dantian in the lower abdomen, until—at the end of your exhalation—it eventually returns to the acupoint of Huiyin, thus completing a Minor Heavenly Cycle.

The removal of the diaphragm is not something that will happen overnight. Generally, it will take a serious practitioner anywhere from one to two years of daily practice to accomplish the task. Therefore, it is very important not to give up during this learning period. Do not lose faith in the method described here. It is the only royal way to success. Do not think that this is mere fiction or a game of imagination as many people do. Have absolute confidence in yourself and in the qigong exercise. The Minor Heavenly Cycle has happened to many people in China, both past and present, and I see no reason why it cannot happen to you. The only thing that can prevent it from coming to you is your own lack of confidence in yourself.

For a confident, persistent seeker of Tao, the time will eventually come when this hurdle will be removed. Once the hurdle of the diaphragm is removed, you will feel a current of air going down the Functioning channel all the way to dantian, unchecked, whenever you exhale, giving you a comfortable sense of warmth, coolness, and internal vibration as a result of the qi movement. As you inhale, you will feel the same current of air going upward along the Governing channel all the way to your head, completing a full cycle of the Minor Heavenly Cycle.

The opening up of the Minor Heavenly Cycle is called *sui-huo-ji-ji*, or the communion between the heart and kidneys, or between the Functioning and Governing channels. This is a milestone in your search for immortality. It is no small achievement for anybody, and you have every reason to be proud of it.

It is advisable that you experiment with the Minor Heavenly Cycle for a couple of years before you attempt the next stage of creating the Major Heavenly Cycle. This is largely out of consideration of the strength of your qi energy, for it takes a much stronger qi energy to create the Major Heavenly Cycle, if only because qi has to travel a longer route in the Major Heavenly Cycle. The entire route of the Major Heavenly Cycle is almost twice as long as that of the minor one. Unless your qi is strong enough, you will not be able to complete the circulation of qi along the Major Heavenly Cycle in a single round of respiration. Therefore, you have to fully prepare yourself in terms of qi strength for the successful launching of the Major Heavenly Cycle. It goes without saying that the longer you circulate qi around the Minor Heavenly Cycle, the stronger will be your qi base, and the greater chance you will have of successfully creating a Major Heavenly Cycle. Keep in mind that everything should come naturally. Only natural results will provide permanent benefits.

The exact length of time spent at this stage of the Minor Heavenly Cycle varies with individual cultivators. It can be anywhere from one year to twenty years, depending on how persistent you are with the training, how many hours you put into it every day, and your health status. After experimenting with the Minor Heavenly Cycle for a while, you will notice many changes. Typically, the qi reserve inside your body will be strengthened, your dantian will be permeated with qi and involuntarily vibrating, and the cycle of your respiration will be significantly prolonged.

If you keep up the momentum, you will be able to experience the wonderful phenomenon of air circulating in your lower abdomen, thirty-six times clockwise and then thirty-six times counterclockwise. This shows that your "sea of qi" has been considerably deepened and enlarged. By the way, this phenomenon is extremely helpful in the process of self-healing. Most marvelous is the sudden, short appearance of a ray of light between the eyebrows. This light is so bright that it can light up an entire room. These are good signs that show that the time is ripe for you to embark on the next stage of cultivating immortality—creating a Major Heavenly Cycle and refining qi into primordial spirit.

To proceed to the next stage, as you exhale, naturally guide your qi flow from your nose all the way down to dantian and perineum, then further down the body along both legs until it reaches the soles of your feet. As you inhale, mentally raise the qi energy from the soles up the legs until both branches of qi merge into one at the perineum, then continue its upward travel along the Governing channel from the per-

ineum to the apex of the head. Eventually, you will be able to circulate your internal qi energy throughout your body along the Major Heavenly Cycle, from head to feet, over and over again. As elsewhere in Chinese natural health care, the guiding principles are naturalness and persistence. Absolutely no force or exertion is allowed. You do not want to help the shoots grow by artificially pulling them upward. By doing that, you kill the shoots. Rather, be patient and let time works out its wonder as was the case with the Minor Heavenly Cycle.

The opening up of the Major Heavenly Cycle is referred to as the "communion between heaven and earth," with heaven representing the head and earth representing the feet. Once this orbit is created inside your body, you are on the highway of refining qi into spirit. You can, consciously and at your will, direct qi energy to any part of the body to heal disease in yourself or others. You can also use it to defend yourself or to attack others, as is often the case with masters of the Chinese martial arts.

For the purpose of self-healing and self-defense, all you need to do is to direct qi energy to specific parts of the body, be it the head, fingers, internal organs, or the abdomen. If you have a stomach ailment, for instance, you can direct your qi to that area to work out the healing. If you direct the qi to your head, you may be able to prop up a stone of 500 pounds with your bare head, and even let others break it in half by hammering it on your head. If you direct the qi to your fingers, you may be able to stand upside down on two fingers as my teacher Wan Laisheng was able to do. If you direct the qi to your abdomen, you may be able to withstand the force of 1,000 pounds in a blow from your enemy. My grandteacher, Dr. Du Xingwu, did this and the force of the blow he received broke his opponent's wrist.

To heal or attack others, you have to release your qi energy out of your body, either through your eyes, fingers, or through your palms. This is called waiqi, or "outflowing qi," in Chinese martial arts. Outflowing qi has been successfully applied to medical diagnosis, anesthesia, healing, and defeating others in physical combat. Of course, anyone serious about immortality is strongly advised against releasing qi energy outside his body. Releasing qi energy means wasting qi energy, the defeat of the very purpose of cultivating immortality.

The Major Heavenly Cycle is exactly the tool for refining qi into spirit, the opening up of which ushers in the next stage of cultivating immortality. Again, the exact length of this stage varies with individuals, depending on many factors such as individual biochemistry, degree of concentration, and not least, whether you have a faithful servant or not. To shorten the length of this stage, and most importantly, to protect the internal elixir already formed, it is vital that you reduce your bodily movements to a minimum at this stage of cultivation. This means you need a devoted servant or friend on whom you can count. Such a servant is needed to help you take care of your daily necessities of life, albeit at this point they are already minimal as compared to ordinary people. The cultivation of immortality requires that at the final stage of training, you reduce your bodily movements to a bare minimum, and completely forget about worldly affairs and daily chores. This allows you to conserve your vital energy, focus your attention as much as possible on the goal of immortality, and speed up the arrival of the final grand moment.

Usually, some common physical changes will happen at this stage, signaling the arrival of the grand moment when one's spirit is totally refined and one is ready to merge one's spirit into the nature. These changes include involuntary vibration and shaking of the body, a burning sensation in the kidneys, a boiling feeling in the scrotum, uproar in the lower abdomen, and air blowing in both ears. Most significantly, you will see a bean-sized luminous ball suddenly appearing in your heart, lingering there for a moment and lighting up all the internal organs before slowly falling down to dantian in the lower abdomen. This is clear evidence that your internal elixir has been created. The ancient Chinese called this phenomenon "male pregnancy" because a fetus-like something is formed in your abdomen. In fact, this luminous ball is simply the internal elixir you have been craving for. Its appearance ushers in the final stage of the pilgrimage towards immortality—merging spirit into nature.

There may be other physiological changes happening during the course of refining qi into spirit. A male seeker of immortality may find that his penis completely withdraws into his body, a phenomenon known in China as both "a horse hiding its penis inside the belly" and "a tortoise withdrawing its head." This is a good sign, showing that he has totally lost his sexual desire, though not his vitality, as a result of qigong exercises. During these exercises, most of one's sexual essence has been successfully refined into qi energy, leaving little room for sexual excitement. This is a natural phenomenon for male cultivators of Tao.

In a similar manner, a female seeker of immortality will, in the course of time, reduce her breasts to a flat level like that of a male. Also, menstruation will cease, even if she is well below the average biological age of menopause. This phenomenon is known as "killing the red dragon," an image derived from the color of both menstruation and nipples. A female cultivator is strongly advised to bring about these physiological changes before attempting to create the Major Heavenly Cycle. Here lies the difference in emphasis between a male seeker and a female seeker of immortality. The former emphasizes the training of qi energy, while the latter emphasizes the transformation of physical shape.

Although the internal elixir is created, it is not strong enough yet to be merged into the Great Ultimate, or nature. It takes time for the internal elixir to become strengthened and perfected. At this stage, your breathing weakens and becomes almost nonexistent. Take it naturally, and never use force. Be patient in waiting for the final moment to come.

At this stage of merging your spirit into nature, your body has returned to that of a baby, full of the most desirable primordial qi and spirit. As time goes by, anywhere between six to ten months from this point, you will notice a bright ball the size of a bean between your eyebrows. The third time this bright ball appears (known as "sunlight breaks thrice"), it is a sign that your internal elixir is perfect, and you should completely put out the "fire" used to refine it.

The process of refining materials in the physical world usually takes fire. Qigong is logically related to fire, as it is the means of refining essence into qi, and qi into spirit. The intensity of consciousness with which you guide the qi to circulate around your body is thus referred to as the intensity and temperature of fire. The more consciously you do this, the greater the fire.

After the "sunlight has broken thrice," you should stop guiding qi with your mind. Otherwise, the already perfect internal elixir will be damaged. You should let the qi energy go its own way without any guidance or interference. Also, no food is allowed except for your own saliva. All you have to do is be patient and wait for the final call of nature.

In plain English, this means the moment of death, but death in a very special sense in the world of xiutao.

Significantly, the Chinese fathers call the entire process of cultivating immortality as "gathering medicines." Here, medicines refer to essence, qi, and spirit, the "three treasures of life," which are the very substance on which the edifice of immortality is built. According to the ancient Chinese, the three treasures of life are not only the basic medicines for all diseases, but are also the vital medicines for the cure of mortal life. In an absolute sense, no three treasures, no cure; no three treasures, no immortality.

While there is a close interdependence among these three treasures of life, they are not equally important substances in the task of seeking immortality. Gathering of essence itself cannot make one an immortal, nor can the gathering of qi. Only the final gathering of spirit can carry the day. However, there can be no spirit without qi energy, and there can be no qi energy without essence. Hence the trinity of the three treasures of life, which is alternatively known as the "three lights of life."

Essence is vital to health and longevity, but is not the ultimate material to be merged into nature to enable one to become an immortal. Rather, it is the material to be refined into qi energy, a treasure of a higher caliber in the trilogy of immortality. In this sense, essence is the basic material for the cultivation of Tao. From a physiological point of view, all living things are constantly going through a process of metabolism. Sexual essence is no exception. Unless refined and stored as something of a more lasting nature, essence will quickly die. That is why seekers of immortality need to refine it into qi energy in a timely manner. Indeed time is life for a seeker of immortality. Moreover, essence can be wasted willingly, as in sexual indulgence, or lost involuntarily as is in the case of wishful sexual thinking (wet dreams), or leaked out of your body without you even being aware of it.

How can this be? There are many ways in which our essence can leak out of our bodies. For instance, urination is one such loophole. We take it for granted that the urinary tract is separated from the semen, so the two won't mingle. As a matter of fact, urination is one common way in which people lose their sexual essence, although only a minute amount each time. Since we all have to urinate frequently, the cumulative effect of such leakage over the years can be significant. Another loophole is thinking about sex, or reading or looking at sexual illustrations. The Chinese sages liken sexual thinking to fire, and sexual essence to water. This image suggests the fire boiling the water. The more you apply fire to the water, the heat increases and the sooner the water evaporates. This is exactly what happens to our essence when we indulge in sexual thinking or pornography. There may not be ejaculation (or orgasm) from such activities, but the loss of essence is inevitable.

Since essence is a vital substance for the production of qi, and the quantity and quality of essence determines the quantity and quality of qi energy we get, it goes without saying that, for the sake of cultivating immortality, the more and better essence we have, the more likely we are to accomplish our goal of immortality. Since life is short and the natural productivity of essence in our body is low, it makes sense to conserve sexual essence and refine it into qi, and to start doing this as soon as possible. Thus, conservation of essence becomes the primary challenge for those devoted to reaching immortality. This means much more than avoiding sex and pornography, although abstinence in sexual intercourse is a very crucial aspect of xiutao.

For most people, especially the young, this can be a gigantic challenge, due to the overwhelming power of libido over human life. No amount of persuasion, no precedents of failed marriages can successfully dissuade a young man from trying to get married. Indeed, sex is a powerful trap designed by nature for the continuation of the species. Even for the elderly who have lost the physical ability to have an erection, forgetting about sex is not an easy task. Their flesh is weak, but their mind is still willing. It is important to point out that this willing mind is another way to waste essence and is harmful to the health, although most people are not aware of it. Only those who have seen through it and realized the Way of Nature can forget about it.

Of course, seeing through life does not mean living through life. The more unlucky and frustrated you are with life, the closer you are to finding a good teacher. By this I mean the teacher of life who will be able to tell you the essences of life deprived of all its vanities and glories. The more you learn about the philosophy of life, the sooner you will come to the grand realization that all is vanity in this temporary life. Tao begins with one's self-imposed effort not to look at beautiful men or women and listen to decadent music. When one can affect deafness and blindness to external temptations, he or she is already on their way toward longevity, if not immortality.

While sexual urges and temptations are the greatest stumbling blocks in the way to immortality, the physical inability to have sex is not good, either. This is because impotent people are lacking some vital essence for the cultivation of immortality. Therefore, impotent people have no hope for immortality. They have to have their disease cured before they can attempt to seek immortality, otherwise, all their efforts will be to no avail.

In addition to total mental focus on qigong exercise, there are some other special secrets taught by the ancient Chinese for the sake of conserving essence. One of these secrets is to imaginatively look inward at your own internal organs and listen to the internal sounds of your body during breathing exercises. Imagine that you are seeing the peristalsis of your internal organs and hearing the sounds generated by it and the qi movement inside the body as you guide your qi to flow by these organs. This is called *nei-shi-fan-ting*, "look and listen inwardly," in the Chinese natural health care system, and is considered a highly effective means of covering up the potential "loopholes" of essence in the body.

As you progress in the art of breathing and meditation, you will ultimately be able to see your own internal organs through your mind's eye, as some Chinese qigong masters have successfully done. This is known as "the heavenly eyes opening up." The very practice of looking and listening inwardly will greatly help you to concentrate on the qigong exercise, thus minimizing distraction. Your heart is the command center of your body, and your eyes are the windows of your heart. Open your eyes and you disturb your heart. Disturb your heart and you waste your spirit.

Another secret is to frequently collect saliva in your mouth and swallow it down to dantian. The Chinese fathers considered saliva to be a precious liquid, which can be directly transformed into essence by due process. To emphasize its vital importance to life and health, they call it by various fancy names, such as "liquid of jade," "water of the flowery pond," "water of the heavenly lake," and "envoy of peace."

The reason saliva is sometimes called "envoy of peace" is because the ancient Chinese believed that it could pacify the mind and primordial spirit. Therefore, conservation of saliva must be undertaken together with conservation of essence. That is why the ancient Chinese are strongly against excess speech, for fear that precious saliva will be wasted as a result. To facilitate the generation of saliva and its transformation into essence, the ancient Chinese taught us to put our tongues slightly against the upper palate as often as we can. Practice shows that this practice can significantly boost the gathering of saliva in the mouth. Another benefit of this is that it can serve as a natural check against excess talking, because you are almost tongue-tied.

To do this correctly, put your tongue slightly against the upper palate as often as you can until saliva fills your mouth. Then close your eyes (if you are not already doing qigong) and swish the saliva in your mouth for a moment, while breathing deeply and naturally, thinking of dantian as you exhale. Divide the saliva collected into three small mouthfuls. With each exhalation, swallow one mouthful of saliva down to dantian.

Actually, not only does sexual essence need to be conserved, but qi energy and spirit should also be jealously conserved. This is a principle that is applicable to seekers of both longevity and immortality. To conserve qi energy, we must minimize our speech. To conserve spirit, we must minimize our thinking and worry, and close our eyes as often as possible. We should also avoid traveling in thunderstorms and going out in the rain, and run no more than ten miles a day. These are important rules regarding the conservation of qi and spirit.

In terms of food, walnuts, pine nuts, hazel, and fresh fruits are strongly recommended as part of the diet of a seeker of immortality. Cultivation of immortality is best undertaken in a dry location, rather than a humid or wet place. The location should be high in altitude, not low and close to water. Dry, high land is close to heaven, which makes the eventual merging of spirit into nature easier. That is why most immortals in China have attained their immortality in the northern part of the country where the weather is dry and the elevation is high. Popular places include the Hua Mountains in Shenxi province, Ermei Mountains in Sichuan province, Sun Mountains in Henan province, Hen Mountains in Shanxi province, and Yanjiao Mountains in Henan province, all having an elevation over 4,000 meters.

According to Chinese sages, the best timing for cultivating immortality is from midnight to early morning. Midnight is the time when the first wave of yang qi energy of the day is generated, in nature as well as in the human body. During this time, the moon is at its brightest, and the first light of dawn breaks. In the body, the primordial yang qi energy is generated from the Gate of Life. This is the most precious yang qi energy of the day, because it is pure and unpolluted by worldly thoughts and environmental disturbances. Practicing qigong around

this time enables you to gather the precious qi energy existing in nature, in addition to the initial yang qi energy inside your body, thus doubling the effect of refining essence into qi, and qi into spirit. Qi and sexual essence gathered around this time will directly nourish the brain and spirit, facilitating the creation of internal elixir. One hour of training at this time is equivalent to two hours at other times of the day. Consequently, you get twice the result with half the effort. That is why Chinese seekers of immortality invariably get up around this time and devote themselves to the gathering of special medicine for immortality. Dr. Wan Laisheng, for instance, used to begin a new day by getting up at midnight and practicing qigong for three hours. He used no alarm clock; his biological clock was accurately set at that time for decades.

In regard to timing, the Chinese fathers put forward the concept of "dynamic midnight." It actually has nothing to do with the time of day, but rather, dynamic midnight refers to the time when qi energy permeates your lower abdomen and you feel like you have an erection. This is the biochemistry "midnight" of the body. According to the ancient Chinese, the natural tendency to erect as a result of permeation of qi in the absence of any sexual stimulation is an indication that the initial yang qi energy inside the body is generated, and you should lose no time in gathering this precious "medicine." This is the most precious and highest quality sexual essence, because it is the result of a harmonious communion between the kidneys and the heart. However, if the erection is stimulated by sexual thought or outside temptation, that is quite different story. The ancient Chinese referred to this difference as "the yang juncture," which is the demarcation between primordial essence and polluted essence. Typically, when sexual thought or temptation leads one to an erection, the essence inside the body is already "polluted," and its quality degraded. By seizing the opportunity of dynamic midnight to practice qigong, you catch both quality and quantity.

There are two basic types of three treasures of life: the prenatal treasures and the postnatal treasures. The task of cultivating Tao is to nourish the prenatal treasures with postnatal treasures, with the aim of completely restoring the three treasures to their prenatal states. Prenatal qi comes from taiji, "the great ultimate," and resides in the Gate of Life, or kidneys. It is the source of postnatal breathing qi. The breathing qi is the complement to prenatal qi, and is the primary tool for creating heavenly orbits and gathering medicines in search of immortality. As such, it is likened to fire for the smelting and forging of iron. Just as when we use fire to forge weapons, it is vital that we regulate the breathing process in search of immortality. This is a delicate issue, for too much regulation will damage the internal elixir, while too little regulation will lead you nowhere. Only when we can regulate breathing in a manner between existent and nonexistent, having and not having, with neither enthusiasm nor aloofness, can we hope to produce the desired result. Of the three treasures of life, both kinds of qi can be used for cultivating immortality. As for essence and spirit, only the prenatal type should be used. Postnatal essence and spirit are turbid and stale, and therefore should not be used.

In summary, the process of seeking immortality involves the following steps: withdraw your mind from external temptations (especially sex and money) so that you can refine essence into qi; concentrate your mind on the task of breathing exercises to the exclusion of all worldly affairs; create Minor and Major Heavenly Cycles; refine essence into vital qi and vital qi into primordial spirit and internal elixir; and eventually merge the primordial spirit into nature.

The earlier you devote yourself to this task, the greater will be your chance of success. This is because we humans all dramatically change the biochemistry of our body and organs every sixty years. Once we reach the age of sixty, our internal organs are deteriorated and worn out, unless we have taken good care of our health throughout our life. For this reason, the Chinese call sixty "the gate of hell," or a full cycle, which is a dangerous time in one's life. With persistent and proper effort and time, internal elixir can be created in the body. It is this internal elixir that will detach from your physical body as you decease, merge into nature and give you an eternal life, either in paradise or in famous mountains.

As you can tell from the above, the voyage towards immortality is a long, arduous, and necessarily painful one. Indeed, nothing can be lasting without pain and sacrifice. It takes great courage, strong determination, extraordinary persistence, good health, and longevity, as well as reliable assistance to get to the other shore. Without great courage and determination, one dares not sail into this uncharted water. Without excellent health, one cannot stand the long ordeal of xiutao. Without considerable length of life, one cannot go through the lengthy process of cultivating immortality. Here, what is needed is not enthusiasm, but persistence. Enthusiasm is like a thunderstorm; violent as it is, it never lasts for long. Persistency is like the drop of water which will, in due time, penetrate a rock. Thus, many factors must be combined for the attainment of the grand goal. That is why the number of people searching for immortality are as many as hairs on an ox, but the number of people who have become immortals are as few as the horns on an ox.

For all its difficulty and rarity, immortality is within the reach of human beings. Indeed, this is one of the basic premises of traditional Chinese culture. Westerners believe that man is created by God, while, in striking contrast, the Chinese ancients believed that gods are made of man. In fact, all the gods and goddesses revered in Chinese culture were once ordinary men and women. This is the case with Gautama Buddha (563–483 B.C.), the founder of Buddhism; with Bodhidharma Dharma, the founder of Chinese martial arts; with Kuan Yin—Bodhisattva of compassion; and with Taoist immortals such as Zhang Shanfeng and Nu Dongbin. By means of persevering self-denial, self-cultivation and self-sacrifice, they successfully elevated themselves to the full level of deity.

Chapter 14

Special Solutions for Special Problems

I n this section, various diseases (listed in alphabetic order), their symptoms and causes, and their corresponding therapies in Chinese natural health care system are discussed in detail. Some advice regarding the use of these treatments is in order.

First, you should see a medical professional when an ailment or illness progresses to a serious level. Second, there is no universally agreed upon order of effectiveness for the therapies listed. A lot depends on the individual. Indeed, some may not even work for some people. This is why I have listed a number of alternative therapies for people to choose. As to where to start, it is the Chinese practice to take one or two therapies at a time, try them for a week or so and see if they work. If you feel better as a result, continue the therapies; if you don't feel better, try something else. If you feel you are allergic to a specific treatment, stop it right away. That is typical of what the Chinese have been doing for centuries.

Third, listing all of the various therapies does not mean that you should try all of them. It is not necessary to do so. It just means that there are different alternatives.

Fourth, there is no strict regulation as to the dose of each therapy. Again, this is an individual matter, depending on each person's needs and tastes. The good news is that since they are all natural remedies, dosage is not so important a factor as in the case of traditional drugs. However, it is always advisable not to overdo anything. Again, it is up to the individual to determine what is enough.

NOTE: It is important to note that for each of the ailments listed in this chapter, if your condition does not improve or if the symptoms worsen, see your physician or a medical professional as soon as possible.

Acne

Description
Acne is an inflammatory disease of the skin, usually on the face, arising from obstruction of the sebaceous glands, resulting in pimples. It occurs most frequently among teenagers following puberty. (It is also known as "Youthful Beans" in China.) A pimple forms when an oil gland in the skin is blocked and secretions and bacteria build up under the skin. It can be itchy and painful, and if not handled properly, scar tissue can form in the affected areas.

Symptoms or signs
Acne includes pimples (small red swellings), whiteheads, or blackheads (swellings that are white or black on the surface).

Causes
An overproduction of sebum, a fatty secretion produced by small glands under the skin, clogs the pores, often leading to a bacterial infection. This overproduction of sebum is caused by eating foods high in saturated fat or sugar, which become saturated fat in the blood. When wastes are retained and the colon is clogged, the body purges toxins through the skin and lungs, where these toxins cause abscesses and acne. The secretion of sexual hormones can also cause acne in teenagers. Other causes include a zinc deficiency, allergies (food and environmental), stress, and oral contraceptives.

Prevention and treatment
It is best to eliminate alcohol and soft drinks from your diet. Avoiding foods that contain processed sugars, dairy products, and saturated fats, which interfere with the liver's ability to function properly as a detoxifying organ, is also important.

- Avoid chocolate and nuts and irritating spicy, fried, and hot-nature foods.

- Eat raw garlic every day. Garlic purifies the bloodstream and purges the body of toxic waste. Garlic ethers get to the skin soon after digestion, killing bacteria there.

- Eat raw cucumbers. Cucumbers are rich in potassium, sodium, and phosphorus, which can neutralize blood acidosis and facilitate the excretion of wastes through the kidneys, so that there is less chance of them going through the skin.

- Green beans, soybeans, raw potatoes, and bitter gourds are helpful.

- Drink a cup of cool honey tea or green tea in the morning.

- Clean a lotus flower and soak it in a cup of boiling water for five minutes while covered. Drink it as tea, twice a day. This has been proven to be highly effective in killing acne.

- Keep regular bowel movements.

- Use clean towels.

- Rub the inside of a banana peel over the affected areas.

- Cut or pull back your hair so that it doesn't hang over your face. Wash your hair every day.

- Place warm, wet towels on the affected skin for ten to fifteen minutes, three times a day, to open the pores and allow for deeper cleaning.

- Get enough sleep.

- Practice breathing exercises twice a day to promote sleep, cleanse your mind, and reduce stress.

AIDS

Description

An acronym for Acquired Immune Deficiency Syndrome, AIDS is a fatal disease for which no effective cure has been found. It is estimated that in America alone, there are 1.2 million people infected with HIV, the virus that causes AIDS.

To understand the disease and its causes, we have to talk about HIV (human immunodeficiency virus) first. HIV is an infectious virus that attacks the body's natural immune system. It makes the infected person especially susceptible to diseases that are rare in healthy people. These diseases often signal the onset of AIDS. Since it is the direct cause of AIDS, HIV is often called the AIDS virus. According to the Centers for Disease Control and Prevention, almost 1 million Americans are infected with HIV and half of them do not know they are infected. AIDS is now the leading cause of death in people between the ages of twenty-five and forty-four. There were more than 500,000 reported cases of AIDS and over 311,000 AIDS-caused deaths, of whom most died of tuberculosis and pneumonia.

It can take more than ten years for someone with HIV to develop the signs and symptoms of AIDS. In other words, a person infected with HIV can look and feel healthy for many years yet still infect other people.

Symptoms or signs

The symptoms of AIDS can be classified into acute infection and chronic asthenia. Acute infection shows signs of a constant high fever, rapid unexplained weight loss, persistent and severe fatigue, persistent diarrhea, unexplained night sweats, and severe numbness or pain in the feet or hands. Chronic asthenia causes symptoms like deep depression, loss of appetite, extreme tiredness, shortness of breath and dry cough, swelling of glands in the neck, armpits, or groin, unusual sores on the skin or in the mouth, or an increased outbreak of cold sores.

Causes

AIDS is directly caused by HIV. HIV destroys the immune system, which makes it impossible for the body to fight off diseases or even minor illnesses. HIV is spread when blood, semen, or vaginal fluids from an infected person enters someone else's body. A high-risk lifestyle is the major cause of AIDS. This includes unprotected sexual intercourse (vaginal, anal, or oral) with someone who is HIV-positive, or sharing injection needles and syringes with someone who is HIV-positive. AIDS can also be contracted by receiving a contaminated blood transfusion or spread to babies born to, or breast-fed by, HIV-positive women. Sharing toothbrushes, razors, or other personal items with others is also a dangerous practice, because these items could be contaminated with infected blood. Such activities abuse the body's metabolic system to a degree that the virus can easily penetrate the immune system cells. The weakness of the immune system is further worsened by improper diet, lack of exercise, and air and water pollution.

Sexual intercourse with someone who is HIV-positive is the "highway" to HIV. It does not matter whether you are a homosexual or a heterosexual. HIV is spread from man to woman, woman to man, man to man, or woman to woman. When you have more than one sex partner, your chances of being infected with HIV increases. The more sexual partners you have, the greater your risk of contracting HIV. The risk is further increased by not using condoms correctly each and every time you have sex.

Sharing infected needles or syringes with an infected person can happen in both hospital and private settings. While mostly occurring among drug users, accidental contact with infected needles can happen when working with hospital patients or medical waste. HIV can also be passed from an infected mother to her child during delivery or while breast-feeding. Blood transfusions can be risky if the donated blood is not pre-screened for the virus. Currently, all blood in the U.S. is closely screened for the virus, even the possibility of it. Prior to 1985, donated blood was not widely tested for HIV.

In summary, HIV can be passed from one person to another in four ways: sexual intercourse, sharing needles, pregnancy/breast feeding, and blood transfusions.

HIV, however, is NOT spread by the following:

- Public toilet seats, telephones, or water fountains.

- Swimming in public pools or hot tubs.

- Mosquito bites.

- Casual contact with someone such as kissing, hugging, crying (tears), or shaking hands.

- Sharing food, drinks, or utensils.

- Being coughed or sneezed on.

- Donating blood (so long as the needle is unused).

Prevention and treatment

In the absence of an effective cure, it goes without saying that prevention is the best treatment. Avoid the risk factors discussed previously, using latex condoms properly every time you have sex, reducing the number of sexual partners, avoiding illegal drugs, and never sharing needles or syringes with others. If you have reason to believe you may have contracted the virus or engage in risky behavior, get an HIV test. Knowledge, in this regard, is life. What you know can save your life. Meanwhile, eat plenty of raw fruit and vegetables, including fruit and vegetable juices. These are foods that can strengthen your immunity without side effects.

Dietary therapies

- Avoid high-sugar, high-fat, and processed foods.

- Boil drinking water long enough to kill any microbes and bacteria that could cause illnesses in people with weak immune systems.

- Cook everything well to ensure that bacteria are killed, especially meats.

- Eat only wholesome vegetables and fruits: carrots, potatoes, yams, beans, nuts, walnuts, brown rice, pineapple, bananas, sweet potatoes, bitter gourd, and sea fish but not shelled seafood.

- Eat only unprocessed, complex carbohydrate foods, plus a lot of fruit and vegetable juices each day.

- *Glossy ganoderma* is a mushroom thought by the Chinese to have the ability to enhance the body's resistance to diseases, help treat cancer and AIDS, strengthen vital qi, and promote longevity. To use it, either boil it in water and drink the soup, or grind it into powder and swallow it with water.

- Garlic and ginger are thought to contain antiviral substances and can boost one's immune system. Therefore they can be extremely helpful in treating AIDS, especially when accompanied by tuberculosis and pneumonia.

- *Astragalus membranaceus* is a plant that has been used in China for thousands of years to enhance the body's natural immunity to disease.

- *Cordyceps sinensis* is another plant that has been in use for a long time in China to enhance the body's immune system, and to nourish the kidneys and the spleen.

Other natural therapies

While still fatal, the AIDS death rate has been declining over the past few years. This shows that AIDS patients are surviving longer. It is believed that those patients who live the longest are most likely those who take it easy and have a positive outlook. In other words, the disease may not be as deadly and hopeless as most doctors suggest. The interesting thing is that the moment you stop worrying about your disease, the disease becomes less deadly. Take care of today, and tomorrow takes care of itself. This is one way of relieving the symptoms of AIDS, and so far, it may be the most effective and powerful treatment.

- Reduce stress.

- Keep an optimistic outlook.

- Control the emotions.

- Get enough sleep.

- Practice qigong at least twice a day, thirty minutes each time. Qigong can cleanse your body and mind and enhance your immune power. (See appendix 1.)

- Soft exercises reduce stress, activate the lymph node system, release toxins, and strengthen the immune system.

- Acupress the Jianjing acupoint several times a day, two to three minutes each time. This can reduce stress and enhance the immune system. (See appendix 7.)

Alcoholism

Description

Alcoholism is defined as the addictive use of alcoholic products. A person becomes an alcoholic if he or she becomes physically and/or psychologically dependent on alcohol. People tend to have an alcohol problem if the use of alcohol interferes with their health or daily living. Habitual and heavy use of alcohol has serious health consequences. Long-term heavy drinking causes liver, nerve, heart, and brain damage, high blood pressure, stomach problems, impotence, and cancer. It can also lead to violence, car accidents, and depression.

Symptoms or signs

They include trembling, delusions, sweating, blackouts, denial (of the problem), and personality changes.

Causes

Alcoholism can be a matter of your mental status and lifestyle, no matter if you're rich or poor. Some people who become addicted to alcohol have problems with their relationships, career, or finances, which they cannot handle, so they resort to alcohol to escape. The result is usually that as the more alcoholic one becomes, the more serious one's problems become. There also may be genetic reasons why some people are more prone to alcoholism than others. Scientists discovered that a sugar imbalance is yet another reason for alcoholism. Individuals with an exceptionally high biological demand for sugar may turn to alcohol because alcohol has the highest sugar content of any food substance. (Ethyl alcohol contains no sugar content, in and of itself. The only alcoholic drinks that contain any significant sugar content are the sweetened drinks, e.g. some cocktails, wine coolers, schnapps, etc. Chronic alcohol abuse can disrupt the body's ability to regulate sugar levels. This combined with the fact that alcoholics often are not compliant with diabetic medications and dietary regimens makes them prone to hypoglycemia.)

Natural therapies:

- Eat a high protein, low carbohydrate diet, with protein preferably in the form of fish and chicken rather than eggs and red meats. By reducing carbohydrate intake, insulin production is limited and thus greatly reduces the body's craving for sugar. The worst foods are candy, chocolate, ice cream, sodas, and refined foods.

- Drink a cup of heavily brewed tea when intoxicated to relieve symptoms quickly.

- Drink a cup of fresh radish juice to relieve intoxication.

- Eat plenty of fresh, juicy fruits.

- Drink some vinegar or ginger juice.

- Drink pear juice, or some salt water, or soda water.

- Eat several olives.

- Drink a cup of juice made of lotus roots.

- Use a cold towel to cover the forehead.

Allergies

Description

An allergy is our immune system's attempt to protect us from something that is usually harmless. What happens is that antibodies search out the invaders, thus triggering special cells in the body to release chemicals, resulting in what is known as an allergic reaction. Allergies take many forms after being exposed to certain substances (plants, dust, pollen) or eating certain foods. An estimated 35 million Americans suffer from various forms of allergies.[1]

Symptoms or signs

They include itching, cramps or diarrhea, swelling of the lips, eyes, face, tongue, or throat, runny nose, and rashes, hives, or other skin irritations.

Causes

Causes of allergies vary with the individual. Scientists have found that the capacity to develop allergies is an inherent trait that affects about one quarter of the population. Some people are born overly sensitive to certain foods such as milk, eggs, fish, and shellfish, or certain animals such as dogs and cats. Certain environmental factors such as heat and humidity, pollution, or areas with high pollen counts can cause reactions as well as many chemicals such as perfumes, paints, and detergents. Asthma patients are more likely to experience food allergies. House dust is a common allergen that often acts as a secondary trigger in people with allergies to pollen, animal dander, etc.

The seasons have a lot to do with allergies. Just as spring is usually associated with hay fever, autumn is the season in which allergies are more common. In autumn, about one-fifth of the population is hit by allergies. Asthma sufferers may find their situation deteriorates to a sometimes dangerous level during fall. Fall allergens are innocent grains of pollen released by plants as part of their reproductive cycles. We just happen to intercept the pollen before a receptive plant does. For some of us, this causes nasal and throat tissues to swell, and a sneezing reflex to erupt.

Prevention and treatment

Avoid polluted air and water, which means stop smoking and avoid smoky areas (secondary smoke). Avoid refined starches and sugars, pasteurized milk, red meats, chemical additives, and coffee. Find out which foods you are allergic to and totally avoid them. Stay inside the house when the allergy season hits. Clean the house often; a thorough cleaning at the beginning of fall, along with regular dusting and vacuuming throughout the season, can significantly reduce the risk of autumn allergies. Change the clothes you wear to work or outdoors immediately after you get home, putting those clothes in a separate, isolated place.

Dietary therapies

- Eat a varied diet. Since the effects of food allergies are cumulative—the more you eat, the more you suffer—it is advisable to eat a variety of foods and rotate them in your diet to avoid taking any single kind of food too often. Thus, instead of having apple cider each day, drink orange juice one day, carrot juice another, and grapefruit yet another.

- Drink plenty of carrot juice and/or potato juice, which can detoxify the liver, blood, and intestinal tract, relieving allergic symptoms.

- Eat raw cucumber to purge blood and kidneys of acids and other toxins, thereby facilitating excretion of wastes and relieving allergies.

- Eat more fish, seeds, fresh fruits, and vegetables because these contain essential fatty acids, which can alleviate allergies.

Alzheimer's Disease

Description

Alzheimer's is a progressive, degenerative disorder that causes structural and chemical changes in the brain, resulting in abnormalities that impair memory, thinking, judgment, and personality. An article in *USA Today* reported that about 4 million Americans are affected by this disease, which is deemed incurable and kills 100,000 Americans each year.[2] It is estimated that by the next century there will be 14 million Americans afflicted with this disease as the size of the elderly population grows.

Alzheimer's disease takes especially heavy tolls on elderly people. Generally speaking, the older one lives, the greater one's risk of being afflicted with this disease. Every one in ten Americans over the age of sixty-five is a patient of this disease, and the toll is even heavier on those who are over eighty-five years of age, where the risk is one in three of the whole population. This disease doesn't care who you are—rich or poor, president or janitor—the toll it takes is the same. China's Mao Tse-tung and Deng Xiaoping both died of this disease. Former president Ronald Reagan is said to have been diagnosed with it right after his eightieth birthday.

Although the disease causes little physical pain to the patients, it is one of the cruelest diseases known because it causes so much mental anguish, both to the patients and to their family members. Memory loss progresses to the point of forgetting names and even faces of family members, and disorientation of time and place, to the extent of becoming lost on their own street and not knowing where they are. Other symptoms include difficulty in performing familiar tasks such as feeding and clothing oneself, frequently misplacing or losing items, paranoia, language disturbances, rapid mood swings for no apparent reason, and becoming extremely confused.

Symptoms or signs

These can include memory loss; disorientation or confusion; difficulty in performing daily tasks such as feeding and clothing oneself; paranoia; difficulty speaking; and rapid mood swings.

Causes

Theories vary as to exactly what causes this disease. Some suggest that it is inherited, others suggest viruses, toxic elements in the environment, as well as deterioration of the body's immune system. Biologically, Alzheimer's disease results from the deterioration of brain cells, which leads to an interruption of communication between these cells. When brain cells are stressed, they do not function properly and the disease occurs. The deterioration of brain cells has many causes. One is an unhealthy diet, especially excess fatty foods, alcohol, and cigarette smoking. Hypertension is yet another cause which, over time, may do irreversible damage to blood vessels in the brain. As a result, some brain tissues are slowly starved of oxygen and die, interfering with the proper communication between brain cells. Another common cause is Parkinson's disease, the patients of which have a 30 percent chance of having Alzheimer's disease at the same time. This is especially true in the later stages of Parkinson's disease. Actually, while not clearly understood yet, these two conditions seem so closely related to each other that they are sometimes regarded as sister diseases.

Prevention and treatment

Alzheimer's disease is a life-long process; it does not develop overnight. Worse still, early diagnosis is very difficult. As such, prevention should start long before the first symptoms appear. This means cultivating a healthy lifestyle in terms of diet, rest, mental discipline, physical exercise, and environmental awareness. My teacher, Dr. Wan Laisheng, used to tell me that the brain functions like a bulb. If you keep the light on for a long time without turning it off, the bulb will burn up sooner than expected. The same thing happens to the human brain. If we abuse or overuse it constantly, we will be punished by nature for neglecting to take proper care of what we have been given.

Alzheimer's disease is just one form of such punishment, as Chinese health care understands it. This is exactly the reason why the Taoist sage Lao Tze advocated the principle of quietness in order to preserve the brain and vital qi. Therefore, qigong, the Chinese breathing exercise, is considered an excellent prevention against Alzheimer's disease. Actually, none of masters of qigong has been found to suffer from this disease, no matter how old they lived. This is proof enough of the benefit and effectiveness of qigong in preventing and curing the disease. Besides qigong, other forms of soft exercises are very helpful to brain health. For one thing, they increase the flow of blood and supply of fresh air to the brain cells.

Our brain, like our bodies, needs adequate nutrition for its growth and proper functioning. Of particular importance are vitamins A and E, and beta-carotene, which are antioxidants that help offset the effect of aging. Make sure that your diet supplies enough of such nutrients to the brain while avoiding anything that can damage the brain such as cigarettes, caffeine, and alcohol.

Dietary therapies

- Avoid coffee, alcohol, and cigarettes.

- Eat animal liver, egg yolks, milk, cod liver oil, tomatoes, mango, papaya, and yams, which are rich in vitamin A and helpful in preventing and treating Alzheimer's.

- Eat plenty of carrots, apricots, cantaloupes, and other deep-yellow vegetables and fruits, because they are rich in beta-carotene.

- Eat plenty of peanuts, walnuts, and green leafy vegetables. They contain rich vitamin E, which has been shown to benefit the immune system of the elderly and may help protect against Alzheimer's.

- Whole grains, particularly whole wheat products such as oatmeal, are rich in vitamin E, so also is corn oil.

- Regularly eating pork marrow can help prevent developing this disease. Chinese fathers believe that pork marrow can help maintain the health and vitality of the human brain.

- Egg yolk is a good nutrient for the brain and can help prevent and treat the condition.

- Vitamin B_{12}, folic acid, and other nutrients are conducive to brain cell regeneration.

Other natural therapies

- Keep the brain active by learning new things all the time.

- Practice qigong on a daily basis. Qigong is an effective natural means to preventing and curing Alzheimer's disease. Clinical experiments in China proved that this Chinese breathing exercise has great preventive and therapeutic effects on Alzheimer's. As will be illustrated in detail in appendix 1, qigong works wonders mainly in three ways. One is to supply the brain with more fresh air and oxygen that is definitely needed in this case. Another is to facilitate the blood circulation to the brain. Yet another is to provide peaceful relaxation for the brain that is equally indispensable for its long, effective functioning. The effect of qigong in treating this special disease will be further enhanced if you can imagine guiding your qi up toward the head.

- Shake your head from side to side several times a day. This improves the vitality and blood circulation of the brain.

- Give your brain a short rest after intense mental work by closing your eyes and taking deep breaths of fresh air, focusing your mind on the lower abdomen (dantian).

- Regularly expose yourself to fresh air. Fresh air is vital to the health and vitality of the brain cells. Make sure that the places where you work and sleep are well ventilated.

- Improve the quality of your sleep so as to replenish your brain energy.

- Avoid stress.

- Knock your head with your forefingers, covering up your ears with your hands. Do this twice a day, once in the morning and once at the bedtime. This will prevent the stagnation of brain cells, enhance their vitality, and prolong their lives. (See appendix 5.)

- Massage the eyes, neck, nose, and face several times a day. These parts of the body are close to the brain. By doing this, it is believed that brain health can be improved. (See appendix 5.)

- Comb your hair with your fingers several times a day to improve brain health.

- Apply finger pressure to the following acupoints several times a day: Baihui, Fengchi, Taiyang, Yintang, and Shangxing. (See appendix 7.)

Anemia

Description

This is characterized by a deficiency in the production of red blood cells, especially the oxygen-carrying element hemoglobin. As a result, the amount of oxygen that the blood is able to carry becomes reduced. This leads to a lack of energy and vitality.

Symptoms or signs

Symptoms can include a pale complexion and lips, white fingernails, cool limbs, low body temperature, jaded (loss of) appetite, vertigo, ringing in the ears, headaches, dizziness, decreased eyesight, indigestion, chronic fatigue, depression, loss of sexual drive, vomiting, and lethargy.

Causes

Anemia results from a significant reduction of blood or red blood cells in the body. Females are more liable to this condition than males due to menstruation, childbirth, and breast-feeding, all of which can reduce blood levels in the body.

Without regard to gender, the following are the most common causes of anemia:

- A poor diet consisting mainly of refined and processed foods and overcooked foods. Such foods are deficient in nutrition, especially iron.

- Chronic indigestion and constipation.

- Kidney, liver, or lung disease.

- Chronic inflammation and extensive cancers may inhibit production of red cells.

- Bleeding from gums, ulcers, and hemorrhoids.

- Deficiency in breaking down vitamin B_{12}.

- The bone marrow may be incapable of producing enough red cells for normal replacement needs.

- Chronic, heavy smoking can damage the oxygen carrying capacity of the blood.

NOTE: Aplastic anemia can be a very serious disease with even more serious causes. Anyone with this disease should be under the close supervision of a physician.

Prevention and treatment

Avoid coffee, tea, cigarettes, and refined and processed foods such as white flour products. Eat a nutrient-rich, healthy diet. Avoid excess work and rigorous exercises. Practice soft exercises in fresh air to increase the intake of oxygen into your blood. Get sufficient rest and sleep and follow the dietary therapies to nourish the blood and liver.

Dietary therapies

- Avoid coffee, chocolate, and alcohol.

- Avoid drinking tea, because tea can hinder the body's absorption of iron from food.

- The following foods are found to be effective in relieving anemia: carrots, longang (a sweet, delicious fruit grown on trees in southern China and Southeast Asian countries), black beans, green vegetables, apples, grapes, animal liver, spinach, beef, chives, day lily, nuts and seeds, and gluten. These foods mainly nourish the liver.

- Regularly consume animal liver and blood as part of a daily meal.

- Stew five ounces of rabbit meat in water together with twenty red dates for an hour. Eat it as a dish to nourish the blood.

- Stew twenty red dates in water with one ounce of ginseng and eat it all. This also nourishes the blood.

- Stew twenty red dates in one cup of water together with two spoonfuls of malt sugar and eat it all to nourish the blood.

- Stew a cup of chicken blood in half a cup of rice wine for thirty minutes. Eat the blood.

- Regularly eat homemade chicken soup.

- Red rice is believed to nourish the blood and relieve anemia, and should take the place of white rice as a staple food.

- Eat plenty of spinach, carrots, peanuts, cabbage mustard, and leaf mustard. These vegetables are rich in iron and other vital minerals. Consequently, they can build strong blood plasma, especially iron-dependent hemoglobin. Of course, they are best consumed in raw form, or only lightly cooked.

- Eat plenty of animal liver, pears, almonds, pineapple, strawberries, oranges, grapes, and raisins. The Chinese believe that these foods are good for the nourishment of the liver and blood.

- Drink the blood of a finless eel and eat its meat. In China, eel is available everyday in the fresh food markets.

- Put half a pound of sweet or brown rice and five ounces of black soybeans in boiling water. Simmer until half cooked, then add two ounces of red dates and continue cooking until well done. Add some brown sugar and eat it once a day.

- Eat steamed or cooked duck each day until you feel better.

- Boil dried red dates and mung beans in water until the beans break. Add some brown sugar, eat everything up, twice a day. Do this continuously for two weeks.

- Soak ten dates and one ounce of Chinese wolfberry in water for two hours. Afterwards, add two eggs. Stew them together for ten minutes. Eat the eggs and dates and drink the soup.

- Eat plenty of grapes or drink plenty of grape juice each day.

- Stew sliced lean mutton together with some dong quai and ginger in water for thirty minutes. Add some salt and brown sugar into it. Eat the mutton and drink the soup once a day.

- Eat pork or beef liver. Clean and cut into small pieces. Slightly fry it together with some onions. Then put in some water and a little bit of sugar to steam it up. Eat it as a meal, two to three times a week.

- For macrocytic anemia (usually caused by a deficiency of folate or vitamin B_{12}): clean a pork kidney and cut it into pieces. Soak it in warm water for half an hour and boil it in water. Add some salt before eating it. Eat once a day for two weeks.

- For aplastic anemia: boil soaked black fungus with twenty red dates with some brown sugar. Eat it twice a day until recovered.

- Black beans, sesame, egg yolks, peas, honey, sunflower seeds, bananas, raspberries, and blackstrap molasses all contain iron in easily absorbable forms.

- Cook two ounces of dansheng (*Codonopsis pilosula*) together with twenty red dates in water for an hour. Drink the soup and eat the dates. Dansheng is a root herb similar to ginseng. You can get it in any Chinese herbal store. Eating this nourishes the blood and liver.

Other natural therapies

- Increase your exposure to sunlight and fresh air.

- Practice Dharma's internal exercises every day. (See appendix 5.)

- Take a cold bath every day, and massage the body right afterward.

- Get sufficient sleep each and every day. Learn ways to improve your sleep (see listing for "Insomnia").

- Apply finger pressure to the following acupoints: Zhongwan and Qihai. (See appendix 7.)

Angina

Description

Known as angina in medical terminology, this is a disease marked by waves of acute pain or discomfort felt in the chest, often accompanied by a sense of suffocation. This is due to an insufficient amount of oxygen reaching the heart muscle, which leads to spasms preventing the heart from pumping the necessary blood to all the body tissues. People with a history of angina have a greater risk of heart attack.

Symptoms or signs

Symptoms of angina include discomfort in the chest, brief attacks of chest pain, and pain in the jaw.

Causes

Angina can be caused by any of the following factors:

- Physical exertion. This leads to a shortage of oxygen due to the increased oxygen demand of the heart.

- Thickened coronary arteries lower the blood flow to the heart muscle.

- Thickened blood, caused by fat, sugar, and cholesterol in the diet, results in a weakened heart unable to pump blood into other parts of the body.

Prevention and treatment

Natural therapies

- Avoid junk food, processed foods, sugar, alcohol, coffee, smoking, and high-saturated fats.

- Eat a lot of fruit, fruit juices, whole wheat bread, yams, carrots, beets, potatoes, corn, beans, and other vegetables. Also recommended are high-protein foods such as fresh fish, chicken, turkey, and eggs.

- Practice qigong twice a day, breathing deeply and naturally to increase the oxygen supply to the heart.

- Massage or rub the chest several times a day as directed in Dharma's internal exercises. (See appendix 5.)

- Make sure that the air you breathe in is fresh and that your house and work areas are well ventilated.

- Apply finger pressure to the following acupoints several times a day: Danzhong, Hukou, Quepen, Ximen, and Xinshu. (See appendix 7.)

Arthritis

Description

Arthritis is the name for a family of 120 kinds of related diseases, all the which have something to do with one or more joints in the body. Simply put, arthritis means inflammation of a joint. According to the estimates provided by the Arthritis Foundation, nearly one out of every seven Americans are affected by arthritis in various forms, with some 8 million diagnosed to have rheumatism and 30 million to have osteoarthritis. Of osteoarthritis sufferers, 80 percent are women.

The very word "arthritis" evokes a specter of fear and pain, if only because 37 million Americans are afflicted with it, resulting in 45 million lost workdays and $35 billion in medical care and lost wages each year.[3] There are two major forms of the disease: osteo-arthritis and rheumatism. Osteoarthritis is a degenerative condition, which often accompanies old age as a result of a lifetime's use of the body's joints. Rheumatism is an autoimmune disorder that is more severe and disabling than osteoarthritis.

With osteoarthritis, as the cartilage becomes weaker, it fragments, and bony, knobby spurs develop at the edges of the joint. The joint becomes stiff and often painful. A bone fracture is often the first sign of the disease. The patient often feels aches and stiffness of the joints. As the case develops, it can deform the joints, and make them swollen. The older one gets, the more painful it becomes. This triggers an inflammatory process leading to stiffness.

Rheumatoid arthritis is a disease of the autoimmune system which overreacts to foreign matter in the joints. This overreaction causes deterioration of the synovial membranes surrounding lubricating fluid in the joints. It causes chronic pain, and this pain usually intensifies during cloudy or rainy weather. Because of the bulk of inflammatory cells in the joint, it becomes swollen, and feels puffy to the touch. The increased blood flow due to the inflammation makes the joint warm. Such cells release enzymes into the joint space and cause further irritation and pain. The syndrome is often compounded by a limited ability to exercise and thus disuse.

Rheumatism is one of the most complicated diseases yet known. Its sufferers notice problems in parts of their bodies other than the joints. These problems include muscle aches, fatigue, joint stiffness (particularly in the morning), and even a low fever. Morning stiffness is often considered a hallmark of rheumatism. After a short period of rest or even just sitting for a while, the whole body becomes stiff and hard to move. The disease works on the erosion of the bone and may even rupture the tendons, possibly crippling the patient. Occasionally, rheumatism may attack other body tissues, including the nerves, small arteries, lungs, and the whites of the eyes.

Symptoms and signs

These can include joint pain or stiffness, muscle aches, and fatigue.

Causes

Rheumatoid arthritis is a condition associated with increased levels of immune complexes in the joint space. Osteoarthritis is caused by immune, physical, nutritional, and congenital factors. Thus, constant and heavy use, as in the case of football players, can lead to weakness in the area and pain, stiffness, and disability. The fact that arthritis comes to most of us who live long enough shows that it is, to a large extent, a natural consequence of usage and time. Usage and time have the natural effect of wear and tear on the chemicals and cartilage of joints and limbs, causing them to become swollen and dysfunctional. This is why many professional soccer players suffer from arthritis. Again, the delicate rule is that of the golden mean— too much is as bad as too little.

In terms of nutrition, this can be caused by a deficiency in the nutrients that form collagen tissue, the material that holds the body together. The support system of the body fails, causing pressure on weakened joints and leading to inflammation. It is believed that one of the most important nutritional causes of rheumatism is zinc deficiency in the synovial fluid of the joints. Other nutritional causes include deficiency in vitamin D and gastric acidity. Both of these substances aid in the normal acquisition of calcium by the bones and thus their healthy development.

Rheumatism is generally believed to be caused by autoimmune problems, mycoplasma infection, and even hereditary factors. More important, arthritis seems to be related to the body's immune system. This is because immune complexes are present in the serum and joint fluids of most arthritis patients. A reasonable diagnosis is that the body is unable to produce sufficient antibodies to prevent the virus from entering the joints. Another theory holds that arthritis may also be the result of an allergy caused by eating certain foods, especially red meat, eggplant, green peppers, potatoes, tomatoes, and tobacco containing the toxin solanaise, which causes inflammation in the joints.

Prevention and treatment

Since obesity and inactivity are two major causes of arthritis, the prevention strategy should naturally include regular exercise and a complex carbohydrate diet as its main components. Of particular importance is a regular standing exercise, such as walking or running, which are the only ways to strengthen the bones. Swimming is an excellent exercise in itself, but not for the purpose of preventing arthritis. This is because it does not train the bones as well as standing exercises. Also, be sure that you wear clothes that are fully dry, do not live in a house that is humid and poorly ventilated, and avoid picnics in the open air (for fear that the moisture or wetness in the air will get into the body).

Dietary therapies

- Avoid salt, ice cream, sugar, white bread, hot peppers, and pasteurized milk.

- Follow a very low-fat and vegetarian diet, which is not only anti-inflammatory, but also weight-controlling. Being overweight put extra stress on joints, ankles, feet, hips, knees, and lower back.

- Cook a snake with some ginger. Eat the snake and drink the soup. Or soak the snake in wine and drink two cups of the wine each day. This helps the circulation of blood and drives out the wetness in the body. (Consult a medical professional in case of allergic reactions to the snake.)

- Consume foods that can activate the acid state in your body, for arthritis is caused when your body system becomes too alkaline. This high alkaline state can be corrected by changing your body to an acid state. Foods that can help establish an acid state include grains, nuts, soy products, black beans, gourd, snake, wax gourd, cucumber, lentils, cider vinegar, fish, and poultry.

- Take ten capsules of fish oil per day. This will decrease the chronic inflammation and the resulting pain of arthritis.

- Take vitamin B-complex and barley.

- Drink the blood of finless eels and eat their cooked meat. This helps the circulation of blood and drives out the wetness in the body.

- Cook dried ginger, towel gourd, and rice together to make a porridge. Eat it as a meal. This helps the circulation of blood and drives out the wetness in the body.

- Mix one pound of fresh cherries and five cups of rice wine in a big jar. Cover it up for at least one week. Drink one to two ounces of the wine, twice a day. This can alleviate numbness of joints and paralysis from arthritis.

- Drink two ounces of hawthorn fruit juice or wine at bedtime to relieve arthritis pain.

- Drink plenty of grapefruit juice and celery juice. This can help relieve the pain.

- A cup of grape wine a day may also help.

- Eat plenty of fresh black grapes each day. They have been found to have a strong therapeutic effect on arthritis pain.

- Boil three fresh figs with three ounces of lean pork or chicken eggs and half an ounce of rice wine. Eat once a day to alleviate arthritis and rheumatism.

- Eat chestnuts at bedtime to relieve numbness and weakness of limbs.

- Eat raw spinach. This vegetable can help dissolve uric acid crystals in the blood.

- Eat carrots, parsley, cabbage, grapes, and cucumbers. These foods can dissolve and neutralize uric acid crystals in the blood, thus relieving rheumatism.

- Boil black soybeans and add some honey when done. Eat it all. This can relieve rheumatism and pain in the knees.

- Apply sesame oil externally to the affected region and massage for ten minutes to relieve rheumatic pain and fatigue.

- Fry one pound of black soybeans until they start to crack. Soak the fried beans in rice wine for thirty minutes. Drink the wine to relieve rheumatic pain in joints. (Better still if one can eat the beans.)

- Eat edible ants or use medicine made of ants such as Ant Rheumatoid Arthritis Medicine, which has been shown in a clinical study in China to be 90 percent effective.

Other natural therapies

- Do soft exercises everyday. Exercises have been proven to increase bone strength and strengthen the joints. It is common knowledge that joints need muscle for support. Exercises strengthen the muscles around a joint, feed the cartilage, and guard it against damage. It helps the joints remain supple and lubricated. Exercise also boosts one's morale and self-confidence in fighting the disease. It is important, however, to strike a balance between rest and exercise. Traditional Chinese soft exercises such as those introduced in the appendix of this book are especially recommended because they are designed to build good muscle tone rather than muscle strength, which is exactly what arthritis patients need. Still, the amount of exercise needed varies with the individual based on his or her condition and feeling. Again, moderation is the best principle. But it is important to continue using the painful joints. Here the motto is "use them or lose them." Joints should be exercised through their full range of motion several times a day.

- Practice Chinese regulated sex. Sex—so long as it is regulated and not excessive— is one of the greatest relievers of pain, and a form of soft exercise in itself. Since there is a strong psychological element to arthritis, the patient's spiritual status can play a significant role in the treatment of the disease. People who take an active and sexual part in life are better equipped to fight arthritis physically and mentally. Both exercise and regulated sex serve well to boost one's morale and self-esteem. Indeed, the best medicine for arthritis is a patient's willingness to combat the disease with an unbending spirit.

- Use your palms to massage the knees. Do this several times a day.

- Rub the soles of your feet frequently. The Chinese believe that arthritis has a lot to do with the humidity that intrudes into our body through the soles. Rubbing the soles frequently can induce the humidity out of the body and prevent it from entering the body.

- Cover the affected area for fifteen minutes, several times a day, with a warm towel or a warm bag containing hot water or melted wax. This can relieve pain.

- Apply finger pressure to the following acupoints three times a day, five minutes each time: Chenfu, Shouwuli, Fengshi, Kunlun, Xiaguan, Hegu, Renzhong, Quchi, Yaoyangguan, Yinlingquan, Tianshu, Weizhong, and Zusanli. (See appendix 7.)

Asthma

Description

Known as a disease of civilization, asthma is a severe allergic disorder which affects 15 to 16 million Americans, and about 4,000 of them die from asthma each year. The medical cost for treating asthma in the U.S. is a staggering $5 billion per year.[4] Latest reports say that the U.S. death rate from asthma has doubled since the last decade, and asthmatic attacks are one of the most common causes of emergency room visits. Children, poor children in particular, are most at risk. The asthmatic rate among American children has increased 74 percent during the period from 1982 to 1994. Indeed, it is the most frightening and life-threatening of the common respiratory diseases.

Characterized by recurring breathing trouble, asthma is a condition that causes inflammation and obstruction of the airways. What happens is that the muscles surrounding the bronchial tubes of the lungs spasm, the mucous lining swells, and secretions build up. As a result, breathing becomes quite difficult. An excess amount of mucus production further narrows the air passages and can aggravate the difficulty in getting the air out. During an asthma attack, the patient may feel short of breath and find it difficult to respire (with or without an audible wheeze). He or she may have a cough, constricted chest, or painfully congested lungs. Air flow in and out of the lungs becomes restricted and the patient may cough, wheeze, and feel chest pressure. The wheezing is caused by the passage of air at high speed through the smaller air passages.

The asthmatic attack may be transient or persistent. In a severe case, the patient has great difficulty breathing, perhaps being able to breathe only while in an upright position, and eventually the skin or mucous membranes become discolored. This disease, if not treated in time, can be life-threatening.

Unfortunately, for most American asthmatics, the only known relief from these debilitating symptoms is a combination of expensive drugs. These drugs provide only marginal and temporary relief, and some have known side effects such as insomnia. Conventional American medicine has no cure for asthma.

Symptoms or signs
These can include itching and discharge from the nose, sneezing and general malaise, rapid constriction of the bronchial passages, followed by breathing difficulties, spasmodic coughing, wheezing, and expectoration.

Causes
Asthma is an accumulation of mucus in the lungs and a consequent blockage of air passages that blocks the outflow of air. (No, asthma is not due to an accumulation of mucus in the lungs. That's merely a result of the underlying cause of the disease.) Asthma is not contagious. Genes and family history may have something to do with it, for it tends to occur in families where other members have this problem. Air pollution is one of the greatest causes. Ozone, fumes from diesel fuel, and smoking are direct causes of air pollution and therefore trigger the disease. Usually the patient is in a hypersensitive state, and many substances, such as hormonal changes, strong odors, animal fur and feathers, fish, shrimp, and other metabolic products may serve as allergens that induce spasms in the bronchial muscles. Medications and emotionally upsetting events

such as excessive laughing and crying, as well as cold temperatures, can contract the airways, causing asthma. Also, strenuous exercise can trigger the incidence of asthma in some people.

In traditional Chinese medicine, asthma is caused by a deficiency of kidney and lung qi energy and accumulation of mucus, which leads to a blockage and disruption of lung function. Again, this can have internal and external reasons. Internal reasons include excess loss of essence due to indulgence in sex and sexual thinking. External factors include cold weather and improper diet.

Prevention and treatment
Avoid cold weather and stress, and perform regular soft exercises; these are the first line of defense against asthma. Also try the following natural and dietary therapies to help strengthen the lungs and respiratory system.

Dietary therapies
- Asthmatics are believed to have low blood sugar. Keeping this fact in mind, the proper diet should exclude canned foods, dairy products, wheat products, and citrus fruits.

- Avoid smoking or at least do not smoke inside the house. Other family members can suffer the same disease as a result.

- Avoid all foods or anything that you are allergic to, especially watch out for seafood and razor clams.

- Avoid cold foods and drinks, especially in the evening. The Chinese believe that cold foods are no good for the lungs and respiratory system.

- Avoid pasteurized milk, white bread, and other foods made of white flour.

- Remove all dairy foods from the diet. Dairy foods can generate mucus.

- Avoid alcohol.

- These foods can help cure asthma: millet, animal blood, peanuts, grapes, sesame, walnuts, green onions, chicken, egg whites, and especially almonds.

- Stew a fresh egg in rice vinegar and eat it. Do this twice a day consecutively for a month.

- Cook a cleaned and sliced pork lung together with some rock sugar in water. Eat the lung and drink the water twice a day.

- Fry four ounces of sesame seeds. Soak the sesame in ginger juice and honey for a day. Take two to three spoonfuls of the mixture twice a day, once in the morning before breakfast and once at bedtime.

- Pound some walnuts, almonds, and ginger together and soak them in honey and ginger juice. Take one to two spoonfuls of the mixture twice a day, once in the morning with an empty belly, and once in the evening.

- Mix some sugar cane juice and fresh hawthorn juice. Warm the mixture and drink it to stop coughing immediately.

- Take six ounces of honey, six ounces of pork oil, (if you can't buy pork oil, forget about this therapy), six ounces of sliced ginger, and a little brown sugar. Cook them all in two to three cups of water until the soup thickens. Mix two spoonfuls of the soup in water and drink it on an empty stomach. Do this twice a day, once in the morning and again in the evening.

- Make a porridge out of a bean curd, one ounce of gingko fruit, and some rice. Cook it with some water and eat it as a meal.

- Clean and slice fifteen ounces of fresh pork lung. Cook it together with two ounces of almonds in two to three cups of water for forty-five minutes. Drink the soup and eat the food.

- Steam some white gourd with rock sugar in water for thirty minutes. Drink the soup and eat the gourd.

- Cook some kelp and green beans together in water for an hour. Add some brown sugar when done and eat it as a meal.

- Steam two ounces of tremella, fifteen red dates, and some rock sugar in water. Eat the food and drink the soup.

- Steam some pork lung (cleaned and cut) in water with some ginseng and tangerine pith. Drink the soup and eat the lung.

- Soak one ounce of green tea in two cups of water for an hour. Cook two eggs in the tea for ten minutes until there is only

- one cup of water left. Drink the tea and eat the eggs. Do this once a week.

- Stew some radishes in water with some honey. Drink and eat everything.

- Stew some chicken with two cut oranges for thirty minutes. Eat it as a dish.

- Stew one to two fresh cleaned sparrows in water with some rock sugar. Eat it as a dish. Do this once a day for a week.

- Cut two pears and one pork lung. Cook them together in water with some rock sugar for about an hour. Eat the pears and drink the soup.

- Cook ten dates and some pumpkin together in water. Add some brown sugar. Eat it as a dish.

- Clean and cut a fresh pork lung. Cook the lung together with one ounce of almonds for an hour. Add some ginger juice when done. Drink the soup once a day or every other day.

- Clean and cut two carrots. Cook them with fifteen red dates in water for about thirty minutes. Eat and drink everything. Do this twice a day.

- Eat a porridge made of almond powder every day.

- Soak one ounce of tremella in water for an hour. Add some rock sugar and stew the tremella for another hour. Eat the tremella and drink the soup. Eat this once or twice a day.

- Use some Lingzhi powder to cook lean pork meat and eat it as a dish. Once a week is fine.

- Stew one ounce of almonds and two pears in water for thirty minutes. Add some rock sugar. Eat the almonds and pears, and drink the soup.

- Fry two eggs with some chives and eat.

- Drink at least ten cups of clean water daily to dilute bronchial mucus. Water can help loosen the mucus in the lungs and make breathing easier.

- Honey is good because it clears the lungs and soothes coughing spasms.

- Lemon juice can dissolve mucus in the sinuses and bronchial tubes and thus relieve the condition.

- Barley water can relieve bronchial spasms. Cook barley in water for twenty to thirty minutes. Drink it like tea.

- Clean a fresh sparrow and cut into pieces. Stew it in water together with some rock sugar for one hour. Eat the sparrow and drink the soup.

- Clean a fresh radish and cut it into pieces. Stew it in water with some honey. Eat the radish and drink the soup.

- Eat radishes and/or drink radish juice twice a day.

- Cook two ounces of almonds and a Chinese francolin (partridge), cut and cleaned, together. Eat it as a meal.

- Grape juice helps clear mucus and phlegm from the lungs.

- Carrots, spinach, and celery are very helpful foods for asthma. Eat them raw or drink their juice.

- Garlic contains potent ethers and enzymes that dissolve mucus in the lungs and kills bacteria in the body, including the air passages. Eat three cloves of raw garlic each day, right before a meal.

- Pineapple and berries are beneficial because they help dissolve mucus.

- Peel three fresh peaches and steam them with one ounce of rock sugar. Eat them once a day for a week.

- Place a slice of onion under your tongue when an asthma attack occurs. Raw onion is so potent that bronchial spasms can often be relieved by simply sucking on a slice of onion.

- Drinking a cup of strong coffee can also help when an attack occurs.

- Steam one ounce of walnuts with some rock sugar and radish seeds for thirty minutes. Eat the mixture twice a day for one week to treat chronic asthma.

- Boil two ounces of fresh chestnuts with five red dates and some lean pork. Eat it all to treat asthma.

- Boil one ounce of sword beans in water for thirty minutes. Add some honey and drink. Do this twice a day. This helps ease the coughing and wheezing.

- Combine half a pound of tofu, three spoonfuls of honey, and five ounces of fresh radishes. Boil them together and divide it into two meals. This helps ease the coughing and wheezing.

- Boil a pumpkin in three cups of water with some honey until soft, then use the condensed pumpkin soup to mix with three ounces of fresh ginger juice. Boil over low heat for two minutes. Drink one cupful with warm water, three times a day. This helps ease the coughing and wheezing.

- Put a little bit of dried orange peel, apricot seed, seaweed, and fennel seed in three cups of water. Boil them until the water is reduced to only one cup. Divide into two servings.

- *Astragalus membranaceus* is a plant that has been used in China for thousands of years to enhance the body's natural defenses to disease, and to strengthen the lungs and relieve shortness of breath or respiratory colds. This can be consumed by cooking it in water or taken in a pill or powder form.

- Soak lotus seeds and a lily in water for two hours. Then add some lean meat and a little salt, and stew together for thirty minutes. Eat the food and drink the soup.

- Edible ants and medicine made from ants are believed in China to be able to relieve asthma and pain.

Other natural therapies

- Do soft exercises every day to strengthen the lungs and the immune system.

- Massage the chest several times a day.

- Qigong is especially helpful to asthma patients. It greatly enhances the function of the lungs and relieves the symptoms of asthma. The average person uses only fifty percent of their lung capacity, wasting a large portion of his or her natural resources. While practicing qigong, imaginatively guide the qi to the chest where you feel uncomfortable as a result of asthma. This method will strengthen your lungs and facilitate the healing of the disease. (See appendix 1.)

- Practice sound qigong and make the sounds of "Shang" or "An." This helps relieve asthma. (See appendix 3.)

- Use your knuckles to lightly tap your spine. This can relieve asthma and other ailments related to lungs.

- Bend your head over a basin of hot water. Breathe in the vapor as hard as you can. This can relieve problems in the air passages of the ears, nose (sinuses), mouth, and throat.

- Apply finger pressure to the following acupoints several times a day: Danzhong, Dazhui, Fengchi, Fengmen, Lieque, Taiyuan, Fenglong, Hegu, Quchi, Taixi, Zusanli, Lianquan, Xuanji, Zigong, Zhongwan, Yutang, Huagai, Jiuwei, and Tiantu. (See appendix 7.)

Bad Breath

See "Halitosis."

Breast Cancer

Description

Breast cancer is the second most fatal type of cancer for women in this country. In fact, it is one of the leading cause of death for women between the ages of fifteen and fifty-four. Each year, more than 182,000 American women are diagnosed with breast cancer.

Symptoms or signs

Those afflicted with breast cancer usually feel a small lump in the breast; many may have nipple discharge. However, whether or not one has breast cancer is not something that can be correctly determined by self-examination alone.

NOTE: For an accurate diagnosis, women should have a mammogram done.

Causes

Recent research shows that diet has a major influence on cancer of women's reproductive organs, and also breast cancer. Alcohol intake is also positively correlated with breast cancer. By contrast, women who consume plenty of soy foods such as tofu and bean sprouts have a significantly lower breast cancer rate than those who do not. This is because all soy foods are rich in phytoestrogens. Unlike estrogen from animal sources, the estrogen from plants protect breast cells from the estrogen made in the body or those received from the environment. This can help explain why Chinese women have a much lower rate of breast cancer than their American counterparts, for soy foods is a major component in traditional Chinese diets. The same phenomenon has been discovered in Japanese women.

Another cause of breast cancer is the unnatural estrogen replacement or surgical measure performed to artificially enlarging the breast. A study completed at Harvard shows that women who take estrogen for more than five years have a 74 percent higher risk of contracting breast cancer.

A 1982 study suggests that chlorinated drinking water may be a factor in breast cancer. Chlorine has been added to city water supplies for more than a century to protect citizens from harmful microbes. According to Dr. Barbara Joseph, a consultant of women's health in Stanford, Connecticut, chlorinated water may be a major contributing factor in breast cancer as well as in a significant percentage of all colon and rectal cancers.

Prevention and treatment

As important and fundamental as regular examination of the breasts is, so is a healthy lifestyle that includes diet, exercise, and mental hygiene. Women should follow a diet rich in vegetables, fruits, soy products, and fish oils (omega-3). A study conducted by Dr. John Glaspy at the University of California's Jonsson Cancer Center reported that women who adopted such a diet for three months experienced an increase in polyun-

saturated fatty acids shown to reduce breast cancer risk, and a decrease in those fatty acids known to promote cancer. Besides a healthy diet, stress management is of vital importance in the prevention and treatment of cancer. Stress can promote and aggravate cancer cells. The longer and more intensely one experiences stress, the greater the risk of developing cancer. Regular exercise helps relieve stress and provides the breasts with more blood and oxygen, reducing the chances of developing breast cancer.

Dietary therapies

- Avoid foods that are rich in methylxanthines such as coffee, chocolate, soft drinks, and strong tea.

- Do not smoke cigarettes and avoid second-hand smoke.

- Avoid foods high in animal proteins. Many studies show that diets rich in animal protein are correlated with a higher incidence of breast cancer.

- Avoid fatty and smoked foods such as bacon, sausage, and hot dogs.

- Eat a lot of soy food products such as tofu, soy beverages, and bean sprouts. Soy contains phytochemicals called isoflavones, which are converted into natural estrogen after digestion, and can prevent breast cancer by deterring normal cells from changing into cancer cells.

- Follow a low-fat diet rich in natural fiber, which increases the excretion of estrogen and decreases the amount of hormones in the blood stream. Fiber also facilitates the removal of carcinogens from the body and keeps the colon and intestines in good health.

- Eat foods rich in beta-carotene such as oranges, carrots, cantaloupe, and apricots.

- Regularly eat sea vegetables such as kelp, bladderwrack, nori, carrageen, dulse, and sea slug.

- Regularly eat garlic cloves, which can strengthen the immune response of cells.

- Regularly use olive oil when cooking.

- Consume plenty of nuts and beans, which are rich in essential fatty acids and good for breast health.

- Eat plenty of whole grains. Whole grains are rich in natural fiber.

- Mix orange juice with rice wine and drink three spoonfuls three times a day. The Chinese believe this can help kill tumors in the breast.

Other natural therapies

- Reduce your stress level. Stress, as has been pointed out, weakens the immune system and therefore the body's ability to fight disease. People who are under chronic stress are vulnerable to getting various types of cancer.

- Practice qigong every day. By inducing rhythmic movement of the breast and more oxygen supply to the area, qigong can be a very effective prevention against and healer for breast cancer. While doing qigong, imaginatively guide your qi to your breast, letting the refined qi directly do its healing work at the diseased part of the body. Qigong also reduces stress. (See appendix 1.)

- Massage your chest two to three times a day as directed in Dharma's internal exercises. (See appendix 5.)

- Expose yourself as much as physically possible to fresh air. Fresh air itself is especially important to the proper functioning of the lungs and breast. I believe fresh air can benefit the breast because polluted air can cause breast cancer.

Bronchitis

Description

Bronchitis is inflammation and irritation of the bronchial tubes in the lungs resulting in excess mucus in the lungs. The inflamed bronchial tubes secrete a sticky mucus, which is difficult for the hairs on the bronchi to clear out of the lungs. As the body attempts to get rid of the mucus, coughing occurs. Bronchitis can become chronic, especially among those who smoke or work in polluted air. In severe situations, it can lead to pneumonia.

Symptoms or signs

Besides coughing, other symptoms include discomfort or tightness in the chest, low fever, tiredness, sore throat, runny nose, and sometimes wheezing.

Causes

Bronchitis is caused by chronic inflammation of the linings of the airways, usually by smoke inhalation. Because the inflamed airways cannot clear mucus, it is far more prone to infection. Bacteria don't flourish on toxins, but on normal bronchial mucus that the body is unable to remove. Bronchitis often occurs after a cold or an upper respiratory infection that does not heal completely. It is usually caused by cigarette smoking. This is particularly the case with chronic bronchitis in which 75 percent of patients have a history of heavy smoking. Chronic bronchitis may occur with chronic asthma or emphysema.

Prevention and treatment

Dietary therapies

- Clean and cut a fresh pork lung. Cook the lung with one ounce of almonds for an hour. Add some ginger juice when done. Drink the soup. Do this once a day or every other day. This soothes the lungs and bronchitis.

- Peel one to two pears. Cut them into pieces and steam or boil it with some rock candy. Drink and eat everything.

- Eat more fish, yams, and seafood instead of red meat.

- Eat porridge made of almond powder.

- Soak one ounce of tremella in water for an hour. Add some rock sugar and stew the tremella for another hour. Eat the tremella and drink the soup. Do this once or twice a day.

- Clean and cut two carrots. Cook them with fifteen red dates in water for about thirty minutes. Eat the carrots and dates and drink the soup. Do this twice a day.

- Use some Lingzhi powder to cook lean pork meat and eat it as a dish.

- Stew one ounce of almonds and two pears in water for thirty minutes. Add some rock sugar into it. Eat the almonds and pears, and drink the soup.

- Cook two ounces of almonds and a Chinese francolin (partridge), cut and cleaned, together. Eat it as a meal.

- Soak one ounce of green tea in two cups of water for an hour. Cook two whole eggs in the tea for ten minutes until there is only one cup of water left. Drink the tea and eat the eggs. Do this once a week.

- Stew some radishes in water together with some honey. Drink the soup and eat the radishes.

- Stew some chicken with two cut oranges for thirty minutes. Eat it as a dish.

- Stew one to two fresh cleaned sparrows in water with some rock sugar. Eat it as a dish. Do this once a day for a week.

- Cook twenty dates and some pumpkin together in water. Add some brown sugar and eat.

- Boil some licorice in water over low heat and eat it as a soup.

- Soak one pound of radishes or pears in honey for a few hours before eating them.

- Cut up two pears and one pork lung. Cook them together in water with some rock sugar for about an hour. Eat the pears and drink the soup. Better still if one can consume the pork lung.

- Eat plenty of carrots, celery, spinach, and lemons. Either eat them raw or drink their juice.

- Insert a peeled grapefruit into a cleaned chicken, add some water and steam the chicken with the grapefruit. Eat the cooked chicken and drink the broth. Repeat this once a week.

- Soak lotus seeds and the lily in water for two hours. Then add some lean meat and a little salt, and stew them together for thirty minutes. Eat and drink everything.

- Clean and cut a fresh pork heart. Fry it in vegetable oil seasoned with a little bit of salt. Eat it as a dish.

- Clean and cut a fresh sparrow into pieces. Stew it in water with some rock sugar for one hour. Eat and drink everything.

- Clean a fresh radish and cut it into pieces. Stew it in water with some honey. Eat the radish and drink the soup.

- Wash seaweed and cut it into small pieces. Cook it in water for a short while and eat it with sugar as a meal. Do this once a day for three weeks. This is effective for chronic bronchitis in the elderly.

- Drink a lot of water (at least ten cups) each day to help thin the mucus in the lungs so your cough can clear.

- Do not smoke and avoid secondhand smoke. Smoking irritates the lungs and slows healing.

Other natural therapies

- Breathe moist air from a hot shower or a basin filled with hot water. The heat and moisture will liquefy the mucus and help cough it out.

- Lie on your stomach and hang your head and chest over the side of the bed for one minute. Do this three times a day. It helps drain the mucus.

- Practice qigong every day. When practicing, imaginatively guide your qi to the chest and lungs. (See appendix 1.)

- Practice Dharma's internal exercises, and massage your chest to increase blood flow to the area and relax the lungs. (See appendix 5.)

- Practice Dharma's morning exercises to strengthen the lungs and breathe in fresh air. (See appendix 4.)

- Sleep well and build up energy to heal.

- Frequently rub your neck with your hands. (See appendix 5.)

- Apply finger pressure to the following acupoints frequently: Shuitu, Fengmen, Neiguan, Hegu, Yutang, Dazhui, and Tiantu. (See appendix 7.)

Cancer

Description

Before AIDS emerged as a disease, cancer was the most fatal and feared disease in the world. Even today, it remains the second biggest killer of Americans after heart disease, responsible for 20 percent of all American deaths.[5] In 1996 alone, cancer killed 547,000 Americans or 1,500 people a day. The 12 million-plus cancer survivors in this country need to remain on constant guard against the comeback of the "old monster."[6] Indeed, there are few American families who have not had personal experiences with cancer, and the direct cost of cancer treatment in the U.S. alone is $30 billion each year. It is estimated that by end of the century, almost half of all Americans will be inflicted with a certain type of cancer.

Cancer is the recurrent injury to the cells in a tissue over a long period of time, which results in the abnormal growth of body cells that spread to other parts of the body and manifest themselves as malignant tumors. In other words, it is the malignant development of tumors in the cells that is capable of killing us if left untreated. These tumors eventually impinge on glands and organs, causing their destruction. The degenerative process of cancers causes the deterioration of bones, lymph and blood systems. When the cell can no longer contain the number of viruses, these viruses attack and invade other cells. Thus, the tumor grows bigger and bigger, and the situation becomes worse and worse if not checked in time. Normally, most cells replicate themselves at a rate synchronous with normal growth and repair. Each cell (with the exception of ova and sperm) contains a full complement of chromosomes; yet each develops in a manner fit for its own purpose. When a cell becomes cancerous, it multiplies faster than it should and disturbs the normal balance of hormones. Studies show that cancer viruses weaken and destroy the DNA of the cells and immune system.

So far, about 250 types of cancer have been identified.[7] In the U.S., the most common forms of cancer among women are cancers of the breast, uterus, and large intestine. Among men, the lungs, prostate, and large intestine are among the most common cancer types. Sites of cancer vary, but its main characteristics are the same, which include an abnormal, seemingly unrestricted growth of body cells, with the resultant mass compressing, invading, and destroying contiguous normal tissues. Cancer cells then break off or leave the original mass and are carried by the blood or lymph to distant sites of the body. There they set up secondary colonies, further invading and destroying the organs that are involved.

Signs or symptoms

Since all cancers work against the cells and the immune system, most will experience unexplained pain, loss of appetite and weight, as well as persistent fatigue and weakness as their early warning signs. (See also "Breast Cancer," "Prostate Ailments," and "Skin Cancer.")

Causes

There are almost as many different causes of cancer as the varieties of cancer itself. Chinese medicine believes that it is the result of long-term poisoning of body cells as a consequence of an unhealthy lifestyle and environmental pollution. Specifically, the following factors are most often blamed for the development of cancer in the human body: smoking; alcohol; high-fat foods, especially red meat; high sodium; eating spoiled foods; eating foods while they are too hot; water and air pollution; exposure to pesticides and other chemicals, radiation (UV rays) and excess sunlight; and stress and depression.

Studies show that at least 90 percent of lung cancer in men and 70 percent in women are smoking-related, which is responsible for 30 percent of all cancer deaths.[8] This is because smoking spoils a mechanism that normal lungs have for cleansing themselves and other organs of poisons.[9] This explains why heavy smokers are also much more vulnerable to cancers of the mouth, throat, kidney, and pancreas than nonsmokers.

Kitchen smoke resulting from frying foods in oil or directly cooking foods in a fire, such as a barbeque, is a direct cause of lung and nasal cancers. A study completed in Zhongsan Hospital in Taipei found that Tai-wanese women have a high lung cancer incidence because they often fry fish at home with little ventilation, because the kitchen smoke contains cancer-inducing elements.

Heavy drinking has been shown to be closely related to cancers of the throat, mouth, larynx, and liver. Alcohol and tobacco taken together increase the risk of intra-oral cancer to fifteen times that of those who neither drink nor smoke. Overexposure to sunlight or heavy tanning is conducive to skin cancer. Air pollution is shown to be a big cause of nasal and lung cancer.

It is estimated that diet is a factor in almost 40 percent of the cancers that develop in men and in 60 percent of cancers that occur in women. A high intake of animal fats is associated with cancer, particularly that of the colon. Smoked and salted foods are also harmful. It is also found that cancer patients share some personality traits, such as pessimism, inactivity, perfectionism, hot temperedness, power-orientated, self-abasing, and overachieving. For instance, Japanese scientists have found that people with a tolerant/tolerable type of personality are less likely to suffer from cancer than nontolerant people.[10] Stress in particular can lower your body's defenses against cancer and other diseases. There is strong clinical evidence pointing to the possibility that chronic stress alone can cause tumors to develop and deteriorate from benign to malign by disturbing the hormonal balance in the body. Dr. A. Panzer of the University of Pretoria in South Africa finds that stress causes disturbances in body functioning. As a result, cancer may happen due to decreased melatonin, depending on individual personality traits.[11]

Prevention and treatment

The guiding Chinese principle of prevention against cancer is to follow a healthy lifestyle. This requires an individual decision as to what and how much to eat, how to handle stress, how to exercise properly, and how to find a healthy environment for living. The good news is that at least 90 percent of all cancers can be prevented with the knowledge of the Chinese natural health care system. This involves, among other things, avoidance of smoked, salted, fatty, fried, and stale foods; avoidance of red meats; effective management of stress and depression; avoidance of sexual indulgence; regular exercise (particularly qigong exercise); stopping smoking; drinking plenty of pure water, and enjoying plenty of fresh air.

On the more proactive side, there are certain foods that can help you prevent cancer. They include tomatoes, oranges, garlic, apples, soybeans, carrots, red peppers, and green tea. These are foods that Chinese people love very much. Modern research confirms that these are cancer-fighting foods because of the nutrients they contain, such as genistein, capsaicin, catechin, allicin, lycopene, beta-carotene, and multiple vitamins.

Dietary therapies

* Follow a high complex-carbohydrate, low-fat diet that includes a lot of raw fruit and vegetables, whole grains, beans, and

nuts, and as little meat and fat as possible. Vegetables contain lots of fiber, especially when eaten raw. A diet high in fiber may protect you against colon cancer. In addition, many vegetables and fruits are rich in phytonutrients and antioxidant nutrients—vitamins A, C, and E, which have proven to be able to protect us against and help cure cancer of the esophagus, larynx, lung, colon, stomach, and heart. According to a study of more than 2,000 Welsh men, those who ate the most fruit had half the risk of dying from cancer.[12] Particularly recommended are carrots, peaches, apricots, squash, broccoli, citrus fruits, cantaloupe, cabbage, cauliflower, strawberries, peppers, and tomatoes. These fruits and vegetables contain strong anticancer compounds such as sulforaphane, lycopene, and allylic sufides. On the contrary, animal fat is hard to digest and easily gets deposited in the tissues, poisoning the cells and contributing to their malignant change.

* The traditional Chinese diet is largely composed of rice, soybean products including tofu, fresh vegetables and sea vegetables, fruits, and some fish, with little red meat or dairy products. Such a diet is low in fat and is therefore helpful in preventing and treating cancer. In particular, both rice and soybeans are known to contain rich protease inhibitors—a substance believed to retard cancers of the breast, colon, prostate, and stomach.

- Eat plenty of cruciferous vegetables including broccoli, cabbage, and cauliflower. These vegetables are rich in sulforaphane that can prevent and treat all kinds of cancer.

- Regularly drink vegetable juices. Juices from some common vegetables such as carrots and cabbage have been found to be able to reduce the cell mutations produced by carcinogens in tobacco smoke and barbequed (burned) meat.

- Eat plenty of fruits and also drink fruit juices, especially grape, lemon, apple, and banana.

- Eliminate all red meat. Meat has a tendency to weaken the immune system. For one thing, animal fat is hard to digest. It produces many poisonous toxins. Protein from animal meat breaks down into a toxic substance in the body, so use as little red meat as possible. In particular, never eat meat or fish that is not fresh.

- Do not eat peanuts that are spoiled or have fungus grown over them.

- Do not eat soup or foods while too hot. This can prevent mouth cancer.

- Stop using tobacco in any form, including passive smoke.

- Stop using alcohol products. Alcohol abuse is the major cause of liver cancer.

- Eat less. Limiting the caloric intake has an inhibiting effect on tumor formation and development.

- The way foods are cooked and prepared matters a lot. Do not eat charred or barbecued foods. Avoid pickled, smoked, and salted foods. Foods prepared in these ways contain nitrosamines conducive to cancer. Try not to fry foods, but instead, boil or steam them.

- Soak half a pound of soybeans in water overnight and then boil them in water together with some garlic cloves for thirty minutes. Then drink the soup and eat the beans as a meal. Do this once a day. The combined properties of soybean and garlic can help deter or suppress the cancerous tumor.

- Eat foods rich in vitamin A and C, such as oranges, green peppers, apricots, peaches, carrots, spinach, etc. Eat these foods raw if you can.

- Eat garlic or onion, olives, and fish oil everyday. Eat apricots, brown rice, cabbage, sunflower seeds, watermelon, and winter squash. These foods contain anticancer substances.

- Bake a crab and grind it into powder. Take a teaspoonful of crab powder together with some rice wine twice a day to help treat breast cancer.

- Drink five glasses of carrot juice daily. Carrots are very helpful in preventing and healing cancers in many parts of the body, such as the lungs, stomach, uterus, throat, prostate, and breast.

- Even more helpful is the consumption of radishes or radish juice. Radishes may be able to kill cancer cells.

- Regular consumption of cauliflower can have a very good effect on preventing and treating cancer.

- Take Lingzhi mushroom powder and make it into a tea. Drink it once a day.

- Regularly drink green tea, which has been proven to possess antimutagenic properties and lower the rate of stomach cancer in regular drinkers.

- Drink plenty of pure water each day. It can cleanse our body of pollutants and other dirty materials.

Other natural therapies

- Exercise regularly. The soft exercises introduced in this book are the most suitable for cancer patients. These exercises reduce your weight, lighten your heart, enhance your immunity, and make you feel better and stronger. Also, it has been shown that exercise can strengthen the cells and promote the release of an anticancer hormones in the body.

- Practice qigong twice a day. While doing qigong, imaginatively guide your qi to the diseased part of the body, letting it heal directly on the spot. (See appendix 1.)

- Keep a light heart and be optimistic. Optimism is one of the most powerful natural treatments for all diseases, cancers in particular.

Cataracts

Description

Cataracts are the result of an opaqueness in the lens tissue of the eye. They usually form in our later years because when we are young, our bodies provide checks and balances to help our eyes maintain their health. In youth, the lens of the eye focuses the light on the retina and allows us to see well. As we age, the lens grows larger, and begins to accumulate scar tissues called cataracts. This accumulation of cataracts attracts water and leads to a swelling of the lens. As a result, the lens becomes opaque, cloudy, and blind spots appear in the middle of the visual field. Consequently, light cannot penetrate through the lens as it should, even when the person is wearing a corrective lens.

Decreased vision, particularly at night, comes first. Ultimately, blindness can result. The same process usually occurs in both eyes, although often one eye deteriorates faster than the other.

There are several types of cataracts: complicated cataracts from ocular disease; irradiation cataracts from exposure to certain rays; traumatic cataracts from a perforating injury; and congenital cataracts due to impaired formation.

Cataracts are extremely costly. In 1994, cataract surgeries performed in the U.S. alone cost consumers over 4 billion dollars. Cataracts seem to be a natural companion of aging. According to the National Society for Prevention of Blindness, 75 percent of people over the age of sixty-five have some degree of cataract development. Cataracts are a leading cause of blindness, even at their early stages, especially among older people.

Symptoms or signs

They can include blurred or double vision, and a general loss of visual acuity.

Causes

Cataracts don't appear suddenly. They are the result of years of age-related changes, oxidative stress, nutritional deficiencies, metal poisoning, eye infections, exposure to ultraviolet sunlight, use of certain drugs such as steroids, and other physiological factors. They can also be caused by the swelling of the lens as a consequence of a deficiency of certain enzymes such as potassium, which deactivates the molecular pumping system of the lens between the sodium and potassium concentrations. As a result, a greater than normal density of sodium accumulates, leading to the attraction of fluid from the humor of the eye into the lens.

Prevention and treatment

We can actually do much to prevent cataracts from happening. This means protecting the eyes by not overusing of them. This can be done by regularly closing the eyes to rest after every hour while working; avoiding direct exposure to sunlight and fluorescent light (by wearing sunglasses) to prevent cataracts and macular degeneration; eating foods rich in vitamins A and E; and regularly practicing eye exercises (see appendix 5, "Dharma's Internal Exercises").

Dietary therapies

- Eat foods rich in vitamins A, C, E, and zinc such as carrots and carrot juice, beets, cabbage, broccoli, onions, and fish.

- Eat pork or chicken liver as a meal, once a day for a week. The Chinese believe that the eyes are closely associated with the function of the liver.

- Eat plenty of apples, blueberries, and coconuts. These are fruits that can strengthen your vision.

- Eat animal livers. The Chinese believe that the eyes are closely associated with the function of the liver.

- Eat zinc, vitamin B_2, and vitamin E daily. (Take these separately as a supplement.)

Other natural therapies

- Close your eyes periodically after reading or working on a computer.

- Rotate your eyes periodically after reading or working.

- Acupress the following acupoints several times a day: Baihui, Jingming, Sibai, Muchuang, Meichong, Jingming, Tianyou, Jujiao, Daling, Hegu, and Zhongzhu. (See appendix 7.)

Cholesterol, High

Description

Simply, it means that the cholesterol level in the blood is high enough to lead to more dangerous conditions such as clogged arteries, heart attack, and stroke. It is a dangerous sign that needs to be addressed quickly.

Two types of cholesterol exist in our body: good cholesterol (high density lipoprotein, or HDL) and bad cholesterol (low density lipoprotein, or LDL). While both kinds of cholesterol are normal in the blood, excessively high levels of LDL create cholesterol deposits on the artery walls, causing plaque formation, which narrows the arteries, restricting blood flow to the heart. The higher the LDL level, the greater the chance of heart disease.

Symptoms or signs

A blood test is needed to accurately determine your cholesterol level. A high cholesterol level is considered to be 240 milligrams or higher.

Causes

This problem is mainly the result of a long-term diet high in saturated fats, compounded by a sedentary lifestyle and excess weight. Saturated fats tend to raise the level of cholesterol in the blood. Cholesterol is found in all animal products but is especially high in egg yolks and organ meats. Smoking is another cause. Last but not least, heredity has a role to play in one's cholesterol level.

Dietary therapies

- Avoid eating beef, lamb, pork, and ham, as well as butter, cream, whole milk, cheese, and egg yolks. Egg whites are good, though.

- Adopt a basically vegetarian diet.

- Make soybeans and soy products a permanent part of your diet. Scientific studies show that soy products can dramatically lower cholesterol.

- Eat plenty of sea vegetables such as bladderwrack and carrageens. These largely pass through the body undigested, and can therefore purify the bloodstream, and prevent the low density cholesterol from becoming deposited in the body.

- Use polyunsaturated oils to replace animal fats. Such oils are usually liquid oils of vegetable origin such as corn, cottonseed, soybean, and sunflower oils. They tend to lower the level of cholesterol.

- Eat garlic, asparagus, oatmeal, peanuts, prunes, and tofu regularly. These foods have been shown to lower the levels of cholesterol.

- Eat a high-fiber diet that will prevent fats and cholesterol from being absorbed by the body.

- Eat fresh fish and seafood which has a larger proportion of unsaturated fat as well as the beneficial fat, omega-3.

Other natural therapies

- Do physical exercises every day.

- Practice sound qigong and make the sound of "High" while exhaling. (See appendix 3.)

Chronic Fatigue Syndrome

Description

It is estimated that three million Americans are suffering from chronic fatigue syndrome (CFS), of whom 70 percent are women. As the name implies, this disease is characterized by feeling chronically tired, lethargic, exhausted, or lacking in energy. Sometimes, it can lead to neurogenic pains. People with chronic fatigue syndrome are not just constantly tired. Their fatigue is debilitating, often keeping them away from work or normal daily activities.

Symptoms or signs

It can be accompanied by a wide variety of symptoms such as mild fever, sore throat, painful lymph glands, muscle pain and weakness, headaches, and insomnia, for three months or more.

Causes

While Western medicine has not determined specific causes for CFS, Chinese natural health care believes fatigue occurs when certain basic human needs are not being met. Examples of this are a lack of enzymes from food due to overcooking, overprocessing, or bad combinations; not getting enough sleep and rest, not exercising regularly, or wasting precious energy by overworking or indulging in sex.

Depression, emotional loss, recent illness, and iron-deficiency anemia can also trigger chronic fatigue syndrome. Stress and depression can contribute significantly to fatigue if they persist for any length of time. Iron deficiency, overwork, low blood sugar, thyroid problems, and chronic illness are often cited as root causes of fatigue.

Traditional Chinese medicine diagnoses this disease as a deficiency of vital qi energy in the body. It is a sign that the energy has run below normal levels, that serious disease may happen at any time, and that it is high time to conserve and build up the "strategic reserves."

Prevention and treatment
Dietary therapies

- It is very important to eat foods that can boost your energy and do not add to the degree of fatigue. This means avoiding foods that are hard to digest and low in nutrients.

- Other avoidable foods include sugary, refined, and preserved foods, microwaveable (prepackaged) foods, smoked and barbecued foods, and dairy products.

- Eat whole grains, nuts, beans, fruits and vegetables, fresh sea fish, and eggs. Drink plenty of fruit juice.

- Pour boiled water into a pan with sliced ginseng in it. Cover for five minutes and then drink it. Drink this twice a day on an empty stomach.

- Eat plenty of tofu and soybean products every day.

- Clean and slice a pork stomach. Cook the stomach with some dry ginger, a dozen of dates, and two slices of ginseng. Eat it as part of a meal each day.

- Eat plenty of walnuts, preferably on an empty stomach. In China, walnuts are considered to be an excellent supplement for vital qi energy.

- Drink a cup of grape wine twice a day to tone up your energy and alleviate fatigue symptoms.

- Eat foods rich in vitamin B_6, which plays a key role in transforming the nutrition one takes in into useful energy. These foods include but are not limited to animal kidney and liver, egg, tofu, peanuts, active yeast, wheat germ, raw grains, fresh fish, and carrots.

- Grind lemon seeds into powder and mix it with grape wine. Drink it every day for a week.

- Mix warm water with some vinegar and drink it as a tea. Drink three times a day.

- Boil one ounce each of rice, lotus seeds, and brown sugar for twenty minutes. Add an egg when the seeds and rice are soft. Eat this every evening for two weeks. This helps build up the qi energy needed for fighting fatigue.

- Sheep's milk, when consumed regularly, can tone up the vital energy and relieve chronic fatigue.

- Regularly drink beef or chicken soup. This helps build up the qi energy needed for fighting fatigue.

- Cook twenty red dates and two ounces of dansheng (*Codonoposis pilosula*) in water for about an hour. Drink the soup and eat the dates. Do this once a day to help build up the qi energy needed for fighting fatigue.

Other natural therapies

- Get enough sleep and limit your sexual activity—if you do not know the art of regulated sex—to conserve your energy. (See chapter 8.)

- Do qigong three times a day. Qigong can boost your energy level and reduce fatigue. (See appendix 1.)

- Practice Dharma's morning exercises and Dharma's internal exercises. (See appendices 4 and 5.)

- After practicing the breathing exercises, rub both hands first to warm them, then rub the soles of both feet twenty times. Immediately afterward, put the warm hands on both knees while at the same time deeply exhaling, making a "Heh" sound each time you exhale. Do this nine times. This method has been around for

2,000 years. It has the effect of nourishing the body's qi and blood, enhancing the functioning of the kidney, liver, and nerve system. Thus, it can strengthen the body and relieve symptoms characteristic of CFS. (See appendix 3.)

- Apply finger pressure to the following acupoints several times a day, for a few minutes each time: Chengshan, Renzhong, Sanyinjiao, Dazhui, Shenmen, Lieque, Yinlingquan, Qihai, Zhongwan, and Zusanli. (See appendix 7.)

Common Cold

Description

This is the most common of all diseases. All of us have experienced the following symptoms at the onset of a cold: a stuffy or runny nose; sneezing; blocked breathing passages; a tickle in the throat; dryness in the nose; weak appetite; and mild fatigue. As the cold develops, we experience red eyes, slight aches and pains, a sore throat, headache, chest discomfort, and coughing. As the cold further progresses, the nasal mucus may thicken.

A cold usually lasts one or two weeks, and the Chinese believe that seven days is a cycle that is the minimum time needed for the recovery of any disease. Colds occur throughout the year, but are most common in late winter and early spring. Sometimes a cold will lead to more serious complications such as chronic sinusitis and bronchitis.

Causes

Conventional wisdom believes that contracting a virus or bacteria is the real cause of the common cold. There are some 200 viruses that can cause a cold. These viruses can come into contact with our body by several means—a kiss, a handshake, using a pay phone, someone sneezing nearby, or sharing eating utensils and towels. Most cold viruses undergo a period of one to seven days of incubation before causing any noticeable symptoms.

Since there is no completely "clean" place, all of us are exposed to viruses all the time. Why do only some of us catch a cold, while others do not, even though we're exposed to the same virus? As the Chinese natural health care system sees it, it is the depletion of energy and the resulting weakened immunity that makes our body vulnerable to viruses. It is our own immune system, not the virus, that determines whether or not we catch a cold.

Prevention and treatment

With so many strains of viruses around that can cause the common cold, you may start to feel outnumbered. But help is easily available, and it comes in a natural way. You can prevent colds by eating well, getting enough sleep, and avoiding stress and depression. Also, if you can, avoid kissing, shaking hands, using public phones, and sharing eating utensils and towels. The ancient Chinese also held that clothing and bedding that is too warm will make you vulnerable to catching a cold. It is important to stay out of the wind while sweating, bathing, or sleeping. Negligence of this rule will lead to severe cold and health problems. Most important of all is to keep a healthy lifestyle. This includes regular exercise, especially rubbing your face with both hands a dozen times each morning as soon as you get up, along with washing the face, drinking plenty of water and fruit juice daily, and chewing garlic cloves once a day.

Dietary therapies

- Stop smoking to avoid further irritating the sensitive tissues of the throat and nose.

- Stop drinking coffee; instead, drink a lot of green tea. The Chinese often drink strongly brewed tea to drive away colds and headaches (and it works).

- If the cold is accompanied by coughing or nasal congestion, avoid dairy products and wheat products. These foods are often described as "mucus-producing" foods, and could aggravate respiratory infections and phlegm.

- The focus should be on strengthening the immune system. In terms of diet, eat foods rich in vitamin C and minerals, because these materials can enhance our immune system. Other foods that can help include orange peel, peppermint, and radishes.

- Fry tofu together with green onions in peanut oil, adding brown sugar and salt. Eat it as a dish. This induces one to sweat, which in turn helps get the cold out.

- Eat plenty of green and orange vegetables as well as fruits.

- Cook one ounce of sliced ginger and two ounces of scallions in water for twenty minutes. Drink the soup hot.

- Alternatively, cook sliced ginger in water together with some brown sugar. Drink the soup hot and go to bed. Cover up the body and let it sweat. You may find the cold has disappeared when you wake up.

- Fry some green Chinese onions in pepper oil. Add some water and noodles. Eat as a meal. This is meant to induce sweating.

- Sip two mouthfuls of fresh lemon juice, three times a day. Lemon helps dissolve and eliminate excess mucus in the respiratory system, restores mucous membranes and tissue integrity in the system, thus preventing mucus excretion through the lungs and nose.

- Mix orange juice and apple juice in a glass. Drink five glasses of it each day to improve immunity.

- Cook noodles in water and add a sufficient amount of pepper. Eat the noodles warm to help induce sweating.

- Mix carrot juice with lemon juice and drink it a couple of times daily.

- Mix orange peel, green tea, and slices of ginger. Add boiled water to make a tea of this mixture. Cover it up for three minutes, then drink the tea.

- Slice two ounces of ginger, and boil it with one cup of water for about three minutes. Then add brown sugar to the soup and drink it all. Go to bed immediately afterward, and cover yourself up with enough blankets to ensure that you perspire.

- Chew several cloves of garlic before each meal.

- Smash five small pieces of peeled garlic, and mix it with some rice vinegar. Then drink and eat it all. Go to bed and let yourself perspire.

- Clean a whole chicken and cook it with some fresh ginger slices in enough water to cover them up for thirty minutes. Drink the soup to help expel the mucus.

- Slightly fry some ginger slices with the white heads of green onions in vegetable oil and mix them with noodles. Eat as a meal. Both improve immunity and induce sweating.

- Crush two ounces of fresh ginger and squeeze out the juice. Mix the juice with a small bottle of warmed rice wine and drink to trigger perspiration.

- Cook an egg together with a glass of rice wine. Add some brown sugar while the egg is half cooked. Eat the egg and drink the soup to relieve headaches.

- Use sweet basil leaves as a seasoning to substitute for parsley or green onion, in case you cannot find parsley or green onion.

- Brew tea and dried loquat leaves (these are the leaves of a fruit tree in China) together. Drink the tea twice a day.

- Drink a lot of pure, warm water (at least ten glasses per day) to compensate for the virus' drying effect on the tissues of the nose and throat. Water flushes the toxins, and helps relieve congestion of the nose and throat by diluting the mucus. Also, water induces sweating, which is helpful for reducing fevers and relieving colds.

- Eat chicken soup. It is even better to add spicy additions such as ginger or pepper, to help thin the mucus in the nose.

- If phlegm sticks in the throat and is hard to expel, drink a cup of warm water containing 1 to 2 percent salt (approximately half a teaspoon).

Other natural therapies

- Get extra sleep and rest to conserve your body's energy in its struggle against the virus and bacteria.

- Rub your nose and neck several times a day, using the back of your thumbs and palms. (See appendix 5 .)

- Practice soft exercises only, avoiding any vigorous exercise. The idea is to enhance the spirit and morale rather than to train the muscles at this time. During this period, rest rather than activity should be the keynote of life.

- Sponging has a cooling effect on the body's temperature. If the cold is accompanied by a fever, you can sponge your-self with tepid water for fifteen minutes to lower the temperature.

NOTE: Fever during a cold is generally not harmful, and should only be lowered if it makes the patient more comfortable or if the fever rises above 104 degrees. Several studies suggest a fever may in fact be protective as the body's natural de-fense against viral infection.

- Soak your feet in hot water for fifteen minutes, and then drink some ginger tea before going to bed.

- Keep your bed warm and let your body sweat.

- Humidify the bedroom and, better still, your whole house.

- Boil some slices of dried ginger in pure water. Inhale the steam when the water boils. Do this several times a day. It will open up congested sinuses and lung pas-sages, allowing you to discharge mucus, breathe more freely, and heal faster.

- Wash your hands often, especially before meals and after exposure to those who have a cold.

- Move your bowels everyday. Regular bowel movements can help get rid of viruses and bacteria as well as the fever.

- Play some light music to amuse yourself and relieve stress. Stress can make colds worse.

- Frequently rub both sides of your nose with your thumbs. (See appendix 5.)

- Apply finger pressure to the following acupoints several times a day: Taiyang, Baihui, Hegu, Lieque, Quchi, Yuji, Waiguan, Yingxiang, Fengmen, Fengchi, Fenglong, Jujiao, and Taichong. (See ap-pendix 7.)

Constipation

Description

Constipation is a chronic problem for more than 4 million Americans, making it one of the nation's leading health annoyances. This ailment is characterized by difficulty in hav-ing a bowel movement, sometimes accompa-nied by cramping and pain in the rectum from the strain of trying to pass hard stools. There may be small amounts of bright red blood on the stool caused by slight tearing as the stool is pushed through the anus. Nor-mally, we need to move our bowels once a day. This is the metabolism cycle, and it is re-quired for physical and mental health.

Stools contain wastes from the foods we eat. These wastes contain lots of bacteria and poisonous elements. It is necessary to get rid of these on a daily basis. If a stool becomes lodged in the rectum, mucus and fluid will leak out around the stool, leading to fecal in-continence and a series of health problems, such as indigestion, insomnia, stomach and intestine diseases, fever, and lack of appetite. However, when the bowels become sluggish, as in the case of constipation, a regular bowel movement is hampered and toxins accumulate in the body, causing imbalances in the bacterial flora of the colon and triggering diseases. It is important to realize that the longer the digested food stays in the colon, the more likely it is that bacteria will grow and release toxic chemicals, leading to colon cancer, which alone kills 55,000 Americans each year.

Symptoms or signs

These include hard, compacted stools, cramping or pain in the rectum, and blood on the stool.

Causes

It is caused by a lack of three things: exercise, which stimulates peristalsis, the wave-like muscle contractions that move food along the gastrointestinal tract; fiber in the diet, which adds bulk to the stool; and fluid, which softens the stool so it can pass without causing pain or tearing anal tissue. Lack of fluid in the colon is what makes the stool hard and bowel movements difficult. Hardness of the stool slows the peristaltic action, causing the waste materials to stay in the bowels. The deficiency of fluid in the colon is in turn caused by an unhealthy diet and lack of exercise. Refined foods with little fiber do little to help the bowels move. Lack of exercise only exacerbates the situation. The more foods you take in, the harder it is to get rid of the waste.

Irregularity in your lifestyle can also cause constipation. For instance, not having a regular schedule as to when to go to bed, when to rise, when to eat, and especially when to have a bowel movement during the day. All of these can lead to constipation. Another instance is travel, which alters the normal bowel rhythms.

It is known that certain drugs can result in constipation, such as narcotics, iron pills, and calcium pills, because these drugs require a high acid environment to be properly assimilated. Mental stress, a heavy workload, and pain due to hemorrhoids can also lead to constipation. Peristalsis also weakens with age, so constipation can be a frequent problem for the elderly.

Prevention and treatment

Follow a high-fiber diet. High-fiber diets not only prevent constipation but may also prevent diverticulosis, hemorrhoids, intestinal polyps, and even colon cancer. Avoid fried foods as well as sugary foods. Drink plenty of water and juice. Exercise each and every day. Develop a set time for a daily bowel movement and answer "nature's call" promptly—do not wait until the urge is over. A bowel movement should be on the top of the daily list of priorities.

Dietary therapies

• Follow a high-fiber diet made of whole grains and oats, brown rice, fresh vegetables, and fruits. Fiber you take in as food is not digested. It moves through the bowels together with other wastes. It draws water into the stool and adds bulk while softening the stool.

- Eat slowly and chew thoroughly, with your mind focused on the meal. This will greatly help digestion, which in turn will facilitate a bowel movement.

- Particularly recommended are sweet potatoes, which have been proven to be highly efficient in preventing and treating constipation as well as other problems.

- Apples, bananas, figs, papayas, and pears are also good for relieving constipation.

- Eat a porridge made of almond powder (available in all Chinese grocery stores) each and every day.

- Soak one ounce of tremella in water for an hour. Add some rock sugar and stew the tremella for another hour. Eat the tremella and drink the soup. Take this once or twice a day.

- Cook lean pork in some Lingzhi powder and water, add some seasoning, and eat.

- Stew one or two figs in water with some honey. Drink the soup and eat the figs.

- Stew one ounce of almonds and two pears in water for thirty minutes. Add some rock sugar. Eat and drink everything.

- To stop bleeding caused by tearing, drink several cups of fresh celery juice each day.

- Mix radish juice with some honey and drink it on an empty stomach. This specifically softens the hardened stool in the bowels and facilitates the movement.

- Clean and cut an eggplant. Mix it with some sesame oil and salt. Stew for thirty minutes and eat.

- Steam two ounces of tremella, fifteen red dates, and some rock sugar in water. Eat the food and drink the soup.

- These foods can relieve constipation: castor bean, sesame oil, apricot seeds, bananas, peaches, soybean oil, walnuts, and watermelon.

- Drink three spoonfuls of fresh potato juice together with some honey on an empty stomach in the morning before breakfast. This softens the stool.

- Sesame porridge or sesame oil are excellent relievers of constipation. Eat sesame porridge as a meal, or drink honey water together with some sesame oil each day.

- Eat two very ripe bananas in the morning on an empty stomach.

- Eat raw walnuts twice a day, one ounce each time.

- Eat one or two fresh figs at bedtime. This is especially good for the elderly.

- Drink fresh milk in the morning on an empty stomach.

- Drink a glass of grapefruit juice first thing in the morning on an empty stomach.

- Drink at least ten cups of water each day.

- Eat prunes or drink prune juice. Prunes contain a natural substance that eases constipation.

- Boil one ounce of plum seeds in water and drink twice a day. Do not eat the seeds.

- Drink a cup of salt water or honey water with several drops of sesame oil first thing in the morning.

Other natural therapies

- Practice some form of soft exercise regularly every day.

- Practice qigong and focus your mind on the acupoints of Yongqiong, located at the center of both soles. (See appendix 7.)

- Walk a mile after eating.

- Massage the abdomen three times a day. Each time, rub the hands against each other until they are warm, then use them alternatively to rub the entire abdomen, thirty rounds clockwise and thirty rounds counter-clockwise. This can be performed either in a sitting or lying position. (See appendix 5.)

- Practice "Shaking the Heavenly Pillar." (See appendix 5.)

- Lie down on your back, with legs bent and the soles of your feet on the ground. Practice breathing exercises in this posture for five minutes, twice a day.

- Alternatively, lie on your back and try to press your legs against the chest. Exert some force. This should also be done twice a day.

- Apply finger pressure to the following acupoints several times a day: Tianshu, Daheng, Zhongzhu, Zhongwan, Quchi, Sanyinjiao, Zusanli, Changqiang, Fenglong, Zhongwan, Qihai, Huiyin, Zhigou, and Shangjuxu. (See appendix 7.)

Coughing

Description

Coughing is the body's way of removing alien materials or mucus from the lungs and bronchial tubes. Such materials or mucus irritate the tender lining of the throat, causing the throat to make rough sounds. Basically, there are two kinds of cough: productive and dry coughing. Productive coughing produces phlegm or mucus and helps clear the lungs of such materials. Dry coughing, on the other hand, does not produce mucus.

Here, I address the ailment of coughing in general terms. It can be coughing accompanied by a cold or flu, or it can also be whooping cough in children. Therefore, the therapies introduced here are considered generally applicable to all kinds of coughing, disregarding its real cause.

Causes

Coughing may be caused by a cold, bronchitis, smoking, or air pollution. In traditional Chinese medicine, dry coughing is believed to be a problem with the lungs, while productive coughing is diagnosed to be a dysfunction of the spleen and stomach.

Prevention and treatment

Avoid coffee, dairy products, and sweet, fried, or greasy foods. Stop smoking and avoid secondary smoke. Keep the chest warm and breathe in as much fresh air as you can.

Dietary therapies

- Avoid milk and wheat products to prevent more throat phlegm.

- Avoid cold food and drinks, because the lungs are "afraid" of coldness. In other words, coldness will hurt the lungs.

- Drink plenty of warm water to help loosen phlegm and soothe an irritated throat.

- Clean and cut two carrots. Cook these with fifteen red dates in water for about thirty minutes. Eat the carrots and dates and drink the soup. Do this twice a day. This will reduce phlegm and relieve coughing.

- Cook one to two ounces of the seeds of a white gourd, with one pear and some rock sugar for thirty minutes. Drink the soup. Do this twice a day, once in the morning and once in the evening. This will reduce phlegm and relieve coughing.

- Eat a porridge made of almond powder (available in all Chinese grocery stores) each and every day. This will reduce phlegm and relieve coughing.

- Soak one ounce of tremella in water for an hour. Add some rock sugar and stew the tremella for another hour. Eat the tremella and drink the soup. Do this once or twice a day. It can help reduce phlegm and relieve coughing.

- Cut two pears and one pork lung. Cook them together in water with some rock sugar for about an hour. Eat the pear and drink the soup. This will reduce phlegm and relieve coughing.

- Drink three cups of pear juice each day. This will reduce phlegm and relieve coughing.

- Steam in water two ounces of tremella, fifteen red dates, and some rock sugar. Eat the food and drink the soup.

- Use some Lingzhi powder to cook lean pork meat and eat it as a dish.

- Stew one ounce of almonds and two pears in water for thirty minutes. Add some rock sugar. Eat the almonds and pears, and drink the soup.

- Make a hole in an apple and pour some honey into it. Steam the apple and eat it.

- Soak one ounce of green tea in two cups of water for an hour. Cook two eggs in the tea for ten minutes until there is only one cup of water left. Drink the tea and eat the eggs. Take this once a week.

- Stew some radishes in water together with some honey. Drink the soup and eat the radishes.

- Stew some chicken with two cut oranges for thirty minutes. Eat it as a dish.

- Stew one to two fresh cleaned sparrows in water with some rock sugar. Eat it as a dish. Do this once a day for a week to relieve chronic coughing.

- Boil two sliced snow pears in water and drink the juice. Snow pears are believed to be better able to reduce phlegm.

- Cut one to two pears into small pieces. Add a little water and one ounce of rock candy. Steam them together for ten minutes. Drink the soup and eat the pears. Do this once a day.

- Cut a ripe pineapple into pieces and slowly chew them.

- Slightly cook a radish and eat it, or drink warm radish juice.

- Boil ginger slices with maltose in water for half an hour. Drink the soup hot, twice a day, for three days.

- Boil fresh ginger in water and mix with some honey. Drink it as a tea.

- Boil lotus seeds in water until they are soft. Add some honey and drink.

- Boil in water some fresh ginger together with some dried orange peel and drink.

- Drink two cups of orange juice and/or carrot juice each day.

- Eat raw garlic cloves. Garlic is powerful in killing bacteria and eliminating mucus.

- Chew seven sweet apricot seeds once a day to cure a chronic cough.

- Clean and cut into pieces a fresh sparrow. Stew it in water with some rock sugar for one hour. Eat and drink everything.

- Mix honey in hot water or green tea to relieve a dry cough.

- To relieve whooping cough in children, take two teaspoonfuls of garlic solution (in water) every two hours. (To make a garlic solution, grind garlic cloves and add some water to the juice.)

- Steam one or two fresh figs together with three honey dates. Eat them to alleviate dry coughing and sore throat.

- Steam a fresh lemon with some rock sugar and eat it. This can lessen the mucus discharge and treat whooping cough in children.

- Steam five fresh olives together with one ounce of rock sugar. Eat the olives.

- Eat oranges along with the peel.

- Steam one pound of fresh papayas. Eat once a day for a week to relieve a chronic cough.

- Steam two pears with some apricot seeds for thirty minutes. Eat twice a day to cure a dry cough.

- Boil two ounces of fresh chestnuts with five red dates and some lean pork. Eat them all as a meal.

- Eat fresh peanuts to relieve a cough with mucous discharge.

- Boil red dates and fresh carrots in water for twenty minutes. Drink the soup to relieve whooping cough in children.

- Eat yellow soybean sprouts as a vegetable.

Other natural therapies

- Massage the chest several times a day as directed in Dharma's internal exercises. (See appendix 5.)

- Practice breathing exercises twice a day, focusing your mind on the chest.

- Apply finger pressure to the following acupoints several times a day: Fenglong, Hegu, Taixi, Fengchi, Waiguan, Taiyuan, Lieque, Shouwuli, Lianquan, Xuanji, Jiuwei, Yuji, and Tiantu. (See appendix 7.)

Depression

Description

Stress has become a way of life for many people today. Indeed, most people experience some form of stress or depression at some point in their life. It is estimated that about 17 million Americans—one in every ten adults—experience depression.

Depression is not just a mental ailment. It is the fourth major cause of death in the world. Each year, more than 30,000 Americans take their own life due to depression.[13] According to a report submitted by World Health Organization, it will become the number two killer worldwide by the year 2020, second only to heart disease. Thus, depression is a serious disease and should be treated as such.

Chronic depression should be regarded as an illness, and a real threat to health. Researchers point out that depression can dramatically boost the blood pressure, worsen hypertension, reduce blood flow, reduce antibody production, and thus weaken the immunity power of our body. This greatly increases the chance of contracting various diseases and cancer. This is because when one is depressed, the brain emits depression hormones that are harmful to our physical and mental health, unless we can find some way to dispel or "consume" these hormones as soon as possible. If the depression lasts more than a few weeks or seriously hampers your ability to cope with everyday life, then it is an illness, not just a mood that you can change easily.

Researchers find that women seem to be more affected by depression. Roughly twice as many women suffer from depression as men. Also, rich, ambitious, and successful people seem to be more vulnerable to depression than poor, easy-going, ordinary people. Indeed, wealth and fame are sources of stress themselves. As the Chinese proverbs say: "Devils keep a close eye on the rich families," and "The higher the tree, the stronger the wind." China's Mao Tse-tung used to suffer from severe stress and often cried during his last years, despite his unchallenged position as the leader of the world's most populous nation.

Symptoms or signs

Depression can range from a minor problem to a major life-threatening illness. When you feel sad, frustrated, discouraged, or hopeless, you could be depressed. Depression can take several forms, including manic depressive illness characterized by extreme emotional lows and highs, and dysthymia, a milder, chronic depression with symptoms of persistent fatigue, sleep disturbances, eating disorders, aches and pains, and a feeling that life is not worthwhile any more.

If you have experienced four or more of the following symptoms every day for more than a week, you may be suffering from chronic depression.

- Feelings of restlessness or irritability.

- Feelings of helplessness or worthlessness that do not go away.

- Persistent feelings of sadness, anxiety, or hopelessness.

- Feelings of guilt or strong remorse.

- Lack of interest or pleasure in normal activities or friends.

- Loss of interest in sex.

- Inability to concentrate, remember, or make everyday decisions.

- Decrease in appetite or an upset stomach.

- Difficulty in sleeping or sleeping too much.

- Difficulty in making normal decisions.

- Unexplained weight gain or loss.

- Insomnia.

- Low energy, fatigue, and general weakness.

- Frequent headaches, backaches, stiff neck, rapid breathing, sweaty palms.

- Losing your temper easily and arguing with others.

- General tiredness of life and its affairs.

- Frequent thought of suicide or death.

Causes

There are numerous causes of depression—physical, psychological, social, medical, nutritional, biochemical, and environmental. Life in the modern world is characterized by stressors on many fronts, internal and external, mental and physical. Examples include a confrontation with the boss, job insecurity, remote feelings toward people, a car accident, strained family relations, separation and divorce, death of a close family member, wayward children, domineering parents, financial burdens, and even weather.

Without a doubt, all these contribute to and aggravate the stress and depression characterizing modern life. An excess intake of caffeine in the form of coffee, teas, colas, or chocolate, and abuse of alcohol, both of which deplete the body of vitamin B, are common causes. In addition, demanding too much of yourself is another risk factor. Researchers find that ambitious people are more vulnerable to depression and heart attack than more easy-going people. Low blood sugar and a deficiency or overproduction of neurotransmitters as a result of an improper diet are also listed as causes.

Another theory holds that depression is closely associated with a dysfunctional thyroid gland. It can be either depression that causes the dysfunction in the thyroid gland, or the other way around, or even a combination. However, it has been observed that depression is often the first early warning sign of thyroid disease, as even the slightest sign of thyroid disease can produce symptoms of depression.

In addition to the above-mentioned causes, women can become depressed due to hormone fluctuations and biochemical imbalances. In fact, many cases of depression in women start with a reproductive event—the onset of menstruation, pregnancy, post-partum, or menopause. Hormonal fluctuations interact with neuro-chemical factors to produce mood disorders.

Whatever the cause, major depression usually involves an imbalance of chemical messengers in the brain. Some people are genetically susceptible to chemical imbalances in the brain.

Prevention and treatment

Some people seek to forget their depression by smoking, drinking, or using drugs. This may temporarily relieve the symptoms, but over the long haul it only makes matters worse. The Chinese have a saying: "Mental illness requires mental medicine." Here the mental medicine is used metaphorically to refer to mental means other than drugs or medication, such as psychotherapy, qigong, and Chinese soft exercises. These exercises, practiced regularly, have been shown to be highly effective in treating depression. Depression feeds on itself, so break the cycle. The following measures can help greatly in the struggle against depression.

NOTE: Above all, if you or someone you know feels suicidal or cannot function normally due to depression, see a medical professional for treatment right away.

Dietary therapies

• The diet for those suffering from depression should consist mainly of complex carbohydrates and sea foods. Eat plenty of fruit and vegetables, beans and nuts, as well as fish and sea vegetables.

• Drink plenty of pure water.

• Eat regular meals. Don't skip any.

• Do not eat when in a stressful mood.

• Stop drinking alcohol and caffeine products. Alcohol and caffeine can cause the excess production of adrenaline that can lead to mood swings.

• Ensure that you are taking in sufficient vitamins and minerals.

• Eat plenty of radishes. You can cook them together with chicken, lean meat, or pork bones.

• Avoid simple sugars in your diet. Watch your blood sugar level. Low blood sugar causes depletion of glucose from the brain leading to dysfunction of brain activity and depression.

- Steam one ounce of sliced ginseng in water for twenty minutes and drink it as a tea on an empty stomach or at bedtime.

- Licorice and lily flower both have a calming effect.

- Boil one ounce of raisins with one ounce of red dates in water. Eat to relieve anxiety.

Other natural therapies

- Practice qigong for twenty minutes, twice a day. Qigong can tranquilize your mind, boost your self-esteem, level out emotional upheavals, and counteract the physiological effects of the body's stress response. (See appendix 1.)

- Practice soft exercises regularly, at least once in the morning and once in the afternoon. These exercises encourage the release of mood-elevating chemicals in the brain.

- Talk to good friends about your situation and let them share your burden. Do not try to hide it and bear the full weight of the situation. Most likely, you will make the wrong evaluation of yourself and the environment when you are feeling blue and lonely.

- Take a walk outside in a garden or woods, or drive to the beach or any other scenic place that can divert your attention.

- Laugh or cry out loud. This is an efficient and effective way to quickly disperse the depression. Laughter, like exercise, can help restore balance to your system.

- Do taich'i or any form of natural health exercises. Since such exercises require your full attention in coordinating your breathing and body movements, you can help get over depression in a very gentle way and regenerate the energy in your body.

- Take a warm bath to disperse the depression hormone. Although showering has a similar effect, it is not as good as a bath.

- Go sightseeing or to a party with happy people. Their positive attitude creates a therapeutic atmosphere that can help.

- Surround yourself with optimistic and sophisticated people. The Chinese have a saying to the effect that making friends with sophisticated people gives you a fallback in times of emergency. Sophisticated, usually older, people have gone through their life and most likely have experienced the same situation that you are in. They know that it is useless to worry or feel depressed. Time will cure everything, and there is a time for everything. Such a view of life is very helpful to help take you out of the mire of depression and give you a good perspective on life and the magnitude of the situation.

- Practice regulated sex. This is an excellent way of relieving depression, all the more so if your sexual partner understands your situation. As a matter of fact, many cases of depression are caused by none other than the unsatisfactory sexual experience itself.

- Press the acupoints of Shaohai, Taiyi, and Yongquan several times a day, two to three minutes each time. (See appendix 7.)

- Use your index finger and thumb to gently tug and pull each toe. Do this a few times a day.

- Hold your foot with both thumbs on top and the fingers wrapped under your foot. Press the sole with the fingers while using your thumbs to massage on top.

- Read related biographies, autobiographies, or history books. History or other people's experiences can be your best teacher. You will find companions in historical figures and may also find solutions to your current problems.

Diabetes

Description

This is a serious disease that can lead to blindness, heart attack, stroke, kidney failure, and amputation. It is the fourth leading disease in this country, with 16 million Americans afflicted and growing.[14] It is predicted that by the year 2007, there will be 21 million Americans diagnosed with diabetes. The current medical costs for diabetes stand at $130 billion per year in the U.S. alone.

Diabetes is a dangerous disease that wastes enormous quantities of essential nutrients through urination. It is a metabolic disorder marked by the decreased ability, or inability, of the body to utilize carbohydrates due to a lower production of insulin. Patients of diabetes may often get thinner and thinner, feel weak in the limbs, and tired and sluggish. This is accompanied by headaches, insomnia, dry or itchy skin, loss of appetite, sour taste in the mouth, and cataracts. When a high level of glucose accumulates in the blood caused by either an insufficient or overproduction of insulin, the glucose spills into the urine.

Diabetics can consume all the carbohydrates they want, but cannot use them effectively. The disease does its dirty work by hampering the body's ability to produce or respond to insulin. This is a hormone that regulates the amount of sugar in the blood, as well as its use by muscles and other tissues.

Carbohydrates in the diet are converted to glucose, causing a slight rise in blood glucose levels which, in turn, triggers the release of the hormone, insulin, from a gland in the abdomen called the pancreas. Insulin is responsible for escorting glucose into various tissues of the body for energy production and for conversion to another form of sugar called glycogen, which is stored in the muscles and liver for future energy needs. Without insulin, glucose cannot be used or stored properly. Diabetes occurs when the body does not produce enough insulin or cannot use it efficiently. Moreover, glucose can enter the cells of nerves, eye lenses, and kidneys. Increased levels of glucose in these cells leads to water retention and cell swelling, resulting in cataract formations, nerve and kidney damage, and vascular problems.

The health consequences of diabetes are devastating—kidney failure, serious nerve damage, hypertension, heart disease, and stroke—all because of the overproduction of insulin. Heart disease is the major killer of diabetes patients.

There are two types of diabetes. One type is insulin-dependent, which occurs when the pancreas fails to produce enough insulin. It is more common among children and adolescents. The other type is insulin-independent, which occurs when the body's cells become resistant to insulin, reducing the amount of glucose that can be used by the cells at any one time. It is more common among adults, especially those who are overweight and over forty years of age. It also often lacks obvious symptoms in the early years of development, making it more dangerous.

Symptoms or signs

Excessive urination, dehydration, extreme thirst, blurred vision, loss of appetite, a constant craving for sugar, persistent fatigue, repeated skin or urinary tract infections, increased appetite with weight loss, frequent or recurring skin or gum infections, slow-healing cuts and wounds, recurrent vaginitis, impotence, and in the later stages, numbness in the legs or feet due to circulatory problems, as well as extreme tiredness.

Causes

In traditional Chinese medicine, diabetes is diagnosed to be a case of a constitutional deficiency of yin qi in the pancreas as a result of the overeating of fatty and sweet foods, or excessive consumption of alcohol, plus emotional stress and depression. Modern science finds that genetics also plays a significant role in the disease.

Like cancer and heart disease, an improper lifestyle is the single most important cause of diabetes according to the Chinese health care system. Lifestyle can include a bad diet, lack of exercise, and an excessive and unregulated sexual life. A regular intake of high-sugar, high-fat, and high-carbohydrate foods that are low in fiber can set you up for serious illness. Researchers at Harvard University surveyed 65,000 women, ages forty to sixty-five, and found that a diet low in sugar and high in fiber, such as whole-wheat bread and unprocessed breakfast cereals, cut the risk of developing diabetes by 28 percent.[15] This is because starches and sugars in the diet are converted to glucose before your body can use them.

Normally the human body produces insulin that enables us to make use of sugars and starches and controls the amount of glucose in the blood. Without insulin, the body cannot use or store glucose, so it stays in the blood. As one grows older, insulin production reduces. If the sugar intake remains the same, the blood sugar will rise. If the rise in blood sugar is unchecked, it will lead to diabetes. This is why the diabetes rate increases sharply after one reaches forty-five.[16] If the diet is rich in fiber, it can help reduce the absorption rate of carbohydrates by the body.

This slowing down seems to ward off the risk of diabetes.

Another cause is a fatty diet. Fat tends to offset the effects of insulin. This is further worsened by not enough exercise, which slows down the burning of fat in the body. Fat is closely associated with hypertension, and hypertension is also a cause of diabetes, thus forming a vicious cycle.

Too much sex is another cause of diabetes, based on the Chinese natural health care system. The result of excessive sex is the weakening of kidney function and a deficiency of qi, both of which are vital to the productivity of insulin. With diabetes, this production system is sabotaged. As a result, we either do not produce insulin at all, or do not produce enough to handle the sugar and starches we take in.

Prevention and treatment

Like all diseases of civilization, the treatment for diabetes begins with prevention, and prevention starts with regular exercise and a low-fat, low-sugar, and high-fiber diet. Exercise helps the uptake of sugar by the cells from the blood. It can also help control weight and blood glucose, improve circulation, strengthen the heart, and reduce stress. Regular physical exercise improves insulin sensitivity and reduces insulin resistance and blood sugar levels. If inactive, the muscle cells lose their ability to respond to insulin. It is insulin that puts blood sugar to work. So exercise enhances the body's ability to use blood sugar by keeping the muscle cells in shape. In addition, it reduces blood pressure, improves the lipid profile, and aids in the health of the heart.

Patients should also follow a diet emphasizing complex carbohydrates such as wholesome grains and vegetables, which prevent sugar from entering too easily into the blood.

Dietary therapies

Proper nutrition is fundamental to every diabetes treatment plan. A proper diet is aimed at correcting obesity and reducing blood glucose. Obesity worsens insulin resistance, whereas weight loss lowers blood glucose levels and blood pressure. Therefore, it is highly advisable that you follow a high-protein, low simple-carbohydrate diet. In addition, abstain from sexual activities to build up your vital energy reserve needed to restore the production capacity of insulin.

Ginseng can reduce the level of blood sugar by as much as 40 to 50 milligrams per 100 milliliters blood, as reported by the International Symposium on the Effects of Ginseng held in the Soviet Union in 1954.

- Avoid caffeine and alcohol.

- Substantially reduce refined carbohydrates, sugar, animal protein, saturated fats, salt, and starch in the diet. Also, significantly limit breads, yams, rice, and potatoes.

- Eat foods with high chromium such as mushrooms, peppers, fruits, chicken, eggs, fish, beef, soy oil, and sesame oil. One study shows that chromium can make insulin more effective.

- Consume high-protein and high-fiber foods: wholesome grains, raw vegetables and fruit. Raw foods stimulate the pancreas. Especially recommended are soybeans, tofu, tomatoes, cucumbers, onions, spinach, molasses, Napa (chinese cabbage), radishes, spinach, grapes, watermelon, gourds, carrots, eggplant, onions, chives, tomatoes, oranges, lemons, strawberries, and bamboo shoots.

- Supplement the diet with iron and vitamins. All cases of diabetes are associated with iron deficiency.

- Use some corn silk to cook with a pig spleen (cut and cleaned). Eat the spleen and drink the soup. If possible, do this once a day for two weeks. This is a very effective treatment for diabetes.

- Clean and cut a fresh abalone. Cook the abalone with some radishes and eat.

- Eat sea plants such as carrageens and bladderwrack.

- Mix red beans and carp together to make a dish and eat it once a day. For preparation, soak the red beans in water for two hours. Cut a fresh carp into several pieces. Put the carp into the soaked red beans and cook for twenty to thirty minutes, adding some ginger slices and salt. Eat it as a meal. This is one of the important traditional Chinese dietary treatments for diabetes and prostate diseases.

- Steam a pork stomach together with gingko nuts and eat as a meal. To prepare, clean the pork stomach and cut into small pieces. Add in one ounce of gingko and soak in pure water for half an hour. Then steam for twenty to thirty minutes. Eat this once a day.

- Slice one pound of dried bitter melon (has bumps on the outside of it) and boil it in water for fifteen minutes. Eat as a soup before each meal. Statistics gathered in China show a significant reduction of both blood sugar and urine sugar levels after doing this for one month.

- Consume onion and garlic on a regular basis. These foods contain natural beneficial hormones.

- Boil half an ounce of fresh corn and eat twice a day.

- Mix half wheat powder and half wheat bran together with eggs to make pancakes. Do not add sugar. Eat it as a meal.

- Bring ten ounces of fresh potato leaves and twenty ounces of wax gourd to a boil in water for fifteen minutes and drink the soup. Eat this once or twice a day.

- Soak twenty ounces of fresh onion in boiling water for one minute, with a little bit of salt. Eat and drink all of it. Do this twice a day.

- Drink one to two cups of mare's milk every day.

- Boil a pork or beef pancreas in water with one pound of yams, seasoned with salt. Eat once a day for three days.

- Fry onions and beef, or radishes and lean pork, to make a dish and eat it.

- Boil fresh watermelon peel in water. Drink it twice a day.

- Soak five ounces of mung beans for five hours, then boil them in water over low heat until the beans break. Eat in a day.

- Cook fresh tortoise meat with two ounces of corn hair in water for forty minutes. Drink the soup and eat the tortoise.

- Drinking coconut liquid is very good for diabetes.

- Crush three ounces of dry guavas, squeezing out the juice, and drink before meals, three times a day.

- Boil dried corn silk in water and drink it as a tea, three times a day. This can lower blood sugar.

- Sheep's milk is considered very helpful.

Other natural therapies

- Chinese fitness exercises can increase the uptake of glucose by the muscle cells which reduces blood glucose. Exercise also increases muscle mass, which in turn creates a greater need for energy, thus bringing down high glucose levels.

- Be abstinent in sexual activities so as to build up the vital qi energy reserve.

- Practice Dharma's internal exercises twice a day. It is especially helpful to massage the neck, abdomen, waist, and calves of the legs. This is because the Chinese fathers believe that these parts of the body are closely related to one's qi energy and discretionary system. (See appendix 5.)

- Reduce stress levels by doing qigong or engaging in some recreational activities. Stress can cause the release of certain hormones that inhibit insulin production and increase the production of glucose by the liver.

- Apply finger pressure to these acupoints several times a day: Gongsun, Lianquan, Hegu, Laogong, Yuji, Lianquan, Taixi, Yangchi, Quchi, Neiguan, Sanyinjiao, and Zusanli. Also, apply finger pressure to the depressions along the hairline on the neck. (See appendix 7.)

Diarrhea

Description

This is a common disease that almost everyone has experienced. Also known as "a loose belly" or "the runs," diarrhea is characterized by an increase in the frequency of bowel movements and the discharge of watery, loose stools. It may also cause abdominal cramps, nausea, and vomiting.

Diarrhea occurs when the intestines push stools through before the water in them can be reabsorbed by the body. It is the body's way of quickly clearing out any viruses or bacteria. Diarrhea, especially chronic diarrhea, can be a great drain on the nutrition reserves of the body. It can make you exhausted while seriously weakening your immune system, thus exposing you to many other diseases. It also increases the risk of dehydration.

Symptoms or signs

Common symptoms of diarrhea include pain in the lower abdomen, an urgent need to move the bowel, blood, mucus, or pus in the stool, very loose stools, three or more movements a day, and fever.

Causes

According to modern medicine, the most important cause of diarrhea is a viral infection of the colon. This is especially the case with chronic diarrhea. Food allergies are another reason why some people develop diarrhea. For instance, some people are allergic to dairy products, especially milk. The very use of milk can cause diarrhea. Drinking untreated water that contains germs can also cause diarrhea that develops one to four weeks after exposure. Of course, indigestion, viral infection, and emotional upset can also cause it. Also, many medications have proven to be conducive to diarrhea. These include antibiotics, gold compounds, blood pressure drugs, digitalis, anti-cancer drugs, and even high doses of vitamin C. Another common cause of diarrhea is a bad combination of foods. Many foods are incompatible with others. For instance, milk does not go well with orange juice. In the same way, bananas and yams should not be consumed at the same time.

In traditional Chinese medicine, diarrhea is diagnosed as a deficiency in the spleen and stomach qi energy, which disables the body's ability to hold and consolidate wastes.

The main health risk of diarrhea is dehydration. During bouts of diarrhea, the large intestine does not reabsorb all the fluid it should. If diarrhea continues, the body's stores of electrolytes (sodium and potassium) become depleted, leading to severe medical problems.

Prevention and treatment

Diet and physical hygiene are the first lines of defense against diarrhea. Develop a healthy habit of washing your hands with soap before eating. Eat only fresh, well-cleaned foods. Avoid undesirable combinations of foods at the same meal.

Natural therapies

- Avoid fried, spicy, or junk foods, which often aggravate diarrhea.

- Avoid alcohol, which is dehydrating.

- Avoid coffee, milk, salads, and fruit juice, which can aggravate diarrhea.

- Drink as much clean, warm water as possible without upsetting the stomach. This is very important to prevent dehydration.

- Cut beef into small pieces and cook it with some rice for about thirty minutes, creating a porridge. When done, add some fresh ginger juice. Eat as a meal.

- Drink lemon juice with some salt added.

- Drink plenty of warm tea.

- Cook carp with chives and eat.

- Eat raw radishes or drink radish juice.

- Eat raw walnuts.

- Bananas, apples, and pineapple are good fruits that can relieve and stop diarrhea. Bananas are also rich in potassium, so they help replenish electrolytes.

- Short-term fasting is another effective cure. Allow your stomach to rest, drinking only clear liquids for the first twelve hours.

- Cook ginger slices, lean beef slices, and some rice together. Eat it as a meal.

- Begin eating mild food the next day, such as bananas and rice porridge.

- Boil half an ounce of chopped garlic cloves and some brown sugar together. Drink the soup several times a day until you feel better.

- To relieve diarrhea due to a weak spleen, stew one ounce of gingko fruit and an egg together. Eat this once a day. (Diarrhea due to a weak spleen is more a contracted disease, not an outbreak as caused by a poor diet.)

- Eat one peeled crab apple on an empty stomach before each meal.

- Drink two teaspoonfuls of rice vinegar on an empty stomach.

- Fry three tofu cakes in peanut oil over low heat. Add a little salt and some rice vinegar, then boil them for a while. Eat this once a day.

- Chew fresh ginger or sip ginger ale several times a day.

- Fry some dry figs and dry ginger separately for a while. Then boil them together. Eat three times a day to cure chronic diarrhea.

- Fry one ounce of dry guavas, boil them in water and drink. This relieves diarrhea in children.

- Cook two persimmon cakes in water with two ounces of sliced dried orange peel and two ounces of rice. Eat with your meal once a day, for a week, to cure chronic diarrhea.

- Boil a yam with some ginseng for half an hour. Eat the yam and ginseng and drink the soup to treat for chronic diarrhea.

- Boil two cups of rice wine for five minutes. Then add some brown sugar and continue cooking for another two minutes. Drink the wine.

- Practice fasting for at least eight hours, but drink pure, warm water.

- Rub the abdomen many times a day, to strengthen the functions of the stomach and intestines. (See appendix 5.)

- Apply finger pressure to the following acupoints several times a day: Tianshu,

Neiguan, Daheng, Taixi, Qihai, Shenmen, Zusanli, Fenglong, Nuxi, Wailaogong, Zhongwan, Juque, Shangwan, Guanyuan, and Quchi. (See appendix 7.)

Ear Ringing (Tinnitus)

Description

Also known as tinnitus, this disease is marked by rhythmic, continuous sounds generated in the inner ear. The sounds are similar to those of a cicada, and can make the sufferer feel dizzy and even faint in severe cases. This is often a symptom of other health problems, such as a deficiency in kidney function, insomnia, and neurasthenia. Usually, people suffering from tinnitus also have other problems such as insomnia, palpitations, incontinence, or night sweats.

Symptoms or signs

This is typically noise in your ear such as ringing, buzzing, or whistling when there is no apparent source.

Causes

In traditional Chinese medicine, the ear is considered to be related to the kidneys, where the primordial energy is stored. Hence, ear ringing signifies a deficiency of the kidney qi energy. This deficiency can be the result of chronic disease, or loss of sexual essence due to indulgence in sex. Ear ringing can also be caused by unchecked liver fire (excessive anger), cold, excessive phlegm, a blood clot, heavy metal toxicity, food allergies, dysfunction of minute nerve endings in the ear, and low blood sugar.

A high-fat and sugary diet can also be a problem because excess fats cause the red blood cells to accumulate, thickening the blood thus causing ear ringing. Sugary foods do their dirty job by producing phlegm in the body, contributing to ear ringing. However, the most important cause is a deficiency of kidney qi energy.

NOTE: Persistent tinnitus should be investigated by a physician to rule out more serious problems, especially tumors.

Prevention and treatment

Dietary therapies

- Avoid sugar, fats, and processed foods.

- Crush one ounce of sunflower seeds with the shells, add one ounce of rock sugar, and boil in water over low heat. Drink the soup twice a day to help relieve ringing in the ear.

- Cook fresh mussels, a preserved egg, and some rice to make a porridge. Eat it as a meal.

- Boil in pure water the nutmeat of a walnut for half an hour. Add some rock sugar and drink. Do this once a day for two weeks.

- Steam in water a slice of ginseng. Drink the soup and swallow the ginseng.

- Use chrysanthemum to boil tea and drink several cups of it every day.

- Clean and cut a fresh pork kidney. Fry the kidney with chives together in vegetable oil until done. Eat everything as a dish.

- Clean some pork or beef kidneys and slice them up. Lightly fry it with some fresh ginger for five minutes and eat it as meal. Do this once a day for two weeks.

Other natural therapies

- Practice Dharma's internal exercises, particularly "Beat the Heavenly Drum," several times a day. One of these times should be at bedtime. (See appendix 5.)

- Accumulate and swallow saliva. The Chinese sages hold that saliva is a precious natural material capable of maintaining and restoring health while killing many kinds of diseases. In particular, saliva contains some essential substances that can directly make up the vital energy stored in the kidney and effectively relieve any health problems resulting from a deficiency of kidney energy. However, there is a secret on how to save it and effect a cure. First, be reticent. While speech is silver, silence is gold. This way you save your saliva. To facilitate the process of saliva accumulation, the ancient Chinese urge people to put their tongue against the hard upper part of their mouth and remain silent. As the saliva fills the mouth, swish it around in the mouth to further warm it up. Then close your eyes and do some deep breathing, with the mind focused on the center of the lower abdomen (dantian). Divide the mouthful of saliva into three equal portions, and swallow one portion down slowly with each exhalation. At the same time, use your mind to mentally send it to dantian in the lower abdomen. This simple method can work wonders.

- Apply finger pressure to the following acupoints several times a day: Ximen, Yifeng, Tianchuang, Tinggong, Tianyong, Zhongzhu, Waiguan, and Fengchi. (See appendix 7.)

Eyestrain

Description

Modernization has introduced a number of new devices into everyday life such as televisions and computers. Both can be the cause of eyestrain. Every day, at home or in the office, more and more people stare at spreadsheets and e-mails on computer screens, or watch television for hours on end. One of the results of the frequent clash between high technology and natural biology is eyestrain.

Symptoms or signs

A stinging sensation that is often accompanied by blurred vision, dizziness, and sometimes headaches.

Causes

Technically, it is not the eyes themselves that are strained but the two sets of muscle systems that help the eyes function—the ciliary muscles, which control the focusing mechanism, and the eye movement muscles, which point the eyes toward whatever you are looking at. When you gaze at the computer screen or TV, the ciliary muscles tense up and contract, turning the lens into a ball-like shape. When you look at the horizon, the ciliary muscles relax and the lens is flattened. During close-up work, the ciliary muscles are always tense and tire quickly. This is most severe while working with computers because this not only requires concentration of vision, but also forces the eyes to receive electric rays coming out from the terminals, which in itself is enough to damage the eyes.

In traditional Chinese medicine, the eyes are associated with the liver. Therefore, eyestrain is diagnosed to be a deficiency of liver energy and a general weakness of the blood. When blood sugar runs low, all the nerves turn to the liver for a supply of glucose. If the liver itself is in trouble, you can expect the glucose to be in short supply, resulting in eye ailments among other problems. That is why traditional Chinese doctors always examine the liver function when treating eye diseases. A holistic treatment strategy, understandably, starts with building up liver energy and restoring the blood balance.

Prevention and treatment

A good lifestyle and work habits, plus proper nutrition, are the most vital lines of defense. Eyesight is one of the most precious endowments we get from nature. Just ask yourself this question: Would you trade your eyesight for a million dollars? I am sure for most of us, the answer is "no." Unfortunately, too many of us neglect its value and take it for granted until it is too late. Eyesight, like the rest of our body, needs constant maintenance to keep it in good shape. Modern life seems to make it harder and harder for us to maintain this natural endowment. Computer skills are one of the more vital skills as virtually every office/business today is computerized. Television sets have also intruded into almost every aspect of daily life, making eye protection more and more difficult.

To prevent eyestrain and related eye ailments, avoid watching television as much as possible. Close your eyes for two minutes after every half an hour of computer work or intensive reading. Do not look or read for extended periods of time without rest. Practice acupressure on the appropriate acupoints and perform Dharma's internal exercises regularly.

Dietary therapies

- Avoid fried, spicy, and hot foods. Such foods add pressure on the liver, damaging its function. Chinese medical theory holds that the liver needs to be cooled to function at its best. This is known as "balancing the liver." Spicy foods directly affect your eyes, causing tears.

- Eat pig, beef, or chicken livers to enhance eyesight and relieve eyestrain.

- Eat the following foods: carrots, sunflower seeds, fish oil, spinach, cabbage, bilberry fruit, mustard, peanuts, and chestnuts. These can enhance the eyesight and nourish the liver.

- Drink chrysanthemum tea frequently. This helps strengthen the eyesight.

- Eat two papaya a day to help strengthen the eyesight.

- Regularly eat abalone as a dish. This helps strengthen the eyesight.

- Cook bitter gourd with a cuttlefish and eat it as a dish to help strengthen the eyesight.

- Use boiled water to brew a Lingzhi mushroom for a cup of tea. Drink this tea twice a week to help strengthen the eyesight.

- Cook some fresh lean pork with bitter gourd. Eat this dish once a day.

- Eat plenty of fresh vegetables, especially those with a cool nature such as bananas, apples, pears, watermelon, and honeydew melons.

- Stew ten dates, one ounce of Lycium chinese, and two eggs in water for fifteen minutes. Add some rock sugar. Eat the dates and eggs, and drink the soup.

Other natural therapies

- The ancient Chinese ask us to close our eyes for a minute after working for half an hour. Master Wan Laisheng used to teach me to cover my eyes with a dry towel for a minute after reading for half an hour, or to look into the distance, preferably a green landscape, for a while. This served to relax the tension in my eyes and restore the balance of my visual energy.

- The Chinese natural health care system also strongly recommends that you rotate your eyes several times, seven times clockwise and seven times counterclockwise, followed by taking three deep breaths with the mind focused on the lower abdomen. This eye exercise should be done at least twice a day, once in the morning and once at bedtime. It can work like magic—keeping your eyesight clear, your mind sharp, and preventing you from myopia and eyestrain. Its value and importance has greatly increased as a result of our frequent and sometimes forced contact with electronic terminals.

- Rotate the eyes seven times in each direction after every hour of working or reading. (See appendix 5.)

- Each morning after you get up, go outside into the fresh air and take three deep breaths. Rub your hands until they are warm. Then cover both eyes with the warmed hands for thirty seconds while continuing to take deep breaths. Uncover your eyes and look into the distance. (I learned this technique from Master Wan. Many of my students have reported clearly improved eyesight after doing this for one month.)

- If you do not have time to massage your eyes, deliberately blink every now and again. Unconsciously, we all blink once every five seconds. However, when we are focusing intensely on our work, we may not blink often enough. The longer we go without blinking, the more dried and tired our eyes become, leading to eyestrain and myopia.

- Avoid reading on the bus or while walking.

- Make sure that your office is well lit so that your eyes will not become too focused on the computer screen.

- Turn on the light or open up the shades while you are watching television programs. The additional sources of light will serve to divert your eyesight from the television screen, reducing the damage television does to your eyes.

- Get up early in the morning. Do deep breathing while gazing at the mild sun. Hold on and avoid blinking for as long as you can. This is a very exceptional situation, designed for the training of the eyes. The Chinese fathers believe that it is a good idea to stare at the morning sun for a while. The reason for avoiding blinking now is to train your eyesight.

- Apply finger pressure to the following acupoints: Chuanzhu, Fengchi, Hegu, Taiyang, Shangxing, Zanzhu, Meichong, Neiguan, Sibai, Taichong, Yuwei, Meichong, Baixie (Yemen), Daling, Zusanli, Geshu, Jianjing, Jingming, Jujiao, and Xinshu. (See appendix 7.)

Flu

Description

Medically termed influenza, the flu is a viral illness that can occur any time during the year. It often affects many people at the same time due to its highly contagious nature. Characterized by symptoms of fever, muscle aches, and chills, it can last three to four days and can progress to more severe conditions such as pneumonia or even death.

Symptoms or signs

The flu can cause a prominent headache, sore throat, severe aches and pains, chills, sneezing, runny nose, chest discomfort, acute fatigue, coughing, and a moderate to high fever which can last three to four days. Vomiting and diarrhea may also develop.

Causes

While triggered by any number of flu viruses, the real cause is our own weakened immune system as a result of energy depletion. This may be due to overwork, lack of sleep, unhealthy diet, sexual indulgence, emotional disturbance, or lack of exercise. While many people are exposed to the same environment, some people develop the flu and others escape unscathed. The determining factor is our own energy level and immunity. In retrospect, most of us can recall that the flu was usually preceded by fatigue, which is a sign of lowered immunity in our body. Stress is another factor that can increase our vulnerability to the flu and the common cold.

Prevention and treatment

Flu is contracted through personal contact and contaminated air in poorly ventilated areas. In flu season, which most often occurs in the spring and winter, make sure that the room in which you work or live is well ventilated to allow the stale air to be replaced with plenty of fresh air. Also make sure that you do not share eating utensils and towels with other people, but instead keeping these daily necessities in a clean place. Also eat good foods rich in vitamin C, such as fresh vegetables and fruits. Ensure that you get sufficient sleep and rest, and exercise regularly. All of these will strengthen your immunity.

Dietary therapies

- Avoid simple sugars and dairy products. These foods are believed to increase the mucus in the throat and nose, contributing to coughs and nasal congestion.

- Avoid coffee, alcohol, and nonfood additives such as synthetic colors and flavorings. These foods weaken the immune system and increase mucus buildup in the throat and nose.

- If accompanied by a fever, avoid eating, but drink plenty of water and fruit juices.

- Eat a well-balanced, nutritious diet with plenty of green vegetables and fruits.

- Drink at least one glass of pure water every hour. The body requires even more fluid when you have a fever. Fluids help to lower the body's temperature, keep the mucus more liquid, and prevents complications such as bronchitis and sinusitis.

- Chew several cloves of raw garlic each day.

- Drink two glasses of chicken soup a day. This helps build up the body's energy against the disease.

- Boil ten ounces of yellow soybeans in water for ten minutes; add some parsley and boil it again for another ten minutes. Drink the soup and go to bed. Make sure that you are well covered.

- Slice one pound of fresh radishes and soak them in some rice vinegar for two hours and eat.

- Cut or mince some garlic or green onion (the white head part) and forcefully inhale the smell of the vegetable.

- In summer time, if the flu is accompanied by a high fever, eat plenty of watermelon.

- Drink plenty of juice made of oranges, apples, carrots, lemons, or celery.

- Drinking two teaspoonfuls of vinegar every day can prevent and cure the flu. The Chinese believe that vinegar can help prevent the ailment.

Other natural therapies

- Apply finger pressure to the following acupoints several times a day: Taiyang, Waiguan, Yuji, and Saoshang. (See appendix 7.)

- Get extra sleep and rest. Rest is one of the best weapons to fight viruses, because it conserves energy that is needed to fight the virus and restore balance in the body.

Gallstones

Description

The function of the gallbladder is to store the bile salts and cholesterol made in the liver. Bile salts are then discharged into the intestines to help digest fats. These bile salts are produced in response to the amount of fat in the diet requiring digestion. Sometimes these salts can become stones within the gallbladder which cause local inflammation. These stones are an accumulation of crystallized cholesterol. If the muscular gallbladder tries to expel them, a blockage of the bile ducts by the stones may cause severe pain and further inflammation, or even jaundice. This condition is most often found in diabetes patients or obese people, as well as women over forty. A gallstone that causes jaundice is also producing a degree of obstruction that should be seen by a physician promptly.

NOTE: Jaundice can herald several more serious diseases and should be immediately checked by a physician.

Symptoms or signs

These can include yellowish skin, dark urine, clay-colored stools, vomiting, nausea, and intense and sudden pain in the abdomen that may radiate to the shoulders.

Causes

The main causes of gallstones are a heavy intake of foods high in saturated fat and cholesterol, which increase the production of bile salt and body weight, a deficiency in vitamin C, or liver dysfunction. Basically, it is a metabolism problem with the liver.

Prevention and treatment

It is important that any treatment program includes a mechanism of strengthening the liver while removing the gallstones. This is because gallstones are the symptom, while the liver problem is the cause.

- Avoid sugar and sugar-laden foods.

- Avoid high cholesterol foods such as red meat, fried eggs, dairy products, and oils.

- Follow a high-fiber diet. Foods high in fiber absorb and eliminate cholesterol and bile by keeping them soluble and slowing down the process of absorption. Foods of this kind include whole grains, brown rice, bran, legumes, apples, cabbage, and oatmeal.

- Eat plenty of vegetables and fruits. Beet juice and pear juice can be very helpful.

- Avoid fried foods, animal fat, coffee, nuts, and wine.

- Take olive oil or lemon juice three times a day.

- Eat pork, beef, or lamb liver once a day.

Gout

Description
This is a disease marked by pain, swelling, and inflammation in the joints, most often at the base of the big toe. Gout is more common in men, especially those with a high IQ and those who are successful. Gout is characterized by a high uric acid content in the blood. This leaves deposits of uric acid crystals in the fluid around the joints, thus causing the pain.

Symptoms or signs
Symptoms of gout include a raised but variable blood uric acid level, and a sudden onset of severe, recurrent acute arthritis.

Causes
Gout is caused by the body's inability to metabolize proteins from food. Uric acid crystals form in the fluid around the joints, leading the body to release harmful chemicals that result in inflammation and pain in the joints. A poor diet, lack of exercise, and obesity are direct causes of gout. Most cases of gout are inherited.

Prevention and treatment
Dietary therapies
- Avoid alcohol and caffeinated products since they impair the kidney function needed to get uric acid out of the body.

- Avoid foods such as sardines, shrimp, organ meats, fried foods, cream, ice cream, spices, and mushrooms.

- A proper diet should consist of natural, organic foods that are high in fiber. Fiber aids in eliminating uric acid by absorbing bile acids in the kidneys. Eat plenty of vegetables and fruits, vegetable juices, potatoes, and fish.

- Parsley is a natural diuretic, which is good for relieving gout.

- Eat at least one pound of pears a day. Pears relieve kidney inflammation.

- Eat plenty of grapes. They are rich in alkali, which offsets the acidity of uric acid and helps eliminate it from the body.

Gum Disease

Description
Also known as gingivitis, this is a very painful disease that affects the gums, directly limiting your ability to chew, thus causing indigestion and malnutrition problems. It can also affect your sleep and mood, adding greatly to your stress level. If not treated in time, it can lead to the loss of teeth.

Symptoms or signs
Symptoms include swollen, red, painful, and bleeding gums, bad breath, or loose teeth.

Causes
This disease is caused by bacterial plaque in the mouth due to a lack of dental hygiene. Chinese natural health care believes it is mainly caused by an unhealthy diet, with an excess of hot-natured foods such as fried

foods, and hot-natured fruits such as lon-
gong, lichee, and mangos.

Prevention and treatment

Natural therapies

- Brush your teeth with toothpaste after
  each meal.

- Eat green beans soaked in boiling water.

- Mix grounded olives with wood ashes
  and apply this combination to the painful
  gums.

- Eat two mangos everyday to relieve gum
  bleeding.

- To relieve chronic gum bleeding, slice
  some leaf mustard in pure water for
  hours and drink the soup each day.

- Eat two plums to stop gum bleeding.

- Drink a cup of juice made of lotus roots
  to relieve gum bleeding.

- Eat one fresh tomato seasoned with
  honey twice a day.

- Brushing teeth with refined salt can stop
  gum bleeding.

Hair Ailments

Description

By hair ailments I specifically refer to the
conditions of premature graying of the hair
and hair loss. It is a biological rule that sooner or later our hair will turn gray and gradually be lost. However, premature gray hair
and hair fallout that are not part of the aging
process are indications of health problems.

The medical term for hair loss is alopecia.
It is estimated that 30 million American men
suffer from hair loss.[17] While largely a problem for the elderly, alopecia is haunting
more and more young people in their thirties and forties. Patients with alopecia areata
(sudden loss of hair that usually grows back
in six to twenty-four months) lose all the
hair in one small area while the scalp itself
remains normal. Some lose all their body
hair, others lose all of their scalp hair, and
still others suffer from patchy hair loss. It is a
disease to be taken seriously, because hair
loss and heart disease are linked.

According to Dr. Peter Proctor, bald men
are more than three times as likely to suffer a
heart attack than men with a full head of
hair. The link seems to be nitric oxide, a naturally occurring chemical that fosters hair
growth and prevents blood clots.

According to researchers at the Boston
University Medical Center, premature graying of the hair may be an important risk
marker for osteoporosis. In their study, they
found that men and women whose hair
turned gray before the age of forty were six
times more likely to have brittle bones later
in life than people whose hair did not prematurely gray. The explanation states that the
gene that codes for early graying is probably
linked to genes responsible for bone loss.

Symptoms or signs

Symptoms of a hair ailment include hair turning gray prematurely, a sudden, premature loss of hair here and there or over the entire head.

Causes

According to Dr. David A. Whiting, professor of dermatology and medical director of the Baylor Hair Research and Treatment Center in Dallas, Texas, most people lose their hair as a result of a genetic predisposition linked to the hormone dihydrotestosterone, the active form of testosterone.

In traditional Chinese medicine, gray hair and hair loss are diagnosed to be a deficiency in blood and kidney qi energy. This is because the hair is closely related to kidney functions.

Another cause is found in malnutrition. Research indicates that a poor diet is one of the biggest causes of alopecia. Vitamin deficiency is often cited as the reason for hair fallout. Iodine deficiency causes the improper production of thyroxin leading to hair loss. Also, a low iron count, excessive vitamin A intake, as well as an excess salt intake can also lead to hair loss.

Hair loss can also be caused by the use of drugs such as birth control pills and special shampoos. Ironically, in an attempt to arrest the loss of hair, many people resort to hormonal drugs for help. But the use of many hormonal drugs has been shown to be the very cause of hair fallout. This is because while hair growth relies on hormones and testosterone, excess hormones and testosterone can lead to the opposite effect—baldness. Excess shampoo, especially the chemicals it's composed of, is another risk factor.

Smoking may play the same role in hair loss as in heart disease. Smoking damages the linings of blood vessels, constricts them, and hinders blood circulation. Damaged blood vessels produce less nitric oxide, and diminished blood flow weakens hair follicles. As a result, hair becomes gray and lost prematurely.[18]

Another major cause of hair loss is stress. Cases abound in which someone's hair suddenly turned gray after a divorce, death of a spouse, involvement in a lawsuit, or bankruptcy. Worry and stress are known to constrict blood vessels in the scalp, and increase the production of androgens, the male sex hormones that can kill hair follicles. When the hair lacks an adequate nutritional supply provided by blood flow, it withers and falls out just like flowers and grass. The greatest Chinese poet Li Bai said the following more than 1,000 years ago: "I have three thousand feet of gray hair, as a result of stress and endless care." Obviously, stress has been the most common cause of premature aging for people throughout the ages.

Yet another cause is sunburn. Sunburn irritates the skin, and makes the hair shafts more fragile, resulting in aged skin, which in turn lets air leak into the hair follicles so that the hair turns gray. Worse still, some of the hair follicles may lose their reproductive power, and the hair thins and falls away.

Prevention and treatment

Prevention should work at eliminating the risk factors outlined above. Such a program should include a healthy diet that limits the intake of salt and increases the amount of iodine and iron. (If a person is already getting the recommended amounts of iron and iodine, the person can ignore this advice.) Smoking and excess exposure to sunlight should be avoided. The use of shampoos should also be limited. Cultivate an optimistic, easy-going mentality, and conserve the kidney vital energy.

To treat this ailment, practice the following natural methods:

Dietary therapies

- Avoid high-fat and high-sugar foods. Sugar converts to fat in the body and fat causes the glands to overproduce oil, which blocks the hair follicles.

- Stop smoking.

- Increase the calcium intake in your diet. Calcium-rich foods include fish and pork bone soup. To make pork bone soup, cook one pound of fresh pork bones in four cups of water plus two spoonfuls of rice vinegar for about half an hour until the color of the bone soup turns white and thick. Drink the soup on an empty belly. Do this once a day for as many days as you want.

- Regular consumption of sea grasses such as kelp and edible seaweed can help the growth of hair and even restore the color.

- Regular consumption of ginger can promote blood circulation and thus help restore hair growth.

- Regular consumption of pork or beef kidneys can nourish the kidneys and enhance their function.

- Cook two ounces of heshouwu and two eggs in water. Drink and eat everything.

- Eat foods rich in vitamins A, B complex, C, E, and zinc, such as green vegetables, fruit, carrots, tomatoes, spinach, fish oil, egg yolks, animal liver and kidney, wheat germ, yeast, peanuts, beans, fish, oysters, lean meat, and longan.

Other natural therapies

- Reduce your stress level by practicing qigong every day, and by engaging in some recreational activities.

- Frequently comb your hair with your fingers. This will nourish your hair, preventing it from going gray and falling out prematurely, and benefit your overall health.

- Rubbing the head regularly can promote blood circulation in that area.

- Rub your scalp frequently with your own warm urine (use it right after you have urinated). This can slow down loss of hair, and help regain hair on bald parts of the head.

- Learn how to improve your sleep. Regular, sound sleep nourishes the mind and may be the best therapy for premature gray hair.

Halitosis (Bad Breath)

Description

Halitosis is the medical term for bad breath. It can be a sign of either an internal or external problem. Perhaps only traditional Chinese medicine regards this as a reflection of some internal health problems that are more complex than the hygiene of the teeth and gums. Unfortunately, halitosis has a negative psychological and social effect on the patient, in that bad breath can drive away people, including close friends and important business clients. As a result, business is affected, relations become remote, and one's stress increases.

Symptoms or signs

These can include a dry or burning sensation in the mouth which lasts for a week or more, a bad smell when breathing against your palm, cracked lips, slits at the corner of the mouth, ulceration of the mouth's linings, constipation, and rampant tooth decay.

Causes

The most frequently cited causes are dirty-looking teeth, swollen gums, a pasty tongue, a hot and dry mouth, alcohol, and tobacco. Gum inflammation develops when bacteria accumulate on the teeth (plaque) and produce toxins that damage the gum tissues. The damaged gum tissues bleed when you brush your teeth. Tobacco and alcohol both dehydrate the body. By robbing water, they contribute to the bad smell in the mouth.

While these are all true troublemakers, traditional Chinese medicine sees deeper into the problem and concludes that halitosis may be a reflection of stomach and lung problems. It is seen as an imbalance between the yin and yang energy, with the yin side taking the upper hand. This can mean indigestion, liver fire burning (which means that the liver is hot due to a poor diet, such as spicy, fatty, and sugary foods), and even a deficiency in the kidneys. The Chinese believe that eating excessive amounts of spicy foods, or foods with a hot nature causes indigestion and bad breath develops. This is because such foods upset the stomach, leading to fermentation of carbohydrates or the putrefaction of proteins in the digestive system. These, in turn, are picked up in the blood and eliminated through the lungs via the mouth.

A very common cause of chronic halitosis is chronic sinus infection.

Prevention and treatment

Dietary therapies

- Avoid spicy foods such as onions, peppers, and chili.

- Avoid red meat, excess sugar, coffee, and fried foods.

- Avoid tobacco and alcoholic products.

- Eat more fresh vegetables and fruits.

- Drink a glass of light salt water first thing in the morning after you get up.

- Drink a lot of water during the day.

- Eat plenty of pears.

- For headaches accompanied by a toothache and eyestrain, eat more oysters, bananas, barley, yogurt, and watermelon. Also, drink green tea with some mint.

Other natural therapies

- Brush your teeth with toothpaste after each meal.

- Have your teeth professionally cleaned once a month.

- Keep your bowel movements regular and smooth. A bad smell inside the body will be picked up by the stool and cleansed out of the body in a more natural way.

Headache

Description

Some people experience frequent or chronic headaches in the absence of a cold, flu, fever, or other causes. A headache is an ailment which may have different forms. It may distend in character, being localized to a certain part of the head or all over it. The pain may be dull, stabbing, drilling, or pulsating. In terms of length, it may be transient, persistent, or recurring in periodic, sharp spasms. In most cases, headaches are accompanied by varying degrees of restlessness, dizziness, nausea, and ringing in the ears.

Symptoms or signs

Common symptoms are frequent, chronic headaches with no apparent cause, accompanied by restlessness, dizziness, nausea, or tinnitus. Other possible symptoms include loss of appetite, inability to fall asleep, and fatigue as a result.

Causes

There are several hidden causes of headaches that are seldom considered. One is exertion, mainly in the form of working too hard, sitting for too long in front of a computer, or exercising too much. Exertion puts excess pressure on the tiny capillaries that feed the brain. As a result, the Chinese believe these capillaries get blocked, depriving the brain of oxygen and glucose. It is important to remind ourselves that the system of the human body needs exercise, but too much exercise—mental or physical—at one time will cause it to become off balance. This is a sign that too much demand has been put on the internal vital energy before it gets a chance to be replenished, according to the theory of Chinese natural health.

Another cause is desperate sex. Desperate sex is the exact opposite of regulated sex. By desperate sex, I mean sex for sensual pleasure without regard to its long-term, negative impact on health, as is the case in which one squanders away one's precious semen. This is especially the case with men. Surveys show that twice as many men as women suffer from headaches during lovemaking—usually right at the moment of orgasm. This is a classical example of the Chinese saying: "Extreme joy begets sorrow."

The third cause lies in poor nutrition, either by eating unhealthy foods or by frequently skipping meals, usually breakfast. Normally we need three meals a day, as required by the law of nature and warranted by thousands of years of human experience. Constant violations of this rule lower the blood sugar in the body, causing a drain on the vital energy. As a result, not enough blood flows to the head, causing a headache or sense of dizziness.

Another cause can be modern office conditions, such as computer screens, air conditioning, fax machines, and many other kinds of electronic equipment. For one thing, the inaudible sounds emitted by the computer and other electronic office equipment can trigger headaches and increase the levels of stress. Working at a computer screen for too long can also cause headaches.

In traditional Chinese medicine, a chronic headache is diagnosed to be a deficiency in blood and qi energy.

Prevention and treatment

Avoid excess work and pressure. Avoid stress and depression. Stay away from alcohol, cigarettes, soft drinks, and spicy foods. Practice breathing and other soft exercises regularly.

Dietary therapies

- If you have a severe headache, sit down and drink a cup of warm water, or lie down, close your eyes, and take some deep breaths.

- Green vegetables, tomatoes, oranges, and sunflower seeds are good for headaches.

- Drinking a cup of apple juice mixed with celery juice can bring quick relief.

- Eat raw garlic regularly. Garlic can clean up our blood vessels and eliminate toxic wastes in the blood and body, thus relieving the symptoms.

- Stew in water for half an hour the head of a fresh, red silver carp, adding some ginger and salt. Eat everything and drink the soup. Do this once a day for two weeks.

- Drink plenty of orange, lemon, apple, and carrot juices each day.

- Fry some cut coriander in vegetable oil for a couple of minutes. Add salt and water. When the water boils, drop in two eggs, cook them together for a few minutes and eat everything.

- Consume eggs every day. Egg yolk contains rich lecithin and organic cholesterol, nutrients that nourish the brain and build up energy. If this therapy works for you, you should stick with it until the headaches stop.

- Eat fresh radishes or drink radish juice.

- Brew green tea together with some red bayberries. Drink the tea.

- Chew ginseng slices on an empty stomach, or drink ginseng tea. Ginseng is recommended by the ancient Chinese as nourishment for the brain, blood, and qi energy.

- Steam a fish oil capsule and a fresh egg together with crystal sugar.

- Break a fresh egg, preferably a goose egg, and steam it together with a little bit of water and one ounce of rock candy for three to five minutes. Eat it on an empty stomach. Have one to two servings a day.

Other natural therapies

- Knock the back of your head several times a day. (See "Beat the Heavenly Drum" exercise in in appendix 5.)

- Practice qigong twice a day, making sure that the environment is quiet and the air is fresh.

- Apply finger pressure to the following acupoints several times a day: Baihui, Baixie (Yemen), Chengjiang, Waiguan, Shangxing, Hegu, Fengchi, Tianzhu, Fengfu, Qianding, Taichong, Yintang, Hukou, and Taiyang. (See appendix 7.)

Hearing Loss

Description

An estimated 28 million Americans are afflicted with hearing loss. This is a condition characterized by a decrease in one's ability to hear sounds or words. It is frustrating not being able to catch what others say to you or being unresponsive in a conversation. You may be considered confused or uncooperative. If you have to frequently turn up the volume of the television or radio, or if you find yourself frequently asking others to repeat what they have said to you, or if you seem to be mumbling more than you used to, you are most likely afflicted with a hearing loss.

Causes

Most cases involving loss of hearing caused by acute diseases suffered in childhood, such as measles, meningitis, typhoid fever, scarlet fever, and inflammation of the middle ear. Exposure to extremely loud, deafening sounds and the use of some drugs, such as quinine, can also result in loss of hearing. The loss may be gradual.

Prevention and treatment

Scientists find that following a low-fat, plant-based diet keeps the heart healthy may also be responsible for keeping the ability to hear in good condition. A nine-year study conducted in Finland concluded that diet is an important factor in the prevention and even reversal of hearing loss. Researchers discovered that the group of people who mainly consumed unsaturated fats had been found to have much better hearing than those who were ten years their junior but consumed a lot of high-saturated-fat diet.[19]

Natural therapies

- Avoid exposure to loud noises.

- Remove dairy foods from the diet. Chinese believe that such foods can exacerbate the condition.

- Eat fresh peanuts on a regular basis to treat minor hearing loss. The Chinese fathers believe that hearing loss is a symptom of premature aging, and peanuts can prevent premature aging.

- Eat pork kidney as a dish. The Chinese believe that hearing is a function of kidney health, and pork kidney can nourish human kidney.

- Conserve the kidney energy through sexual continence, or better still, through regulated sex.

- Frequently pull and rub your ears since the ears are believed to be linked to the kidneys and, therefore, hearing function.

- Practice Dharma's internal exercise "Beat the Heavenly Drum" several times a day. (See appendix 5.)

- Apply finger pressure to the following acupoints several times a day: Earlobes, Hegu, Waiguan, Quchi, Qihai, Taixi, Zusanli, Huizhong, Zhongzhu, Lianquan, Fengchi, and Yifeng. (See appendix 7.)

Heartburn

Description

Medically known as gastro-esophageal reflux disease (GERD), heartburn is a disease characterized by a painful or burning sensation in the chest or a bitter taste in the mouth. This occurs when the acid in your stomach (gastric acid) backs up into the lower esophagus, the tube that leads from the mouth to the stomach. The acid produces a burning sensation and discomfort between the ribs just below the breastbone. Normally when we eat, our body generates acid to help digest the food. The stomach has a special lining that acts as a shield against this acid, but the esophagus does not have this lining and is very sensitive to gastric acid; that is why we feel the burn when the acid springs up from the stomach.

Symptoms or signs

Symptoms of heartburn include pain or burning in the chest, sour or bitter taste in the mouth, a sore throat, or belching.

Causes

An unhealthy lifestyle is the root evil of heartburn. This includes bad eating habits such as overeating, smoking, drinking alcohol, and eating foods that are irritating to the stomach. A heavy meal can fill the stomach so much that acid can leak from it, especially when you bend over or lie down. Heavy drinking causes your stomach to produce more acid and makes it easier for the acid to overflow back into the esophagus. Foods such as coffee, tomatoes, and citrus juices can also be irritating to your stomach.

Smoking stimulates acid production and weakens your natural defense against acid. Stress can also cause your stomach to produce too much acid. Heartburn can also be a reaction to some medications.

Prevention and treatment

Dietary therapies

- Eat small but more frequent meals. Stop eating when you feel 70 to 80 percent full. Remind yourself everyday of the Chinese motto: "Eighty percent full makes you one hundred percent healthy."

- Avoid alcohol, coffee, tea, and other irritating foods.

- Avoid orange and tomato juices and fatty or fried foods.

- Avoid foods that you find irritating to your stomach or hard to digest.

- Avoid overeating and big meals.

- Avoid eating or drinking for two hours before going to sleep.

- Quit smoking, or at least cut down the amount you smoke.

- Drink plenty of water each day.

- Clean half an ounce of fresh ginger and chop it into small pieces. Put it in a cup of water and boil it for twenty minutes.

Drink it warm. This can calm the stomach and neutralize the stomach acid.

Other natural therapies

- Avoid tight clothing or belts that put extra pressure on the stomach.

- Exercise regularly to control and reduce your weight and prevent obesity. By reducing your weight, you reduce pressure on your stomach at the same time.

- Massage the stomach frequently, accompanied by deep, natural breathing. (See appendix 5.)

- Practice qigong at least twice a day, driving away all stress in the mind. (See appendix 1.)

- Keep a light heart and take it easy.

- Do not lie down after a meal. Acid leaks up more easily when you are in a reclined position. Try to stay upright at least two hours after each meal. Also raise the head of your bed higher than normal.

- Acupress the following acupoints several times a day: Xuanji, Huagai, Yutang, Zigong, Tongli, Zusanli, Sanyinjiao, Shenmen, Neiguan, Tonggu, Daling, Jiuwei, Juque, and Ximen. (See appendix 7.)

Heart Disease

Description

Coronary heart disease is the number one killer in America today, taking over half a million lives each year, and representing about 40 percent of all deaths each year. Already, 58 million Americans have been diagnosed with some form of cardiovascular disease, ranging from congenital heart defects to high blood pressure, to the clogging of the arteries. Countless others have heart disease but do not realize it. Generally speaking, men of any age are more vulnerable to heart disease than women. Currently, half of the American population will develop cardiovascular disease in one form or another during their lifetime.[20]

As we know, the heart is the organ that pumps blood through the arteries. Healthy arteries are elastic and have smooth internal surfaces, ensuring the delivery of blood to various parts of the body. However, if the arteries become hard and the internal surfaces lined with deposits, blood clots will form in these narrowed arteries. This can completely interrupt the flow of blood. In the absence of blood, tissues will die. This is the consequence of heart disease.

Symptoms or signs

Symptoms can include pressure, tightness, fullness, squeezing, or a burning pain in the chest, irregular (extra slow or rapid) heart beat, low blood pressure, pain radiating down the left arm or up the neck, sweating, nausea, vomiting, shortness of breath, anxiety, fainting, or irregular contraction of the heart. Unfortunately, the first indication of heart disease in many people is a heart attack, which is often a fatal symptom.

Causes

This is considered a "disease of civilization." As Western civilization advanced into the twentieth century, it dramatically changed our lifestyle into one characterized by processed foods high in fat and cholesterol, sedentary habits with little need for physical effort, and ever-intensifying stress as a way of a modernized lifestyle.

The result is that lesions of fatty plaque form in the coronary arteries, damaging the lining of the arteries that deliver blood from the lungs to the heart muscle, and obstructing blood flow to the heart. Thus, as the bad cholesterol or fatty deposit accumulates, it causes the muscle cells to migrate inward from the artery walls, mixing with the engorged white cells to form greasy, fibrous plaques, which can harden and crack the artery's lining, causing blood clots to form. A blocked blood flow causes a deficiency of nutrients and oxygen to the muscle tissue, and the pumping heart suddenly falters.

The causes of heart diseases can be any one or more of the following factors:

- Diet: A high-sugar and high-fat diet resulting in an excess intake of cholesterol. Our liver is able to produce all the cholesterol we need. We do not need to take in extra amounts from meat, dairy products, and eggs.

- Obesity: Being overweight causes increased blood pressure leading to excess strain on the heart. People who are 30 percent overweight are prone to heart disease.

- Diabetes: Over the years, a high blood sugar level causes tiny scars to form in the heart muscle, and changes that result in the narrowing and eventual destroying of the smaller arteries that supply the heart with blood. No wonder more than half of people with diabetes die from diseases affecting the heart or blood vessels. Diabetics have about a three times higher chance of being afflicted with heart disease.

- Aging: The older you are, the greater your risk of coronary heart disease. In general, the risk begins to rise in men over forty and in women over fifty.

- Physical inactivity: Physical inactivity, especially when coupled with an unhealthy diet, is bound to lead to excess weight, higher blood pressure, and increased cholesterol levels. This all contributes to poor heart and vascular conditions and a weakened cardiovascular system, thus increasing the risk of heart disease. Studies show that sedentary people are almost twice as likely to develop heart disease as physically active people.

- Hypertension: High blood pressure is believed to contribute to heart disease by damaging the artery walls, making it more susceptible to cholesterol deposits. Hypertension is a sure sign that the heart is working too hard. Thus, it has to push blood against greater pressure. Even slightly higher blood pressure can affect the function of the heart over time. This may well be the most important risk factor in both heart attacks and stroke.

- High cholesterol: Two types of cholesterol exist in our body: good cholesterol (high density lipoprotein, or HDL) and bad cholesterol (low density lipoprotein, or LDL). While both kinds of cholesterol are normal in the blood, excessively high levels of LDL create cholesterol deposits on the artery walls, causing plaque formation and narrowing of the vessels. The higher the LDL level, the greater the chance of heart disease.

- Smoking: Cigarette smoking plays a notorious role in heart disease, causing more than 100,000 American deaths each year because of damages inflicted on the coronary arteries. Tobacco use directly affects your whole circulatory system, and leads to a decrease of oxygen supply in the blood. It also causes cellular damage, resulting in increased oxidation of the tissues, which in turn leads to increased plaque formation. This is largely because cigarettes contain carbon monoxide, which can deprive the heart of the oxygen it needs to function properly. Smoking causes the blood vessels to narrow, which increases the risk of heart attack and stroke. It is a major risk factor for heart disease. Already it accounts for 21 percent of all deaths from coronary heart disease. Smokers have two to four times as high a risk of heart attacks as nonsmokers.

• Stress: Stress adds pressure to your heart, raises blood pressure, exacerbates high cholesterol levels, lowers your immunity, and secretes large amounts of kidney hormones, which pile up in the blood vessels.

• Genetic background: A close relative in your family who has or has had a history of heart disease will increase your own risk.

• Magnesium deficiency: This can lead to high blood pressure and an increase in calcium along the muscle cells of the arteries. Magnesium is also important for the control of an irregular heart beat.

In summary, it is the consequence of a lifetime of bad habits.

Prevention and treatment

Maintaining the health of the heart is, arguably, the single most essential component to a long, healthy life. Therefore, prevention is the first line of defense against heart disease.

First of all, quit smoking as soon as possible and avoid secondhand smoke. Cigarettes decrease the oxygen supply in your blood, thus leading to increased heart damage.

Watch your weight and keep it down if necessary. This is more important than re-

ducing the cholesterol level in your body. Being overweight increases the blood pressure and puts excessive strain on the heart. Control your body weight through proper diet, which means eating only low-fat, low-cholesterol foods such as vegetables and fruits, wholesome grains and bread. You should also replace red meat with fish, remove poultry skin before eating, and limit yourself to no more than two eggs a week. Fruits and vegetables are rich in magnesium and bioflavonoids, which can help reduce arteriosclerotic plaques and decrease the risk of heart attack and stroke. Of particular help are the following foods:

• Pineapple contains bromelain, a form of proteolytic enzyme shown to be able to decrease the risk of blood clots and break down the formation of fibrin in the blood.

• Strawberries contain flavonoids which are conducive to increased coronary blood flow, decreased blood pressure and heart rate, and improved contractility of the heart.

• Grapes contain resveratrol, a substance capable of reducing cholesterol as well as preventing and decreasing arterosclerotic plaque.

• Green tea contains flavonoids catechins capable of lowering cholesterol, preventing platelet aggregation and therefore heart disease and stroke.

- Ginseng contains ginsenosides and sterols shown to be able to lower blood pressure, reduce cholesterol, and pacify the heart.

Dietary therapies

Diet is the single most important factor for the prevention of heart disease, since an unhealthy diet is the greatest cause of heart disease. A good diet is one that is low in saturated fat such as fruits and vegetables and whole grains and legumes. A low-fat diet and other lifestyle changes may actually reverse the progress of heart disease and help reopen arteries that are clogged.

- Avoid eating and drinking too much at one time.

- Limit the intake of salt, high-fat, and high-sugar foods such as desserts, chips, and soft drinks. Such foods easily convert to glucose and thus cause weight gain.

- Limit the intake of high-cholesterol foods such as red meats, eggs, animal brain and liver, fish eggs, and so on. Chicken is a much better alternative to red meat, but make sure that you remove the skin before you eat it. Eat no more than four eggs a week.

- Avoid coffee and alcohol.

- Drink green tea. Green tea has been shown to prevent arteriosclerosis. This is believed to be the reason why the rate of heart disease is much lower among the Japanese who smoke more than people living in other industrialized countries.

- Follow a plant-based diet with plenty of fresh vegetables and fruits every day.

- Eat plenty of potatoes. This is because potatoes contain rich potassium, a mineral which can regulate your heart rate and lower your blood pressure.

- Stew seven ounces of fresh sea slug with two ounces of rock sugar for thirty minutes. Eat it for breakfast.

- Drinking a cup of beer or grape wine each day can be good for your heart.

- Cook twenty lotus seeds, ten longangs, twenty peach kernels or walnut meats, and ten wide jujubi kernels (dates) together. Eat everything except the kernels and drink the soup once a day.

- The following foods are highly recommended for diabetes patients: rice soup, porridge made of rice and red dates, oatmeal porridge, milk, fish, and grape wine.

- Cook boneless fish slices together with rice to make a porridge for a meal.

- Eat plenty of soy products such as tofu and soy beverages. Soy contains a number of phytonutrients that can help reduce the risk of heart disease.

- Whole grains and nuts are considered healthy foods for heart disease, because these foods contain rich vitamin E, which can slow the oxidation of LDLs so they will be less likely to stick to the coronary artery walls. Oatmeal and whole-wheat bread should be staple foods for patients of heart disease.

- Eat whole-grain bread, bran, wheat germ, and oysters regularly. These foods contain plenty of chromium, a mineral that can help cut down on plaque buildup in the arteries.

- These foods are also beneficial to the heart: garlic, ginger, celery, carrots, bananas, bitter gourd, red beans, lotus seeds, sunflower seeds, currents, blueberries, cayenne pepper, olives, and sunflower seeds.

- Cook eggs in water for ten minutes with some tea, mint, and salt to make "tea eggs." Eat one egg a day.

- Fry some pork heart, soy sprouts, and hotbed chives together to make a dish. Eat it once or twice a week. Hotbed chives are yellow and taste better. It is a common dish in China.

- Eat pineapple daily. Pineapple contains bromelain, a form of proteolytic enzymes, which can reduce the risk of blood clots.

- Eat plenty of grapes. Grapes have been shown to have a nourishing effect on the heart muscles and valves as well as the blood cells.

- Regularly eat sea grasses such as edible seaweed, kelp, and bladderwrack. These sea vegetables largely pass through the body undigested, thus purifying the bloodstream, and eliminating the lower density cholesterol from the heart walls.

- Eat more seafood and fish instead of red meat. Fish and seafood are low in saturated fat, lower in calories, but high in vitamins, minerals, and protein. Most important, fish oil can prevent heart attacks and reduce the risk of heart disease. When scientists induced heart attacks in laboratory rats, they found that those on a diet high in fish oil had fewer heartbeat irregularities associated with the attacks.

- Eat plenty of nuts such as walnuts, peanuts, almonds, and cashews. Nuts may lower bad cholesterol and help keep the arteries clear. Therefore, eating nuts four times a week can cut the risk of heart disease by a quarter, according to researchers at Loma Linda University in California. The researchers found that women who ate nuts more than twice a week could cut their heart trouble by 60 percent.

- Drink a cup of honey water twice a day.

- Cook two ounces of small red beans in water until beans are fully softened like a porridge. When it is ready, add in some brown sugar. Eat it as a meal, once every other day.

- Cook two ounces of lotus seeds in water until the seeds are fully softened like a porridge. When it is ready, add some rock candy and sesame oil. Eat as a meal.

- Steam in water ten walnuts and ten dates for thirty minutes. Add some honey. Drink and eat everything.

- Regularly eat a porridge or tea made of lotus root starch. Add some honey into it.

- Boil one ounce of hawthorn fruit slices in water and drink it as a tea daily.

- Boil yellow soybeans in water for one hour. Add a little salt for seasoning and eat. Do this every day.

- Boil some hawthorn fruits in water; add some sugar and eat it every day.

- Eat eggplant regularly. Eggplant contains vitamin P or bioflavonoids, which can prevent the hardening of blood vessels and is helpful in the treatment of arteriosclerosis and heart disease.

- There is more evidence that vitamin C benefits the artery linings, helping the blood vessels relax and widen.

- Drink some red wine every other day. Moderate consumption of red wine has been shown to prevent arteriosclerosis.

- Eat high-fiber foods to absorb and eliminate cholesterol in the body. Foods rich in fiber include whole grains, raw vegetables, beans, nuts, fruits with peels, beets, carrots, and so on.

Natural therapies

Exercise increases the arterial circulation and thus protects and enhances the heart. Exercises strengthen the heart muscle and makes it more effective in extracting oxygen from the blood. Traditional Chinese soft exercises are particularly good. The rhythmic movement and deep breathing improve the health of the cardiovascular system, increases stamina, helps reduce body fat and weight, decreases total cholesterol, and lowers blood pressure and the sugar level in the blood. Also, such moderate exercises are excellent stress relievers. While moderate exercise is very helpful to the health of the heart, strenuous exercise is harmful. This is because they raise the blood pressure and put excess pressure on the heart muscle and oxygen supply.

The ancient Chinese believed that the palm of the hand was intimately associated with the functioning of the heart. Therefore, rubbing your hands frequently (five times a day, three to five minutes each time) can help prevent heart disease and relieve the symptoms.

- Practice qigong twice a day. Qigong can greatly reduce stress, promote blood circulation, and enhance your immunity and digestion. While practicing qigong, imaginatively guide your qi to focus on your heart. This will greatly facilitate the healing process. (See appendix 1.)

- Practice sound qigong by making the sounds of "Zhen," "Xu," "Ha," and "Deng." (See appendix 3.)

- Massage the chest several times a day according to the principles described in Dharma's internal exercises. (See appendix 5.)

- Keep regular habits to ensure you get enough sleep each day. Go to bed early and get up early. Take a short nap after lunch whenever possible.

- Learn healthy mental discipline methods so as to maintain a light heart, reduce stress, and go easy with life. Excess stress will increase the chances of heart disease or aggravate the situation if you have one.

- Apply finger pressure to the following acupoints several times a day, two to three minutes each time: Tongli, Yutang, Neiguan, Shenmen, Ximen, and Danzhong. (See appendix 7.)

Hemiplegia

Description
This disease is characterized by a sudden paralysis of one side of the body with a twisted or crooked mouth and eye, stiff tongue, and sluggish speech. The paralysis is spastic, although flaccid in the early stages. It may be accompanied by an entire or partial loss of motion and sensation.

Symptoms or signs
Symptoms include sudden weakness or numbness in the hand or leg, sudden dimness or loss of vision, particularly in one eye, sudden difficulty speaking, dizziness, unsteadiness in standing or walking, an extended tongue that bends to one side, and a slanting head that leans to one side.

Causes
Traditional Chinese medicine holds that hemiplegia is mainly due to a deficiency of qi and blood with yin-yang derangement of the heart, liver, spleen, and kidney. It is further aggravated by stress and depression, alcohol use, an unhealthy diet, and indulgence in sex.

In most cases, hemiplegia is triggered by cerebro-vascular accidents, but it can also be caused by other brain diseases or injuries. When a blood clot obstructs a cerebral artery, hemiplegia happens, just like a stroke.

NOTE: For those who are experiencing symptoms, see your physician or go to an emergency room immediately. Therapies listed here are meant to be supplementary measures—not first aid.

Natural therapies

- Eat two ounces of unshelled fresh peanuts, including the skin, three times a day for one week.

- To remove an obstruction from a collateral (branch of a channel) and promote blood circulation, press the following acupoints: Quchi, Jianyu, Hegu, and Zusanli. (See appendix 7.)

- Learn mental discipline and keep anxiety and anger at bay.

Hemorrhoids

Description
Hemorrhoids are the inflammation and swelling in the veins around the anus. They may be inside or outside the anus. Straining to pass hard, compacted stools irritates these veins, causing severe pain and bleeding.

Symptoms or signs
Symptoms include itching, tenderness, pain, or bleeding in the rectal area; and possibly a small lump at the anal opening.

Causes
Hemorrhoids are dilated veins, which can be associated with poor blood flow. When there is a slowed flow of blood in the veins around the anus, painful blood clots may develop. This is a particular type of hemorrhoids called "thrombosed hemorrhoids." The majority of hemorrhoids do not become thrombosed however.

The most common cause of hemorrhoids is an unhealthy lifestyle. This includes chronic, excessive alcoholic consumption; irregular eating habits; excess consumption of fatty, spicy, or fried foods; insufficient intake of high-fiber foods such as vegetables, fruits, and whole grains; sedentary lifestyle; walking long distances while carrying a heavy load; and a short temper. Obesity can also slow down the blood flow. Another risk factor is constipation, which leads to irritation and inflammation as the hard stool passes through the rectum and anus. Pregnancy also increases the risk of hemorrhoids. Indulgence in sexual pleasures, pneumonia, and a weakened body after a long illness are also risk factors that the Chinese believe need to be kept a close eye on.

Prevention and treatment
Regular exercise is the best prevention, because it keeps the body toned and the blood flowing briskly. Stand up every half an hour to an hour and exercise, such as some light walking.

Another preventive measure is to clean the anal area every day before going to bed. This is best done through a hot bath, which not only decreases the risk of inflammation, but also increases blood flow and the healthy development of tissues. Equally important is to eat a high-fiber diet, which includes plenty of fresh vegetables, fruits, and whole grains.

Dietary therapies
- Avoid highly sugared and refined foods such as white bread and cookies. Such foods stress the body and cause tension in the organs, muscles, and glands, and disturb the metabolism process.

- Avoid alcohol, smoking, and spicy, fatty, and fried foods.

- A high-fiber and low-sugar diet is recommended for the prevention and relief of hemorrhoids. Fiber is essential for the digested material to have enough bulk to cause a bowel movement. Fiber enhances the absorption of fluid into the stools, thus making them easier to evacuate.

- These foods are highly recommended for the condition: green beans, oranges, walnuts, papaya, figs, and persimmons.

- Steam five dried persimmons and eat them in the morning.

- Drink a lot of water and orange juice each day.

- Drink plenty of juice made of celery, carrots, or spinach. Such juices contain rich organic sulfur, iron, and calcium, and can help eliminate the sticky wastes from clogging anal capillaries, and benefit the colon and intestines.

- Eat one or two bananas, with peel, on an empty stomach first thing in the morning.

- Peel two bananas and cut them into pieces. Stew the banana together with two ounces of rock candy for twenty minutes. Eat the banana and drink the soup.

- Eat one to two figs on an empty stomach fist thing in the morning.

- Cook two ounces of day lily in water together with some brown sugar. Drink it in the morning on an empty stomach. Do this for four days. The day lily can be fresh or dried.

- Cook pork lung and eat it as a dish. This can relieve any bleeding resulting from hemorrhoids.

- Fry lean pork meat in vegetable oil with towel gourd, add some salt, and eat.

- Soak five dried persimmons in water for an hour. Stew them with two ounces of rock candy for forty minutes. Drink and eat everything once a day, for five days.

- Cook some freshwater mussels together with some lean pork meat to make a dish.

- Cook spinach and pork blood together to make a dish, add some sesame oil, and eat.

- Stew four ounces of fresh fish maw (white sticky part attached to the fish meat) or two ounces of dried fish maw in water with three ounces of rock sugar. Eat it on an empty stomach.

- Steam two ounces of dried figs in an adequate amount of water with three ounces of lean pork. Eat it once a day for two weeks.

- Eat two fresh figs in the morning and evening to alleviate pain and bleeding from hemorrhoids.

- Boil some fresh olives in water together with some ginger. Drink the juice three times a day.

- Fig leaves used externally are also very good in treating hemorrhoids. Cook the leaves in water for about half an hour, then pour the "soup" into a pan to cool a bit. Use the warm soup to gently wash the anal area.

- Take ten fresh figs and some water and bring to a boil, then simmer over low heat for half an hour. Eat them up in two servings, with about three hours in between.

- Cook some freshwater mussels together with some lean pork. Eat the dish.

- Clean and slice one eggplant, and mix it with some sesame oil and salt. Stew for thirty minutes and eat.

- Boil one ounce of black fungus with twenty red dates over low heat. Eat once a day for two weeks.

- Use some peanut oil to fry up eight ounces of clams and add some sliced fresh ginger and water. Simmer until the clams are soft. Add a little salt. Eat it one hour before a meal, preferably after dinner. Do this once a day for one week.

- Peel two bananas and steam them with an adequate amount of brown sugar and water. Eat twice a day for seven days.

- Boil two persimmon cakes until very soft. Eat them twice a day.

- Cook black fungus until very soft and eat it as a soup to relieve hemorrhoids.

- Eat cooked wax gourd on regular basis.

- Eat raw water chestnuts twice a day. Or drink a mixture of water chestnut juice and rice wine daily.

- To stop anal bleeding, grind into powder some cuttlefish bones. Swallow two spoonfuls of the powder each morning before breakfast with warm water. (The best cuttlefish bones are those taken out of dried cuttlefish, which is available at a Chinese food market or in a Chinese herbal store.)

Other natural therapies

- Practice qigong three times a day. Let the air travel down to the abdomen area and cause movement in that area. Qigong has been proven to strengthen the muscles in the anal area and enhance the system. (See appendix 1.)

- Do not sit for more than thirty minutes at a time. Sitting for too long restricts blood flow to the anal area.

- Try not to strain during bowel movements. Try to take it easy and never hold your breath.

- Take warm baths, especially sitz baths of hot water, to soak the anal area.

- Wear cotton underwear and loose clothing.

- Practice anal contracting and relaxing exercises several times a day.

- Frequently massage the calves of the leg. Chinese fathers believe that this can help relieve hemorrhoids.

- Apply finger pressure to the following acupoints regularly: Erbai, Huiyin, Baihui, Tianshu, Neiguan, Zusanli, Xialian, Chengshan, and Changqiang. (See appendix 7.)

Hiccups

Description

Hiccups are due to a spasm contraction of the diaphragm. This involuntary reflex action happens in two stages. First, the diaphragm contracts sharply when the phrenic nerves become irritated. Then, as soon as you inhale, your larynx snaps shut, making a clicking sound known as a hiccup.

Symptoms or signs

If you experience repeated, uncontrollable contractions of your diaphragm resulting in clicking sounds, you have the hiccups.

Causes

Hiccups are often caused by eating too fast or too much, a sudden inhalation of cold air, stimulation of the intestines, or emotional upset. They also occur in elderly people of weak physique, during a chronic or severe disease, after a surgical operation, or during a heart attack.

Prevention and treatment

Avoid eating too quickly or talking while eating. Try not to mingle water with food while swallowing. To relieve hiccups, try the following natural methods.

Dietary therapies

- Mix half rice vinegar and half cold water and drink slowly.

- Mix two spoonfuls of fresh ginger juice with a cup of warm milk. Add some sugar and drink.

- Drink several spoonfuls of lemon juice with some salt added to it.

- Cook several persimmons in water. Drink the soup.

- Drink a cup of fresh chive juice.

- Take one ounce of fresh ginger and squeeze out the juice. Mix it with some honey and drink.

- Boil one ounce of sword beans in water and eat as a soup.

- Burn some hair of a goose. Use warm water to swallow the ash of the goose hair.

- Chew a fresh ginger slice.

Other natural therapies

- Massage the abdomen and calves of the legs. My teacher told me that this will relieve hiccups.

- Press the following acupoints several times a day, two to three minutes each time: Tiantu, Zusanli, Tianshu, Zhongwan, Shanzhong, Tianzhong, Taichong, Quepen, and Neiguan. (See appendix 7.)

High Cholesterol

(See "Cholesterol, High.")

Hoarseness

Description

This ailment is characterized by the inability to speak in a normal tone of voice. The sound one makes is either hoarse or too soft to be heard by others, no matter how hard one tries to talk. This is often accompanied by pain in the vocal cords and throat. In most cases, the vocal cords have been hurt, and the lost voice usually takes days, sometimes weeks, to fully recover. For some people, this can be a very embarrassing situation. Just imagine the plight of political leaders who lost their voices in the heat of their campaign, or a singer unable to perform at some important event. You can guarantee they are willing to try whatever methods are available to recover their voice.

Symptoms or signs

Any abnormal voice change can be a symptoms of this ailment. When hoarse, the voice may sound breathy, raspy, strained, or there may be changes in the volume (loudness) or pitch (how high or low the voice is).

Causes

The most common cause of this ailment is talking for long periods. This is typical of public speakers, political leaders, singers, and sometimes school teachers. Occasionally, these people speak for long stretches and, at times, at the top of their voices, literally making themselves hoarse. In traditional Chinese medicine, this is diagnosed to be an excess loss of qi energy as a result of excessive speaking. In fact, the ancient Chinese often warned people against excess speaking as an essential part of natural health, for they strongly held that speaking too much would hurt one's precious qi energy. They also believe that certain hot-natured, spicy foods can also cause hoarseness of voice.

Another common cause of hoarseness of voice is found in acute laryngitis, which usually occurs due to swelling on the vocal cords from a common cold or upper respiratory tract viral infection. It should be pointed out that smoking is also a major cause of hoarseness. Sometimes, allergies or trauma to the voice box can lead to hoarseness, too.

Prevention and treatment

Natural therapies

- Avoid hot-natured foods such as fried or spicy foods.

- Slightly cook a whole egg. Take it out as soon as the water boils. Eat the egg white until all the white is gone. This method can cure loss of voice and hoarseness due to excessive speaking. This treatment has been in existence for quite a while in China.

- Clean ten to fifteen pieces of *Fructus scaphigerae* fruit. Put them in a cup and brew them in boiling water with some rock sugar for twenty minutes. Drink the tea three times a day.

- Take a fig and cook it with two ounces of rock sugar. Drink the soup and eat the fig.

- Peel one or two pears and cut them into pieces. Steam them together with some rock candy and a little bit of water for ten minutes. Eat and drink everything.

- Cook three ounces of fresh soybean dregs—the white remains of soybeans in the process of making tofu—for a few minutes. Season it with three spoonfuls of honey. Eat it once a day until the voice is recovered. This is good for either loss of voice or a hoarse voice.

- Clean and cut into pieces an equal amount of both water chestnuts and carrots. Cook them together in water for twenty minutes and eat.

- Drink plenty of carrot juice or the combination of carrot juice and apple juice.

- Drink plenty of celery juice.

- Mix some hawthorn fruit and green tea together and brew them with boiling water for ten minutes. Drink the tea and eat the fruit.

- Soak one ounce of tremella in water for an hour. Add some rock sugar and stew the tremella for another hour. Drink the soup and eat the tremella.

- Eat fresh radishes raw, or drink a lot of radish juice.

- Take a fresh egg and make two small holes on both sides of it. Suck and swallow the entire egg through one hole. Do this every morning for a week.

- Eat plenty of watermelon.

- Put your tongue against the upper palate as much as possible, so as to accumulate saliva in the mouth. Once your mouth is full of saliva, close your eyes, do some breathing exercises, accumulate saliva in the mouth, and finally swallow it down in three small mouthfuls.

- Press the following acupoints several times a day: Shousanli, Chengjiang, and Kongzui. (See appendix 7.)

Hypertension

Description

Hypertension is another name for high blood pressure. It means the blood is travelling through the arteries at a pressure that is too high for good health, putting increased pressure on the heart and arteries. It is estimated that nearly 60 million Americans have high blood pressure.

Under ideal conditions, your blood pressure reading should be 120/90. The upper reading is called systolic. It occurs when the pressure of your blood against the artery walls is higher than normal as the heart contracts and forces blood through the circulatory system. The lower reading is called diastolic and occurs when the heart fills with blood and the blood pressure is at its lowest. This is also known as the resting state. The diastolic reading is more significant since the heart and the arteries are in the expansion phase most of the time. When your blood pressure exceeds 140/90, you are diagnosed with hypertension.

Although high blood pressure itself is not necessarily a bad thing, it can damage the heart, kidneys, and blood vessels. This is because when blood pressure rises, the increased power of the blood pounding against the artery walls makes them swollen or crooked over time, slowly choking off blood flow to the kidneys, heart, brain, and eyes. Eventually, the condition increases the risk of heart attack, stroke, kidney failure, and serious eye ailments. More than half of the individuals who have experienced angina pectoris, an aneurysm, or intracerebral hemorrhage have hypertension. When hypertension combines with obesity, smoking, or diabetes, the risk of heart attack or stroke increases several times.

Symptoms or signs

These can include a persistent elevated blood pressure over 130/85, dizziness, especially when climbing up to high places, headaches, ear ringing, sweating, a feeling of pressure in the head and being lifted up while walking, blurred vision, insomnia, palpitations, shortness of breath, amnesia, numbness in the fingers, a sense of stuffiness in the chest, and irritability and lassitude. In severe cases, there may be difficulty in breathing, nausea, vomiting, and even shock.

Causes

High blood pressure is caused by a constriction of blood vessels. As blood vessels tighten, the blood has difficulty passing through. This puts pressure on the heart, which is the measure of blood pressure. The single biggest cause of hypertension is an unhealthy lifestyle: a diet that is high-fat, high-salt, high-sugar, high-sodium, and low-fiber; lack of exercise; smoking; and drinking.

As is now clear, fat raises blood pressure by increasing the thickness of the blood and the weight of the body, and by stimulating hormones that cause the blood vessels to constrict. The case is worsened by a lack of sufficient exercise, which causes fat to store up inside the body and slow down the metabolic process. Hence, obese and overweight people are highly susceptible to hypertension.

Smoking and drinking can significantly elevate the blood pressure and greatly increase the chance of a stroke. Smoking constricts all arteries and capillaries, causing the heart to pump harder to force blood through them.

Consumption of alcohol destroys liver cells which produce chemicals that act as a check on blood pressure.

Stress is another important cause of hypertension. It, along with depression, can increase the adrenaline production leading to hypertension. Stress also constricts blood vessels in your arms and legs while increasing your heart rate. Stress and emotional stimulation can disturb the regulatory function of the vessels in the cerebral cortex, increasing the pressure on the vessels and thus the blood pressure.

Recently, it has been suggested that a deficiency of calcium may be yet another cause of hypertension. The Framingham Heart Study, which tracked 432 men for eighteen years, found that those who consumed the highest levels of calcium had a 20 percent lower risk of developing hypertension than those who consumed the lowest levels.

Environmental factors loom larger and larger as a cause of hypertension. Dr. Ron Kennedy suggests that the toxic heavy metals in the air we breathe and the water we drink are one of the major causes.[21] According to Dr. Kennedy, patients of hypertension have been shown to have toxic cadmium levels four times greater than people with normal blood pressure.

Normally, blood pressure tends to increase with age. Surveys also find that until the age of fifty-five, men have a higher risk of developing hypertension than women. However, after sixty-five, women have a greater risk of developing hypertension than men.

Prevention and treatment

Since weight loss has the greatest significance in controlling hypertension and lowering blood pressure, regular exercise on a daily basis is especially important. Studies based on clinical surveys in China show that regular practice of qigong and Dharma's internal exercises, combined with sufficient sleep, a healthy diet, and mental discipline to manage stress, can all successfully prevent and treat hypertension.

Dietary therapies

- Eliminate all or significantly reduce alcohol, coffee, soft drinks, and sugary, salty, spicy, fatty, and processed foods such as pork, hot pepper, mustard, desserts, and so on.

- Strictly limit the intake of red meat.

- Stop smoking, or at least significantly reduce the amount you smoke, and avoid secondhand smoke.

- Avoid foods with high cholesterol levels such as egg yolk and animal livers and kidneys.

- Eat plenty of fresh vegetables and fruits.

- Sea grass and kelp are effective in reducing blood pressure.

- Cook celery and twenty red dates together to make a dish. Eat it once a day. This can effectively lower the blood pressure.

- Regularly drink tea made of chrysanthema to lower blood pressure.

- Put tomatoes in some boiling water. Peel the tomatoes and eat them.

- Stew seven ounces of fresh sea slug with two ounces of rock sugar for thirty minutes. Eat it for breakfast.

- Clean and slice one eggplant, mix it with some sesame oil and salt. Stew for thirty minutes and eat.

- Cook some fresh mussels, a preserved egg, and some rice together to make a porridge. Eat it for supper.

- Cook some fresh kelp and green beans in water for an hour. Eat them as a meal.

- Fry together over moderate heat some fresh scallops, celery, onion, garlic cloves, water chestnuts, and tomato. This dish is especially effective for persistent hypertension defiant to other treatments.

- Yams or sweet potatoes are especially effective in lowering blood pressure and keeping it at a normal level.

- Use vegetable oils such as sesame, peanut, and corn oil instead of animal-based oils to reduce the level of cholesterol.

- Drink plenty of lemon, orange, apple, celery, beet, and carrot juices.

- Eat fresh bitter gourd and/or towel gourd once a day as a meal. These vegetables are especially effective in reducing blood pressure. To prepare, take out the seeds and cut the gourd into small pieces. Slightly fry it in olive oil and then steam it in some water for two minutes. Eat the dish as a meal.

- Eat garlic, fish oils, celery, hawthorn fruits, and persimmons. Green tea can help a lot, too.

- Take in more calcium (abundant in dairy products and sardines) and magnesium (rich in soybeans and almonds).

- Garlic, onions, watermelon, and cucumbers are good, natural diuretics.

- Boil fifteen ounces of dried peanut plants in water to make a tea. Drink a cup daily for three weeks.

- Eat plenty of bananas each day—at least seven.

- Eat plenty of sea vegetables such as bladderwrack and nori.

- Use chrysanthemum to boil tea. Drink several cups each day.

- Drink a cup of cool honey water together with some sesame oil each morning after getting up and before breakfast.

- Soybeans are very helpful for hypertension. Soak half a pound of soybeans in water overnight, then boil them in water for thirty minutes the next day. Drink the soup and eat the beans as a meal. This helps reduce cholesterol levels.

- Eat one or two ounces of sunflower seeds or pumpkin seeds each day. Eat them in fresh or slightly fried forms.

- Soak two ounces of peanuts in a cup of vinegar overnight. In the morning, drink the vinegar and eat the peanuts. Repeat this for two weeks, once a day.

- Take one pound of fresh celery and squeeze out the juice. Mix the juice with some honey and slightly warm it. Divide it into two equal servings, drinking it one hour before lunch and dinner. The Chinese theory holds that celery can cure hypertension because it affects on the liver and therefore the blood system.

- Eat one to two fresh tomatoes on an empty stomach first thing in the morning for two weeks.

- Chop one pound of water chestnuts and one pound of radishes. Squeeze out the juice and drink it with some honey twice a day.

- Boil seaweed and some rice together with mung beans to make a meal.

- Boil one ounce of hawthorn fruit slices in water and eat as a soup daily. Hawthorn fruit can digest fat and prevent it from entering the blood stream by getting rid of it through bowel movements. Traditionally, the Chinese use it in cooking to facilitate the softening of meat and chicken.

Other natural therapies

- Keep a light heart and a regular daily schedule. Avoid anger and other emotional stimulation.

- Practice Dharma's morning exercises each day before breakfast. (See appendix 4.)

- Reduce the frequency of your sexual activity. Sex has been shown to accelerate the heart rate and elevate blood pressure. Too much sex could worsen the case.

- Practice qigong every day. Qigong has been proven to be very effective in lowering the blood pressure and stress level. This is because in the Chinese natural health care system, qi is held to be the driving force of blood. Qigong exercise, by means of inducing the qi to flow downward through the body, lowers the blood pressure. Scientific observation shows that patients with hypertension have their arteries expand during and after qigong exercise, meaning that their blood pressure has been lowered. (See appendix 1.)

- While doing qigong, think of the acupoint Yongqiong at the center of the soles. Focusing your mind on this acupoint while doing qigong can double the effect of lowering blood pressure. It is held by the ancient Chinese to be able to lower the heart fire and blood pressure. (See appendix 7.)

- Practice sound qigong and make the sounds of "Ha," "Xu," or "He." (See appendix 3.)

- Massage both soles several times a day, preferably after a warm foot soak.

- Frequently pull the ears with your fingers in both directions, i.e., up and down.

- Frequently contract and release the toes. The ancient Chinese say this exercise has multiple therapeutic effects, including lowering blood pressure and boosting sexual vitality.

- Take a warm, not hot, bath. It is highly recommended for the sake of inducing the blood to flow down the body.

- Apply finger pressure to the following acupoints several times a day, two to three minutes each time: Baihui, Fenglong, Earlobes, Fengchi, Guanyuan, Fengfu, Hegu, Qihai, Quchi, Shenmen, Hukou, Taichong, Zusanli, Fengchi, Taiyang, Yongquan, Yintang, and Zusanli. (See the appendix 7.)

Impotence

Description

Impotence is characterized by a man's persistent inability to sustain an erection sufficient for sexual intercourse. This is usually accompanied by a lack of energy or weariness, dizziness, soreness, and weakness in the loins and knees. Thirty million American men have a chronic impotence problem.[22] It doesn't only affect the man, but his partner as well. According to Chinese natural health, sex is an essential contributor to good health and happy relations, married life in particular. The inability to function sexually can be so embarrassing that the Impotence Information Center in Minneapolis, Minnesota, reports 40 percent of impotent men wait one or two years before their first visit to the clinic. Some will even suffer for a decade before seeking help. No wonder many people say that impotence is a man's worst nightmare.

Causes

Impotence is the result of a reduced blood supply to the penis, or a decreased ability of the blood vessels to hold blood. In Chinese medicine, this is diagnosed as a symptom of extreme weakness in kidney yang energy. Typically, this is due to a reckless indulgence in unregulated sex, leading to an enormous loss of vital semen and kidney vital qi energy. Masturbation is another cause often blamed for impotence, because masturbation can cause a severe drainage of the male sexual essence.

Causes of impotence can be physical, psychological, dietary, genetic, environmental, and pharmaceutical (a side effect of medications). Physically, if you are exhausted or seriously sick, sex may simply not be on your mind. Surgery, prostate surgery for instance, can injure nerves and arteries near the penis, causing impotence. Injury to the penis, prostate, bladder, spinal cord, or pelvis can cause impotence by damaging nerves and arteries of the male reproductive system. One common example of such an injury is found in long-distance bicycling.[23] Peripheral nerve compression after long distance cycling afflicts both experienced cyclists and novices.

Research led by Irwin Goldstein at the Boston University Medical Center found that between 10 to 15 percent of all impotence cases are caused by injury during intercourse. Pressure due to weight or exerted bending of the penis can lead to chronic impotence by damaging the lining of the erection chamber. The most common situation in which such injuries happen is when the female partner is sitting or lying on top of the male. Such a position violates the Chinese principle governing male-female relations, which states that man is yang (heaven—top) and woman is yin (earth—bottom). Impotence is just one of the consequences resulting from violating this ancient Chinese philosophical principle.

Of course, impotence can also be the result of other diseases such as heart disease, prostate problems, diabetes, and obesity. It is an interesting observation that the fatter a man, the weaker his sexual ability. Obese people are more likely to suffer from hardening of the arteries and diabetes, which significantly lower the vessel's ability to hold blood in the penis. Chronic constipation can be another reason.

Psychologically, emotional upsets such as stress, anxiety, depression, fear of sexual failure, fear of sexually transmitted diseases, such as AIDS, excessive excitement, guilt, lack of self-confidence, as well as strained sexual relations are all factors that frequently lead to a man's inability to erect. Experts believe that psychological factors cause 10 to 20 percent of impotence cases.

Chronic stress is a "killer" of sexuality. Stress works on two fronts. It triggers the "fight-or-flight" reflex, which sends blood away from the penis and out to the limbs to supply those muscles involved in self-defense or in escaping from the stressful situation. Stress also stimulates the secretion of cortisol, a natural chemical that suppresses production of male sex hormones, leading to impotence.

Some medications taken long-term can lower your libido and sexual vitality. Actually, many common drugs cause impotence as a side effect. These include high blood pressure drugs, appetite suppressants, ulcer drugs, antihistamines, and tranquilizers.

Environmentally, a lack of privacy can also cause impotence which, if persisted, can have a long term dampening effect on male sexuality. This is because of the nervousness created by the lack of privacy. This is especially the case with the male partner who should take a more active role in order for the intercourse to happen.

Genetically, some people are born with a greater sexual drive than others. Some are even born impotent. A well-known example of this was Pu Yi, the last emperor of China (1908–1911). It is believed that Pu Yi was born impotent because his ancestors had indulged in too much in sexual pleasure. Biologically, this depleted the sperm quality and quantity that went into the making of the last emperor—Pu Yi.

In terms of diet, too much alcohol and cigarette smoking can seriously reduce the sexual vitality of a man to the point of impotence. Alcohol is probably the most sexually dampening drug of all if taken in excess. Excess alcohol consumption depresses the central nervous system, impairs the functioning of the libido, dampens sexuality, causes loss of body hair, and decreases testosterone levels. Researchers also found that abusers of alcohol have luteinizing hormone levels 20 percent lower than nondrinkers, and have smaller testes. This suggests that alcohol inhibits the pituitary and has a direct toxic effect on the testes.[24]

Cigarettes also have a dampening effect on sexuality, especially so if smoked chronically and heavily. Heavy smoking constricts small arteries in the gonadal area, leading to a reduced supply of blood to that area and consequently lower sexual ability. A smoker with heart disease has a seven-fold greater risk of impotence than a healthy nonsmoker. Also, chronic drinking of strong tea, especially in the evening, can also lead to impotence. This is because tea also contains caffeine, which has been shown to have a dampening effect on sexuality.

Prevention and treatment

The search for aphrodisiacs has been ongoing for thousands of years in China. A number of foods and herbs have been found to be potent healers of male impotence. Examples are ginseng, asparagus, oysters, mussels, bearded clams, chili peppers, onions, garlic, fennel, hops, pollen, honey, human placenta, and pig testicles. Ginseng, oysters, and animal penises are especially powerful in stimulating the flow of male hormones, creating quick aphrodisiac effects.

Again, a healthy lifestyle is important. Stop smoking and avoid alcohol and caffeinated products. This is important in both preventing and curing impotence. Men who eat a healthy diet and exercise regularly tend to function well sexually as they age. Be moderate in your sexual activity, especially if you do not know the ancient Chinese art of sexual yoga. It is also important to avoid excess and vigorous cycling over long distances, an activity that puts great pressure on the sexual organs and has been shown to be a common cause of impotence.

Oysters are one of the major traditional Chinese dietary remedies to impotence. Oysters contain zinc, an essential substance of the prostate gland function, sperm generation, and sexual libido. It is told by the ancient Chinese that regular consumption of oysters can stimulate the growth of the penis. Men with moderate to severe zinc deficiencies may suffer impaired libido and low sperm counts. Consequently, it is helpful to eat fresh oysters (uncooked) regularly as part of your diet. Try eating half a pound of fresh uncooked oysters each day for one week, and see if you notice a difference. One of my students used to suffer from impotence, and I asked him to try eating half a pound of fresh oysters every day for a month. He did it, and as a result, his sexual vitality changed dramatically. His stamina increased as well as the size of his penis.

Dietary therapies

- Avoid refined sugar, coffee, strong tea, saturated fats, and processed foods. Such foods all have a negative impact on the libido and your sexuality.

- Oysters are one of the main traditional Chinese dietary responses to impotence. Try eating half a pound of fresh uncooked oysters each day for one week.

- Fry some walnuts and silkworm cocoons in peanut oil. Eat as a dish on an empty stomach. You can also stew them in water for half an hour and eat. This can strengthen the kidney function and boost sexuality.

- Stew a fresh beef penis or a couple of beef testicles together with one ounce of Chinese wolfberries and several slices of ginger in water for an hour.

- Cook mutton and garlic cloves together and eat it as a dish. This can strengthen the kidney function and boost sexuality.

- Fry chives together with one or two eggs together in vegetable oil and eat. This can boost sexuality and relieve impotence.

- Seafood, lean meat, and whole grain products are also Chinese solutions to impotence.

- Fry some fresh shrimp in peanut oil together with some Chinese chives. Eat it as a dish for dinner.

- Pumpkin and sunflower seeds are also believed to be able to boost male sexuality and relieve sexual dysfunction. Eat two ounces of fried sunflower seeds or pumpkin seeds each day.

- Soak the meat of a sparrow in water with some rice wine and sugar. Steam them all and eat. This is very helpful to kidney energy and therefore impotence.

- Fry some fresh, sliced sheep liver together with some Chinese chives in peanut oil. Eat at dinner time.

- Eat dove rice. Clean a fresh dove and throw away the innards. Cut the dove meat into small pieces. Add two ounces of rice, two red dates, three pieces of dried mushroom, two slices of ginger, and one glass of water. Cook together on a mild heat for forty minutes. Eat as a meal once a day or once every other day.

- Alternatively, cook dove meat together with pork or beef testicles plus some ginger. Eat it as a meal, twice a week.

- Soak cleaned turtledove slices in sesame oil, salt, sugar, and water for one hour. Then add an egg and cook them together. This will have the same effect as eating dove rice (above).

- Fry garlic or onions together with pork or beef kidneys and eat as a dish.

- Raw garlic itself is a sexual booster. Eating it regularly, on a daily basis, can help relieve impotence.

- Regular consumption of the following foods can greatly facilitate the treatment process: honey, earl tea, ginseng, deer antler, sweet potatoes, animal protein, raisins, lotus seeds, walnuts, and black fungus, particularly white fungus.

- Clean some pork kidneys and some celery. Slice both and fry them together. This builds up kidney yang energy.

- Eat plenty of bananas each day. Bananas contain enzymes and multiple nutrients such as sodium, potassium, tryptophan, and magnesium, which are helpful for sexual vitality and the nervous system, and can help boost the libido and cure impotence.

- Grapes, grape wine, and raisins all have beneficial effects on one's sexuality. For instance, drinking a small cup of grape wine at bedtime can promote sexuality and sleep.

- Eggs, especially raw egg yolks, can greatly boost your sexuality. It is better still if the eggs are prepared with pork or beef testicles. Eat once a day for two weeks.

- Eat corn every day to boost sexuality.

- Beef, lamb, and chicken kidneys are used in China as a yang tonic to improve sexual vitality and cure impotence in men. To cook, slice a kidney and boil it with some rice. When done, add the white heads from six green onions. Eat as a meal.

- Sheep's kidney is warm and is widely used in China to strengthen and nourish the human kidney and cure impotence.

- River or pond eel is another strong aphrodisiac. Clean the eel, cut it into pieces, and steam in water for thirty minutes. Add some rice wine. Drink the soup and eat the eel. The effects can be immediate.

- Fry fresh, unshelled shrimp with garlic cloves and eat once a day.

- Another way to use shrimp as a sexual tonic is to wash live shrimp and put them in a pot; pour in rice wine and cover for two minutes until the shrimp are intoxicated. No cooking is involved, but the shrimp must be fresh and clean. Eat the shrimp and drink the wine. Do this once a day for two weeks. This is both effective and delicious.

- The Chinese believe that mussels can enhance the body's temperature, particularly in the genital area, promoting erections and healing impotence.

- Raspberries also have a similar effect as mussels.

- Take seven ounces of cayenne pepper and one pair of pork kidneys and clean and slice them all. Pour some vegetable oil into a hot pot, and fry them together for three to five minutes, adding some salt. Eat as a dish once a day for two weeks.

- Other foods that are beneficial to patients of impotence include yams, which can stop seminal emissions in men and vaginal discharge in women; walnuts which tone up the kidneys and build yang energy; and bitter gourd seed which is helpful to yang energy.

- When you get up in the morning, take a glass with you to the bathroom. Dividing your first morning urine into thirds, collect the middle third of your urine in the glass (letting the first and last thirds pass). Drink the glass of urine right away. This can strengthen the kidney function.

Other natural therapies

- Save and swallow saliva. Saliva is thought by the ancient Chinese to contain precious substances, which can enhance the immune system, promote vital energy, tone up the kidney, and thus strengthen sexual vitality. In order to save saliva, you have to limit your speech and refrain from spitting. The Chinese have discovered some efficient ways to facilitate the accumulation of saliva in the mouth in order to swallow it in considerable amounts. One of the secrets is to "sweep" your teeth with your tongue three times to generate whatever water you can as a starting point to accumulate more saliva. Then put your tongue against your upper palate for as long as necessary for the saliva to fill the mouth. Once the mouth is full of the liquid, rinse the mouth for a while with the saliva without losing a single drop of it. Finally, close your eyes and take deep breaths. As you exhale, swallow one third of the saliva down to the lower abdomen. Do this three times until all the saliva is swallowed and imaginatively stored in dantian. Do this exercise as many times a day as you can. It can greatly boost your sexual ability.

- Clench your teeth gently, several times a day. This is because the teeth are thought to be connected with the kidneys. (See appendix 5.)

- Pull your ears and earlobes several times a day, since they are also thought to be connected with the kidneys.

- While doing breathing exercises, use your hands to rub both soles of your feet twenty times. Then use your warm hands to massage the kidneys twenty times. Do this twice a day. The Chinese sages believe that the soles, like the teeth, are directly related to the kidneys. Therefore, by rubbing the soles (and also clenching the teeth), you can promote the vital kidney energy and boost sexual vitality over time.

- Contract and relax the toes three times a day. It was believed by the ancient Chinese that the toes are related to your kidney system and therefore sexual function.

- Rub the neck up and down with warm hands thirty-six times, from the back of the ears to the shoulders. Do this three times a day. This is one of the Chinese sexual, and also longevity, secrets (for sexuality means longevity). (See appendix 5.)

- Practice sound qigong three times a day, making the sound of "Hay" while exhaling. (See appendix 3.)

- Practice the mobile qigong exercise "Hands Rising and Falling" regularly, three times a day. (See appendix 2.) You will find greater confidence in your sexual ability, feel less stress, and a build a stronger physique as a result.

- Regularly massage the lower abdomen, waist, and soles of the feet at bedtime.

- Take a cold sitz bath at bedtime during the summer. This has been shown to improve the kidney function, enhance sexual performance, and relieve impotence.

• Find an understanding and encouraging sex partner. Practice regulated sex together with patience and coordination. This is particularly effective if impotence is due to an excess loss of semen in the past or a fear of bedroom failure. Regulated sex can make up for the previous losses in sexual essence while an understanding partner is the best cure for performance apprehension.

• Apply finger pressure to the following acupoints several times a day, two to three minutes each time: Yongquan, Zhongji, Zhishi, Yinlingquan, Tianyou, Yaoyangguan, Guanyuan, Guanzhong, Juque, Mingmen, Weizhong, Qihai, Shenshu, Zusanli, and Sanyinjiao. (See appendix 7.)

Incontinence

Description

Incontinence is the involuntary and uncontrollable leakage of urine, either while awake or asleep. One common myth about this disease is that it is a "nursing home" problem. While incontinence can be a reason why some people end up living in nursing homes, the fact is that about 15 to 30 percent of older people living at home have an incontinence problem.[25]

Incontinence is not just a problem for older people. Almost one in every ten women has an occasional incontinence problem, and their ages range from twenty to sixty. In fact, some 50 percent of young women have complained of occasional light bladder control problems during exercise, after coughing, or even a hearty laugh. In addition, ten percent of all children older than four experience wetting the bed.

As well as being a physical problem, incontinence can also seriously affect one's mental health as well as social life. Chronic depression, reduced self-esteem, fear of or a sense of insecurity about the future, withdrawal from public life, or problems with relationships are common consequences of the disease. Indeed, these troubles are often a more serious threat to health and the quality of life than incontinence itself.

Symptoms or signs

These include involuntary urination or a loss of urine due to pressure from sneezing, coughing, laughing, jumping and so on. Dribbling or leakage of urine can occur when you cannot get to the bathroom fast enough, when you drink even a small amount of liquid, when you hear or touch running water, or when you get up from a chair or out of bed.

Causes

From the viewpoint of Chinese medicine, incontinence is a problem of kidney deficiency, or deficiency of yang-qi, the vital energy residing in our kidneys—the Gate of Life. Due to a deficiency in kidney energy, one is unable to control urination, just as a man is unable to control ejaculation.

Modern medicine considers it to be caused by a urinary tract infection, vaginal infection or irritation, a side effect of medicine, weakness of muscles that hold the bladder in place, hormone imbalance in women, pressure on the bladder, and weakness of the bladder itself. Whatever the explanation, one thing remains clear, the patient must have a weak urinary system.

Incontinence can be triggered by different causes: aging, pregnancy, prostate problems, and long-term illness. Without a doubt, age has a lot to do with incontinence. The Chinese believe that as we grow older, our qi energy declines. This cannot but reduce our control of the urinary system. For women, the pelvic floor sags with age due to a weakening of the muscles. This changes the angle at which the urethra exits the body and predisposes the person to leakage. Pregnancy is another cause. Half of all women have bladder control problems during their first pregnancy, especially during the last trimester. This percentage increases with each additional pregnancy. For male patients, the disease is closely associated with prostate problems, especially after prostate surgery, and prostate problems increase with age. Benign enlargement of the prostate gland tends to block the passage of urine from the bladder until finally the bladder overflows. Small-sized bladders can also cause the problem.

Prevention and treatment

Strong kidneys full of vital yang-qi energy are the best insurance against incontinence. Therefore, the first thing you need to do is to conserve and build up your kidney energy.

This means avoidance of sexual indulgences and practicing breathing exercises and exercises specially tailored toward the kidneys. You should also eat the right foods.

Natural healing methods are especially valuable and helpful for incontinence. For one thing, due to the social stigma associated with the disease, most patients are reluctant to talk about their condition with family members, friends, or even their own physicians. As such, self-help therapies becomes all the more valuable.

Dietary therapies

• Cook five ounces of Gorgon fruit as porridge and eat it as meal. Take this twice a day, once in the morning and again in the evening. Do this for a week and you will see the effect.

• Better still, make a porridge of Gorgon fruit, seven red dates, and one ounce of walnuts.

• Raspberries can check urination and relieve incontinence.

• Soak sliced sparrow meat in rice wine, adding some water and sugar. Steam them together and eat as a meal.

• Cook a cake of bean curd, one ounce of gingko fruit, and some rice together to make a porridge. Eat it as a meal, either in the morning or in the evening. This can relieve incontinence.

• Cook Gorgon fruit to make a porridge and eat it once a day.

- Fry some walnuts and silkworm chrysalis in peanut oil. Eat as a dish on an empty stomach.

- Fry some fresh, sliced sheep liver together with some Chinese chives in peanut oil. Eat as a dish at dinner.

- Fry chives with some fresh shrimp in vegetable or peanut oil and eat as a dish.

- Soak 3 to 5 ounces of dried bean curd in water overnight. Then cook with some rice to make a porridge. Eat as a meal.

- Use salt and water to clean some fresh chicken intestines. Cut into pieces and fry in oil for ten minutes, adding some salt. Pour in some rice wine and eat as a dish.

- Soak ten red dates and one ounce of Chinese wolfberries in water for two hours. Then break two eggs into it, adding some rock sugar and salt. Stew for fifteen minutes and eat. This can strengthen kidney function and relieve incontinence.

- Clean a fresh dove, throwing away all the internal organs, and cut the meat into small slices. Steam or cook the meat in water together with some rice, two red dates, three pieces of dried mushroom, and two slices of ginger for about forty minutes. Eat as a meal once a day or once every other day. This can strengthen kidney function and relieve incontinence.

- Clean a pork stomach and soak it in water together with one ounce of gingko with the shell taken off. Steam them together for twenty minutes, and eat as a meal once a day for a week.

- Fry sliced pork kidneys and celery together and eat them as a meal to strengthen the kidneys and urinary system.

- Steam cleaned pork tail together with black beans. Eat them as a meal.

- Boil some yams with ginseng and walnuts until soft. Eat it once a day for a week.

Other natural therapies

- Practice qigong at least twice a day. (See appendix 1.)

- Contract the anal muscles several times a day, fifteen contractions each time. Contract while inhaling and relax while exhaling.

- Gently clench your teeth several times a day. The teeth are associated with the kidneys and, therefore, this easy exercise can have an amazing effect.

- Pull the ears and earlobes several times a day.

- Contract and relax the toes several times a day.

- Massage the abdomen and waist three times a day as directed by Dharma's internal exercises. (See appendix 5.)

- Frequently massage the calves of the legs.

- Apply finger pressure to the following acupoints several times a day: Zusanli, Fengmen, Changqiang, Guanyuan, Gongsun, Qichong, Sanyinjiao, Shenshu, Weizhong, Yaoyangguan, and Zhongji. (See appendix 7.)

Indigestion

Description
Indigestion can be many things. It is usually a burning sensation in the stomach, often accompanied by bloating or nausea. Whatever you eat seems to be eliminated immediately after eating, either through a bowel movement or nausea.

Symptoms or signs
Symptoms include discomfort or a feeling of fullness in the abdomen; heartburn; nausea; and bloating.

Causes
There are several types of indigestion. One type is known as nonulcerative dyspepsia, which is caused by excess stomach acid. Dyspepsia can indicate a more serious problem, especially if you lose weight, are unable to finish a full meal, or vomit. These can be symptoms of more serious diseases. Another type is known as gastroesophageal reflux disease, which is caused by stomach acid moving back up into the esophagus, causing a sour taste in the mouth or a burning chest sensation that worsens when you lie down or lean over immediately after eating. Indigestion can also be caused by an ulcer, which is an open sore in the stomach lining caused by excess stomach acid. Psychological factors such as stress and depression also contribute to indigestion. Stress causes the overproduction of hormones, which deactivate certain areas of the body including the stomach and the intestines. It interrupts the digestive process, leading to indigestion, flatulence, and hiccuping.

Prevention and treatment
Dietary therapies
- Avoid processed and refined foods. These foods contain chemical additives that are hard to digest.

- Eat slowly and chew thoroughly before you swallow your food. It also generates saliva needed for digestion. Eating too fast without fully chewing adds pressure to the stomach.

- Eating an apple every day can relieve indigestion and constipation, and also boost the appetite.

- Do not eat cold foods or foods taken right out of the refrigerator. Cold foods cause the contraction of the stomach lining and reduce the amount of digestive juices produced.

- Do not overcook foods. Eat them raw as often as you can. Raw foods contain natural enzymes that are helpful to digestion, but are easily destroyed by overheating and artificial processing of foods.

- Do not eat fatty foods, which consume a large amount of hydrochloric acid in the stomach.

- Do not talk while eating. Concentrate on the meal. This mental status will bring out the best in your digestive system so it will absorb the foods you take in.

- Do not drink liquids immediately before, during, or after a meal. Liquids dilute the stomach enzymes needed for digestion.

- Do not drink tea while eating protein foods.

- Do not eat foods that are not compatible at the same time, such as banana and sweet potatoes, or milk and orange juice. Do not eat starchy foods and protein foods at the same time.

- Eat onions, red peppers, green peppers, ham, apples, coriander, hops, malt, papaya, pineapple, plums, radishes, sweet basil, tomatoes.

- Chew slices of fresh ginger, or drink the soup of ginger root. (Squeeze the ginger in a juicer to make ginger soup.) Drink on an empty stomach. This can greatly stimulate digestion.

- Cut a papaya and some fresh ginger into slices. Soak them in rice vinegar for at least two hours. Eat the papaya and ginger on an empty stomach twice a day.

- Eat one or two fresh figs in the morning and again in the evening, to stimulate the appetite and relieve indigestion.

- Cut some beef into small pieces. Cook the beef with rice to make a meal. When done, pour in some ginger juice. Eat it once or twice a day.

- Drink three cups of apple juice a day.

- Drink one teaspoonful of vinegar after each meal. This can promote digestion.

- Drink a cup of beer every day to aid digestion.

- Eat one grapefruit three times a day.

- Drink plenty of hawthorn fruit juice to treat indigestion and abdominal pain.

- Eating some lemon with your meal can help indigestion.

- Eat a few fresh kumquats to relieve indigestion.

- Eat one to two ounces of sour papayas daily.

- Eat fresh pineapple or drink pineapple juice everyday. This can help digestion.

- Eat two fresh plums in the morning and evening to help digestion.

Other natural therapies

- Form a habit of regularly accumulating saliva and slowly swallowing it down to the lower abdomen (dantian). Saliva contains an enzyme that starts the digestive process and enhances the immune system.

- Regular exercise remains the most effective means of fighting indigestion. Of special importance are morning exercises that stimulate the appetite and keep the stomach in high spirits throughout the day.

- Keep bowel movements as regular as possible, at least once a day.

- Apply finger pressure to the following acupoints several times a day, two to three minutes each time: Neiguan, Zhongwan, Chengjiang, Earlobes, Tianshu, Wailaogong, Shangwan, Xiawan, Shangjuxu, Zhigou, Qihai, Zusanli, Shenshu, and Sanyinjiao. (See appendix 7.)

Infertility

Description

Continuation of the species is the "law of nature." In Chinese tradition, not having children is considered the severest example of filial impiety. Unfortunately, one in every six American couples is infertile.[26] Filial piety may not be a concern in modern society any more, but infertility remains a frustrating experience. It is a stressful condition for most couples, often causing anxiety, depression, and fatigue.

Symptoms or signs

An inability to conceive after two years of normal sexual relations in the absence of birth control is a clear sign of an infertility problem.

Causes

Causes of infertility are manifold and complicated. Both sexes can be infertile. On the female side, the underlying reasons for infertility can be irregular menstruation or the absence of menstruation due to a hormonal imbalance triggered by emotional stress or the use of birth control pills. It can also result from the improper development of ovaries, or the presence of a fibrous cyst. Scarring or closure of the fallopian tubes, due to swelling or adherence of the tube walls resulting from infection in the upper reproductive tract, can be another cause. Uterine problems such as a small uterus, uterine cysts, endometriosis, and an abnormal growth of polyps on the interior of the uterus can lead to infertility, too.

Vaginal problems may also cause infertility: vaginal scarring or a cyst; a double vagina or a closed vagina; and vaginal fluid which is too acidic or too alkaline for the sperm to survive. A deficiency of tryptophan, a vital amino acid involved in the reproductive process, is a major nutritional cause of infertility for both sexes. Deficiency of calcium is another nutritional cause. Another common but hidden cause of infertility is cigarette smoking by either or both parties.

In men, sperm may be too scarce to ensure fertility. In other words, the semen does not contain enough vital sperm to ensure fertilization of the female's egg. Scarcity of semen is largely due to deficiency in kidney function, resulting from indulgence in sexual pleasure, chronic nocturnal emissions, or masturbation.

Traditional Chinese medicine regards deficiency of kidney qi energy, depression of the liver qi, and coldness of the blood and the womb as the root causes of infertility in women. These factors can lead to an imbalance of the Functioning and Governing channels, making a woman unable to conceive. A male can be infertile by his deficiency of kidney qi. Kidney qi deficiency will lead to cold sperm, low sperm count, low volume or low density of sperm, or a high percentage of abnormal sperm, which all increase the difficulty of conception.

Prevention and treatment

In Chinese health care, infertility is viewed largely as a deficiency of kidney qi energy. To prevent and treat this condition, one needs to build up and preserve enough kidney qi energy. This should be done through both a proper diet and a healthy lifestyle that includes regulated sex and regular exercising. The foods recommended below are believed to be good for preventing and treating infertility, because they help build up the kidney qi energy needed for fertility.

Natural therapies

- Regularly (once a week) eating chicken or pork livers can stop continuous miscarriages, because these foods nurture the blood system and strengthen the ability to conceive. To eat, fry or cook them with some salt and red dates.

- Mix one ounce of cleaned dong quai with chicken and some water and cook together. Eat this once a day for one month.

- Eat plenty of raw cabbage and green vegetables, which contain a lot of calcium needed for fertility.

- Eat plenty of bananas, which contain tryptophan, a nutrient vital for fertility in both sexes.

- Eat plenty of apples, grapes, pears, and nuts, which contain boron, a substance essential to the absorption and utilization of calcium from food.

- Eat plenty of cucumbers. The ancient Chinese think that the seeds in cucumbers represent the human embryo.

- Eggs, especially fish eggs, contain rich lecithin, which promotes semen production and semen vitality. Eat two (chicken) eggs per day, only slightly steamed; eat fish eggs twice a week. If you can cook the eggs together with pork or beef testicles, they will be more effective.

- Eat raw oysters and raw fish. These foods are strong boosters of male hormones.

- Carrot, celery, and asparagus are also good foods for this condition, because they all have the ability to cleanse the kidneys and strengthen the sexual and reproductive systems.

- Apply finger pressure to the following acupoints several times a day: Qimen, Qixue, Mingmen, Longmen, and Yongquan. (See appendix 7.)

Insomnia

Description

If you consistently have trouble falling asleep after lying in bed for thirty minutes, or if you are easily wakened during the night and unable to fall asleep again, or your mind is still active while asleep, you may have insomnia. Roughly two out of every ten Americans are afflicted with this problem.[27]

Everyone has insomnia at one time or another. Though not physically painful, insomnia can throw your entire system off. Without enough sleep, people become irritable and low-spirited. Insomnia weakens the immune system and lowers the appetite, thus subjecting you to more ailments. It also can elevate your stress and emotional levels, and can even lead to a mental breakdown.

Symptoms or signs

Symptoms include the inability to sleep through the night, trouble falling asleep, or repeated awakening at night.

Causes

Traditional Chinese medicine holds that insomnia is caused by digestive, respiratory, urogenital and endocrine systems, as well as the spleen, heart, and great vessels. It is a deficiency of qi and blood energy in the body as a result of either severe disease, sexual indulgence, or chronic emotional upset or stress, all of which can disturb the yin-yang balance in our body as well as our peace of mind. For instance, people recovering from surgery or serious diseases usually have a harder time getting to sleep. This is because the qi or energy reserve of the body has been significantly drained, according to the theory of Chinese medicine. Also, constipation can cause anxiety and therefore insomnia. It is a well-known fact that physical exercise promotes sleep. That helps explain why very few physical laborers are bothered by insomnia. Also, prolonged, intensive mental activity is a common cause of insomnia. Many intellectuals seem to suffer much more from this disease than others.

Psychological factors such as stress, worries, anxiety, and depression can lead to insomnia. According to Chinese theory, stress and depression add oil to the fire of the heart and liver, leading to unrest of the spirit and therefore insomnia. Some foods can also produce the same result as emotional distress. For instance, spicy and stimulating foods such as peppers, fried foods, coffee, and strong tea taken shortly before going to bed can all contribute to difficulty in falling asleep. Environmentally speaking, an uncomfortable or new bed, noises, or a room that is too hot or too cold are factors affecting one's ability to sleep. Long-term insomnia, which can last for months, is most often caused by general anxiety, depression, or physical weakness, i.e., a deficiency of vital energy.

Prevention and treatment

Dietary therapies

- Stop smoking and eliminate alcohol and coffee.

- Avoid spicy, irritable, and fried foods as well as foods of a hot nature, such as hot pepper, onions, and mangos.

- Avoid drinking tea in the afternoon and evening.

- Avoid high-sugar foods because they can cause the blood sugar to plummet, leading to improper sleep patterns.

- Avoid a big meal before going to bed.

- Eat more mushrooms, soy milk, white radishes, lotus seeds and roots, and tofu. These foods can cool the mind and promote sleep.

- Use a lotus flower to brew a cup of tea. Add some honey and drink it at bedtime to induce sleep.

- Eat plenty of ripe bananas each day. Bananas can promote sleep and relieve insomnia because it is rich in sodium, magnesium, potassium, and tryptophan, all of which are valuable nutrients to the nervous system.

- Soak some lotus seeds and lily in water for two hours. Then add seven to ten ounces of lean pork meat. Stew them together for thirty minutes, and eat it as a dish. Do this once a day for a week.

- Drink a cup of honey water after getting up in the morning. Honey is considered to be of a cool nature and can nurture the liver and balance the nervous system, thus inducing better sleep.

- Drinking apple juice and orange juice can also help relieve insomnia.

- Cook kelp and green beans together in water. Eat them at dinner.

- Clean and cut a fresh pork heart. Stew the pork heart together with one ounce of lotus seeds in water for one hour. Drink the soup and eat the pork heart. (Eating the pork heart is optional as long as you drink the soup.)

- Drinking a cup of warm milk at bedtime can help promote sleep.

- Drink plenty of carrot and/or celery juice each day.

- Eat oatmeal, honey, dates, and sweet potatoes. These foods can soothe the mind and promote sleep.

- Drink plenty of water during the day, but stop drinking it one hour before going to bed (unless you are really thirsty). This to avoid having to urinate during the night.

- Fry one ounce of wheat until it becomes yellow; add fifteen red dates and a little licorice. Boil them together in water over low heat for fifteen minutes. Drink this once a day for seven days.

- Eat one or two cooked egg yolks a day for two weeks.

- Crush some green onions and put it in a jar. Inhale the vapor through the nose while in bed to induce sleep.

- Steam white fungus until very soft, and add some rock sugar. Eat it before going to bed. This can nourish the brain, soothe the mind, and promote sleep.

- Boil one ounce of red dates with the white heads from five green onions. Eat it right before going to bed. This can nourish the brain, soothe the mind, and promote sleep.

- Boil two ounces of fresh lily flowers and half an ounce of rock sugar in water for thirty minutes. Drink the soup before going to bed.

- Boil one pound of fresh mussels in water. Drink the soup and eat the mussels for dinner.

Other natural therapies

- Take a warm sitz bath or soak both feet in warm water for ten minutes immediately before going to sleep. This will greatly reduce the blood level in the brain and thus "inactivate" it so you can sleep better.
  NOTE: this is not recommended for patients of hypertension.

- Practice thirty minutes of qigong before going to bed. Qigong gives you a sense of restfulness after a day's work and calms your mind for a sound sleep. (See appendix 1.)

- Massage the soles until they are warm immediately before going to bed. (See appendix 5.)

- Take a fifteen-minute leisurely walk in the fresh air before going to bed.

- Relax your mind thirty minutes before bedtime by either engaging in some light conversation, watching television, or listening to some soothing music.

- Regularly exercise, especially practicing any of the forms described in this book. (See appendices 1 through 6.)

- Sex is believed to be one of the most powerful catalysts for sleep. As a matter of fact, many people with a long history of insomnia found that it mysteriously disappeared once they got married. A satisfactory sexual experience can be the single most powerful medicine for insomnia, because sexual activities can greatly reduce the stress levels and make you feel relaxed and tired enough to fall asleep shortly afterward.

- Keep a regular schedule as to when to go to bed and when to get up. Keep a record of your sleeping hours and your waking spiritual level as well as how many hours you work efficiently during the day, so you know how much time you really need to sleep. You may lie in bed longer than you really need. If that is the case, you will be awake part of the time while lying in bed. The idea is not to have too much, but just enough sleep each day.

- Use the counting technique to induce sleep while lying in bed. This works by concentrating on very simple numbers, such as 1, 2, 3. This is so that you will not think of more complex or troubling thoughts.

- Apply finger pressure to the following acupoints several times a day, two to three minutes each time: Qihai, Tongli, Neiguan, Zhongwan, Chenfu, Fengchi, Baihui, Qianding, Shenmen, Sanyinjiao, Taiyang, Xingjian, Yintang, Fenglong, and Zusanli. (See appendix 7.)

- Make sure that you have a bowel movement every day. Constipation adds to the stress level and creates discomfort in the abdomen, thus affecting sleep.

Irritable Bowel Syndrome

Description
Technically called gastrointestinal neurosis, this ailment is characterized by abnormal secretions and motor functions of the intestinal tract. This is due to functional disorders in the nervous system, although there is no organic lesion in the gastrointestinal tract itself.

Symptoms or signs
Symptoms include belching, vomiting, diarrhea, abdominal pain which may be accompanied by a headache, insomnia, acid regurgitation, and heartburn. A patient of gastrointestinal neurosis is often lean with a weak constitution. He or she may also experience changes in bowel habits such as constipation, diarrhea, as well as abdominal gas.

Causes
The main causes include chronic stress, anxiety, and an improper diet including eating spoiled or contaminated foods, fatty or sour-tasting foods, and other foods that are hard for the stomach to digest.

Prevention and treatment
Dietary therapies
- Drink grape wine or grape juice.

- Fast for one day, and only eat fresh grapes whenever you feel hungry.

- Boil hyacinth beans in water until soft. Eat this twice a day.

- Boil sweet basil, fresh ginger, and licorice in water. Drink the soup.

- Eat cabbage on a regular basis to relieve gastric ulcers. This is because cabbage is rich in vitamin U, which is effective in treating ulcers.

- Mix lemon juice with soybean oil and drink two teaspoonfuls first thing in the morning on an empty stomach. Do this for a week.

- Steam half a cup of honey and eat it on an empty stomach, twice a day for two weeks. This can relieve gastric and duodenal ulcers.

- Grind some tea leaves and dried ginger into powder. Mix them together and take one teaspoonful with warm water on a regular basis to cure acute gastroenteritis.

Other natural therapies

- Massage the abdomen and the waist twice a day. (See appendix 5.)

- Apply finger pressure to the following acupoints several times a day: Qihai, Taichong, Tianshu, Zhongwan, Guanyuan, Burong, and Zusanli. (See appendix 7.)

Jaded Appetite (Loss of Appetite)

Description

This ailment is a loss of the desire to eat. In America, this is called anorexia nervosa, the now well-known eating disorder primarily of young females. Patients just do not feel hungry and have no desire to eat. Since food is the primary source of energy and vitality, it goes without saying that such people do not have high spirits and vitality. Their work efficiency is low, and they do not have a strong drive for life. They are happiest sitting on the sofa or lying on the bed doing nothing.

Symptoms or signs

These include a dark and yellow complexion and a thick, white coating on the tongue. Those afflicted with this ailment are often in low spirits, fatigued, and underweight.

Causes

There are dietary, physical, as well as mental causes for this ailment. In terms of diet, excess consumption of fatty, sugary, and fried foods can dampen the appetite. Lack of zinc in the diet is another reason why people lose their appetite. Chronic use of drugs rich in iron and calcium can also interfere with the body's ability to absorb zinc in the diet.

Physically, a lack of exercise, physical exhaustion, sexual indulgence and waste of sexual essence, fatigue, as well as conditions such as ulcers and diarrhea all can lead to a jaded appetite. Mentally, stress and depression can have the same consequences. An irregular lifestyle can be another vice. If you do not eat when you are hungry, you may lose your appetite over time.

Prevention and treatment

The best prevention is to keep a regular schedule for meals and follow an active lifestyle. Exercise at least twice a day. Learn to handle stress and pressure so that depression can be avoided. For treatment, therapy should be targeted at the specific causes that lead to the ailment. Thus, if a jaded appetite is caused by depression, treatment should focus on how to lift one out of depression.

NOTE: There are many different causes of depression. Go to the listing on depression, to find out more about its causes and corresponding therapies.

Dietary therapies

- Avoid sugary, fatty, and fried foods.

- Eat pineapple, ginger, basil, radiccio, and onions to boost the appetite.

- Regularly drinking a moderate amount of grape wine can stimulate the body's ability to absorb zinc in the diet.

- Eat plenty of foods that are rich in zinc, such as oysters and other seafoods, raw rice, soy products, walnuts, peanuts, watermelon, and sunflower seeds.

- Eat plenty of radishes or drink radish juice to boost the appetite.

- Eat one to two fresh figs twice a day to stimulate the appetite.

- Eat two fresh tomatoes a day before lunch. This can help digestion and boost the appetite.

- Fry green or red peppers as a dish and eat it to boost the appetite.

- Eating fresh olives will also greatly boost the appetite and help digestion.

- Drinking a small cup of red wine before meal can stimulate the appetite.

- Cook two ounces of dansheng (*Codonopsis pilosula*) together with twenty red dates in water for an hour. Drink the soup and eat the dates. This can strengthen the function of the spleen and stomach and, therefore, boost the appetite.

Other natural therapies

- Regularly practice soft Chinese fitness exercises outdoors. Doing these exercises in the morning is especially helpful to boost the appetite and enhance the spirit.

- Practice sound qigong and make the sounds of "Gong" and "High" while exhaling. (See appendix 3.)

- Apply finger pressure to the following acupoints three times a day: Chengjiang, Shangjuxu, Tianshu, Xiawan, and Zhigou. (See appendix 7.)

Kidney Inflammation (Nephritis)

Description

Commonly known as kidney inflammation, nephritis is a kind of kidney ailment. The most common type of nephritis is glomerulonephritis. Left untreated, nephritis can lead to renal failure. Usually, children between the ages of sixteen months and five years old get it, and it occurs twice as often in boys as in girls, though children of all ages and adults can get it.

Symptoms or signs

These can include swelling around the eyes in the morning, which may last all day, swelling in the ankles, feet and belly, feeling tired and irritable, loss of appetite, frequent and often painful urination, fever, and false obesity accompanied by a pale complexion.

Causes

Although in the majority of cases the exact cause of nephritis is not known, it is believed that long-standing hypertension can cause kidney disease, and accelerate the natural cause of any underlying kidney disease. Also, years of heavy use of headache compounds can slowly produce kidney failure. Certain other medications, toxins, pesticides, and drugs (heroin) can also cause kidney damage.[28]

NOTE: See a medical professional if the condition doesn't improve.

Prevention and treatment
Dietary therapies

- Avoid fresh garlic, green onions, chives, red peppers, nicotine, strong coffee, and alcohol.

- Avoid salt, high-sodium foods, and shellfish.

- Eat corn on the cob, watermelon peel, lily flowers, radishes, sea grass, cucumbers, eggplant roots, small red beans, and black soybeans.

- Cook an equal amount of peanuts and broad beans together in water for about forty-five minutes. Eat this once a day for two weeks.

- Crush cucumbers to squeeze out the juice. Warm the juice and drink it as a tea. Or, boil dried cucumbers in water to make a soup.

- Boil dried watermelon peel in water and drink it as a tea three times a day.

- Boil three corncobs in water and drink it as tea.

- Eat plenty of asparagus. This vegetable contains asparamid, which is one of the most effective natural kidney diuretics. Asparagus can eliminate the body of excess uric acid through the urine. It breaks up uric acid crystals in the kidneys. Steam it and eat it hot before a meal.

- Eat plenty of raw watermelons and cucumbers. These can be used together with asparagus to make a complete meal at least once a week.

- Drinking carrot juice and apple cider vinegar also helps relieve the symptoms.

- Eat plenty of grapes and cabbage.

- Prepare a large carp by removing the internal organs; use a cloth to dry the fish. Boil the carp in water with one cup of small red beans without salt and eat.

Kidney Stones
Description
Kidney stones are one of the most common disorders of the urinary tract, and the most painful besides cancer. This disease is marked by an excess accumulation of mineral salts in the kidneys. Three types of kidney stones can be identified: stones formed from calcium oxalic acid, stones formed from uric acid, and stones formed as a result of consuming too much protein.

Kidney stones cause acute pain in the lower back, radiating to the bladder area in the lower abdomen. The pain is excruciating as the stone is exiting from the kidney into the urethra. The intensity of the pain can be compared to that of the final stages of childbirth. Many patients lose consciousness as a result of the pain.

Some types of kidney stones grow to such a large size that they are unable to exit through the kidneys. Consequently, the filtration mechanism in the kidney will be blocked and surgery becomes necessary to remove the stones. Stones can take from twenty minutes to one-and-a-half months to pass from one end of the urinary tract to the other. They can also lead to bladder and kidney infections. Men tend to be more susceptive to this disease than women.

Symptoms or signs

Usually, the first symptom of a kidney stone is extreme pain, which often occurs suddenly without any prior problems. Typically, it is a sharp, cramping pain in the back and side, in the area of the kidneys or in the lower abdomen. Sometimes, nausea and vomiting occur with this pain. Later, the pain may spread to the groin. In later stages, as the stone grows or moves, blood may be found in the urine. As the stone moves down the ureter closer to the bladder, one may feel the need to urinate more frequently, or feel a burning sensation during urination. Sometimes, fever and chills may accompany any of these symptoms. In this case, there is a great possibility of infection and therefore an urgent need to contact a doctor.

Causes

Diet is the chief cause of the disease. About 80 percent of kidney stones are formed of calcium and oxalate due to an excess intake of calcium, plus improper circulation and insufficient exercise. Typically, the excess calcium comes from dairy products, sardines, and dark green leafy vegetables such as chard, kale, and spinach. Researchers at Yale Renal Stone Clinic looked at the diets of 282 kidney-stone patients and found that those who consumed the highest amounts of salt tended to have the highest levels of calcium in their urine.

Other causes of kidney stones include urinary tract infections or blockage, family history of kidney stones, cystic kidney diseases, gout, excess intake of vitamin D, renal tubular acidosis, and metabolic disorders such as cystinuria (excessive urinary excretion of cystine arising from defective transport systems in the kidneys) and hyperparathyroidism (an increase of secretion of the parathyroids causing elevated serum calcium).[29]

Prevention and treatment

Knowledge is power. Knowing the causes of the disease, we can effectively prevent and treat it by means of natural health and healing. Limiting your salt intake can reduce your risk of developing kidney stones. Do not drink more than two glasses of milk a day because this causes more absorption of calcium by the system. Drink plenty of water each day to flush the kidneys.

Dietary therapies

- Drink half a cup to one cup of fresh radish juice each morning on an empty stomach. This can usually dissolve even the most stubborn kidney stones by passing them out of the body through the urine.

- Substantially reduce the intake of protein, sugar, caffeine, and alcohol.

- Avoid or greatly limit your salt intake, shellfish, and other seafoods.

- Avoid foods with a high oxalic acid content such as dark green leafy vegetables, chocolate, tea, nuts, and seeds.

- Eat plenty of bananas, papayas, watermelon, pears, day lily, and canned cranberries. These fruits have a healing effect on the kidneys.

- Eat only watermelon and asparagus for a meal, one day a week. Asparagus contains asparadid, an effective kidney diuretic which gives urine a strong odor of ammonia, a sign that excess uric acid is being expelled.

- Consume just enough protein to keep calcium dissolved. Average adults need four ounces of pure protein each day. Make sure you take in at least that much.

- Clean and cut half a pound of ginger; crush it to squeeze out the juice; soak ten ounces of red dates in water for an hour until soft; crunch them after peeling and removing the seeds. Combine the ginger juice and crushed dates in a pan; then add ten ounces of brown sugar and steam until they become like a pudding. Eat them up in three days.

- Take some watermelon and boil it with a little sugar over low heat until the juice thickens. Eat one spoonful on an empty stomach twice a day. This can relieve the pain caused by kidney stones and the condition itself.

- Stew some maize corn hair together with some freshwater mussels. Eat the mussels and drink the soup. Do this once a day for two weeks.

- Clean a mandarin duck and cook it with water chestnuts and some ginger until soft. Eat it within two days.

- Fry four ounces of walnuts in vegetable oil until crunchy. Mix the walnuts with sugar and water to make a syrup. Eat twice a day, for as long as it takes for the symptoms to disappear. Walnuts are considered effective in dissolving the stones.

- Boil corn leaves or corn silk in water and drink as a tea twice a day.

- For those whose system is too alkaline, drinking apple cider vinegar regularly can help dissolve the calcium in the body and relieve kidney stones.

- Drink more water and eat less salt. This is the motto that all patients of kidney or urinary stones must keep in mind.

Liver Disease

Description

This is a general name for ailments and dysfunctions of the liver. A swollen liver, cirrhosis, and hepatitis are the major forms. The liver is one of the most important organs of the body. Its function is to generate and filter blood, and remove the toxins we take in.

Symptoms or signs

Symptoms include various degrees of pain in the liver, vomiting acidic fluid, headaches, loss of hearing, ear ringing, dizziness, low flexibility in fingers and toes, a pale complexion, and a tendency to get angry easily.

Causes

According to traditional Chinese medical theory, liver diseases are caused by a blockage of qi and blood energy in the liver. This blockage can be caused by an unhealthy diet, depression, or stress. Alcohol and fried, fatty, and spicy foods are detrimental to the liver. The ancient Chinese held that liver qi should be kept light and smooth; that stress, depression, and emotional outbursts are especially harmful to the liver. People who are susceptible to anger and stress frequently suffer from liver disease.

Prevention and treatment

To prevent liver disease, learn and practice methods of mental hygiene, avoiding emotional upsets, especially anger. This is because the liver favors peace of mind and happiness, but fears anger and tension. There-fore, it is especially important to learn how to control anger and stress, and take life as it comes. Improve your digestion first before you eat the appropriate foods to nourish the liver. Avoid alcohol, coffee, and cigarettes as well. Get plenty of rest; avoid fatigue and overwork. To relieve and cure the disease, try the following:

Dietary therapies

- Avoid fried, spicy, and fatty foods.

- Stay away from coffee, alcohol, and cigarettes.

- The following foods are considered to be healthy and helpful for patients with liver disease: beef, lean pork, tofu, fish, animal livers, Napa (chinese cabbage), dates, ginger, sunflower seeds, green onions, honey, carrots, watermelon, pears, apples, Chinese chives, and soft-shelled turtle.

- Eat plenty of carrots or drink carrot juice.

- Cook 100 grams of fresh mushrooms and 100 grams of lean pork meat together in water with a little bit of salt. Eat as a dish. This can promote the liver function and relieve the ailment.

- To relieve extra water stored up in the stomach due to cirrhosis of the liver, cook three ounces of garlic cloves with one pound of watermelon. Eat it on an empty stomach.

- Stew fresh fish with garlic cloves. Eat it as a dish once every day. This can promote the liver function and relieve the ailment.

- Cut two tomatoes and 100 grams of fresh beef. Fry them together in oil for a few minutes. Add some salt and water and cook for another five minutes.

- Cook celery and ten red dates together. Eat it once a day.

- Use some dried rose flower to brew tea. Drink it twice a day.

- Eat raw tomatoes. They are very potent in reducing the inflammation of the liver due to cirrhosis and hepatitis.

- Cook celery and some red dates together. Eat it once a day.

- Soak in water ten dates and one ounce of Chinese wolfberries for two hours. Add two fresh eggs and stew them with some rock sugar and salt for fifteen minutes. Eat and drink everything.

- Eat beans, spinach, sunflower seeds, cabbages, and beets.

- Eat chicken, pork, or beef liver once a day to nurture your own liver.

- Eat plenty of watermelon, which is especially good for jaundice.

- Use one ounce of sesame seeds, one ounce of sunflower seeds, five dates, one ounce of rock candy, plus enough pure water to cook together until it looks like porridge. Eat as a meal.

- Drink chrysanthemum tea several times a day.

- Dress radish slices with white sugar, rice vinegar, ginger slices, and sesame oil. Eat everything. This can kill bacteria in the liver and help relieve the ailment.

- Clean and cut Napa (Chinese cabbage), carrots, and radishes. Fry them in vegetable oil over moderate heat. Add a little bit of salt and eat as a dish.

- Stew some maize corn hair together with some freshwater mussels and water. Eat the mussels and drink the soup. Do this once a day for two weeks. This can help strengthen the liver function and treat the ailment.

- Use cuttlefish, fresh ginger, mushroom, salt, and sesame oil to make a dish.

- Clean two ounces of pork or beef liver and cut it into small pieces. Take the juice of the liver and mix it with an egg. Steam it over moderate heat for ten minutes, add some salt and sesame oil and eat as a dish.

- Wash one pound of fresh celery and squeeze out the juice; boil the juice with some honey over low heat for five minutes and eat it warm. Repeat this every day for two weeks.

- Mix three cups of rice vinegar, one pound of pork spare ribs, five ounces of brown sugar, and an equal amount of white sugar. Boil these for twenty minutes without using any water. Eat one spoonful of the juice three times a day.

- Cut a cuttlefish, sea slug, and fresh ginger into small pieces. Cook some rice in plenty of water until the water is boiling. Into the rice add the cuttlefish, sea slug, and ginger pieces. Cook for another fifteen to twenty minutes to make a porridge. Eat everything as a meal once a week. This can help strengthen the liver function and relieve the ailment.

- Boil two ounces of malt sugar with some orange peel in water. Drink as a tea to relieve acute and chronic hepatitis.

- Boil three cups of rice vinegar, three ounces of white sugar, and one pound of pork bones together for half an hour. Divide the soup into three equal parts and drink it three times in a day. Repeat this for three weeks. This is effective for treating contagious hepatitis.

Other natural therapies

- Practice qigong every day, imaginatively guiding your qi to the area of your liver while exhaling. (See appendix 1.)

- Avoid highly vigorous exercising and any cause of fatigue.

- Practice sound qigong several times a day, making the sounds of "Ge" and "Xu." (See appendix 3.)

- Massage the liver and abdomen area several times a day. While so doing, casually think of your liver.

- Massage the first section of the index finger. This portion is called "the wind hole"

in Chinese acupuncture, and is considered to be related to the liver. The ancient Chinese held that massaging this area will induce the liver qi energy to flow smoothly and dispel the blood blockage of the liver.

- Apply finger pressure to the following acupoints several times a day: Ganshu, Zusanli, and Taichong. (See appendix 7.)

- Frequently rotate your eyes. The ancient Chinese also held that the eyes were associated with the liver. Rotating your eyes frequently can thus help promote the qi circulation around your liver, improving its health.

Loss of Appetite

See "Jaded Appetite."

Menopause

Description

Menopause is a biological change that women experience later in life. While a natural and inevitable biological event, menopause can cause many health problems for women if not handled well. It occurs for most women between the ages of forty-five and fifty-five, with fifty-two being the average age.

As the name implies, menopause is the cessation of menstruation. This is when ova production begins to decline, and menstruation becomes lighter and irregular before it completely stops. The production of female hormones (estrogen and progesterone) also goes through periodic fluctuations in intensity and quality. Eventually, the follicles cease to produce eggs, leading to a decrease in estrogen production.

A decreased estrogen level is responsible for the four major menopausal conditions: vaginal dryness, cessation of menstrual periods, hot flashes, and osteoporosis. Osteoporosis occurs because as the estrogen levels lower, loss of calcium in the bone becomes greater, leading eventually to osteoporosis. Since estrogen is also responsible for stimulating the production of the natural lubricants in the vagina, vaginal dryness occurs. This may lead to irritation and itching as well as soreness during and after intercourse.

Menopause also increases the risk of heart disease because estrogen has a protective effect on the heart. In addition, menopause is a risk factor for hypertension and elevated blood cholesterol which, in turn, increase the risk of heart attack. These are some of the more nasty side effects of menopause. Modern scientists find that menopause's greatest effect on health and longevity has to do with the fact that estrogen appears to be a "fountain of youth" for the arterial linings in women.

Symptoms or signs

They include lighter, heavier, or irregular periods, vaginal dryness, dry and burning eyes, heart palpitations, panic attacks, lethargy, insomnia, depression, fear of loss of sexuality, and hot flashes. Sudden mood changes that come without warning can also occur.

Hot flashes are experienced by more than half of menopausal women. They are characterized by a sudden feeling of intense heat in the upper body with sweating, and sometimes accompanied by heart palpitations followed by chills. The episodes usually lasts two to three minutes and occur in the evenings. Most women complain about hot flashes for more than one year, and at least one-fourth of women have them for more than three years. Nearly one-fifth of women have a severe problem with hot flashes, experiencing as many as ten or more occurrences per day or sleep interruptions, leading to fatigue, anxiety, and emotional swings.

Causes

According to traditional Chinese medicine, women reaching the age of fifty experience a deficiency of blood and kidney qi energy, with an imbalance of yin and yang and, hence, menopause takes place. Menopause comes to all women at a certain age as the natural aging process, a deficiency in hormones from the pituitary gland, and a disturbance in the metabolic process of calcium. It occurs because the ovaries' production of estrogen and progesterone, the female hormones, is suddenly greatly reduced.

Prevention and treatment
Dietary therapies

- Avoid all caffeine and alcohol products.

- Make soy products such as tofu and soybean sprouts a constant part of your diet.

Soy products have been shown to significantly reduce menopausal side effects in Chinese women.

- Regularly eat eggs, carrots, and yams. These foods have a high folic acid content and can therefore increase natural estrogen production, and as such, protect the bones, heart, and vagina.

- Increase your daily calcium intake. Eat more tofu, skim milk, orange juice, almonds, and canned salmon or sardines. More importantly, eat plenty of fresh fruit and vegetables, such as cabbage, apples, pears, grapes, nuts, and other fresh vegetables. Cabbage is rich in calcium, while such fruits contain boron that is instrumental in the absorption and utilization of dietary calcium. Moreover, these foods can greatly enhance the estrogen level in the blood, according to a study conducted at the Human Research Center in Grand Forks, North Dakota.

- Soak three ounces of black beans overnight. Mix them with one ounce of dong quai and some sliced garlic cloves and cook for twenty minutes. Drink the soup in two equal servings, twice a day. Do this for three days after each menstrual cycle. This can warm the blood, boost energy, and relieve menopausal ailments.

- Fry eight ounces of cuttlefish in vegetable oil with some sliced fresh ginger, adding some salt. Eat it twice a day to relieve hot flashes.

- Eat plenty of soybeans and tofu. Soy contains isoflavones which are powerful weapons against menopausal ailments and breast cancer. Tofu is easily digested and absorbed.

- Boil one ounce each of fresh ginger, red dates, peach kernels, and rice wine in some water. Drink it twice a day, once in the morning and again in the evening.

- Drink a mixture of egg white and rice vinegar to relieve the symptoms of menopause.

- Cook mussels with rice wine, ginger, and black soybeans to regulate the menstrual flow. This is because an irregular menstrual flow is often caused by coldness in the womb, and mussels prepared this way can warm it up.

- Eating sunflower seeds regularly will help produce estrogen.

- Ginseng has earned a reputation as a natural alleviator of hot flashes. It can be American ginseng, Korean ginseng, or Chinese ginseng.

- Drink plenty of water and juices.

Other natural therapies

- Dress lightly to make yourself as comfortable as possible.

- Keep your home and workplace cool.

- Wear layers of loose clothing that can be easily removed.

- Practice qigong and other Chinese fitness exercises every day to help stabilize hormones, strengthen the bones, and reduce depression. Qigong and other exercises have helped many women find relief from hot flashes.

- While practicing qigong, breathe deeply but naturally, and focus your mind on the acupoint of Ruzhong, the midpoint between the nipples. (See appendix 7 for the acupoint location.)

- Regularly pressing the following acupoints has the effect of nourishing the kidney yin energy and reducing the risk of menopausal symptoms or signs: Zusanli, Sanyinjiao, and Neiguan. (See appendix 7.)

Menstrual Dysfunction

Description

Women of childbearing age—normally from thirteen to fifty years old—experience a regular monthly discharge of blood inside the body called the menstrual cycle or period. This serves both to cleanse the body and blood of its waste, and to help release eggs necessary for conception. However, various factors can disturb this cycle and make periods irregular, missing some months or coming earlier or later than normal.

Symptoms or signs

Women with irregular periods report a lowering in their mood and energy levels, reduction in sexual vitality, food cravings, water retention, breast tenderness, as well as night sweats and frequent fatigue. Other symptoms may include excessive or deficient menstruation, a foul odor during menstruation, darker blood than normal, abnormal discharge, and severe pain and cramps.

Some women also experience premenstrual syndrome (PMS), which causes undesirable and uncomfortable physical and psychological changes one to three days before the period. Mental symptoms of premenstrual syndrome include mood swings, mild depression, and difficulty in concentrating.

Causes

Obesity, excessive dieting, strenuous exercise, emotional as well as physical stress, use of birth control pills, hormone imbalances, or problems in the reproductive system—all of these can cause missed or irregular menstruation. Scientists do not have the complete answer yet for the causes of premenstrual syndrome, but it is found that it is closely related to a disorder of an endocrine gland and dysfunction of the outer portion of the largest portion of the brain. Thus, high blood sugar, depression, and a low level of endorphins—a brain chemical that helps you feel good—are considered among the causes.

In traditional Chinese medicine, menstrual dysfunction is attributed to a problem in the woman's blood system. Menstruation is considered to be a variation of blood, and therefore, the blood system has a direct impact on menstrual functions. Excessive bleeding during menstruation is considered to be a symptom of deficient blood qi, whose main function is to control the flow of blood throughout the body. Painful menstruation is considered to be a sign of blood "hotness," and irregular menstruation is considered to be a result of an interruption of blood circulation in the body.

Indeed, Chinese medicine sees blood as the most important life energy for the female. What blood is to a woman is what sperm is to a man. For this reason, all traditional treatments for menstruation ailments start with mending the blood system.

Prevention and treatment

Avoid excess weight and severe dieting. Regularly practice soft Chinese fitness exercises—avoid vigorous exercise or exertion. Keep a light heart by learning the techniques to cope with stress and depression. Regular practice of Chinese breathing exercises can be helpful for this. Avoid alcohol, which is a depressant and can disturb the proper functioning of the blood. In addition, control your blood sugar, and cut back on caffeine and refined sugars.

To relieve the ailments, try the following methods:

Dietary therapies

- Avoid cold foods and drinks such as ice water and ice cream.

- Avoid smoking and secondhand smoke.

- Stay away from irritating foods such as hot peppers and chili.

- Stew some sliced lean mutton together with some dong quai and ginger slices for thirty minutes. Add some salt and brown sugar. Eat the mutton and drink the soup. This is an effective treatment for amenorrhea, i.e., the absence or abnormal cessation of the menses.

- Cook some freshwater mussels in water. When done, add some rice wine and ginger juice. Drink the soup and eat the mussels. This can relieve all symptoms related to menstrual dysfunction.

- Drink fresh lotus root juice. Take this once a day on an empty stomach for a month. This can relieve irregular menstruation and menstrual pain.

- For menoxenia (abnormal menstruation), take two egg yolks and break them into a large glass. Boil some rice vinegar in a pot and add one ounce of moxa leaves. (Moxa is a Chinese herb that is often used with acupuncture.) Cook the moxa leaves in the vinegar for a while, then add some water and boil. Pour the juice into the glass of egg yolks. Mix and drink the egg soup. This can relieve irregular menstruation and menstrual pain.

- Soak one pound of garlic cloves in thirty-two ounces of rice wine (high alcohol content) in a jar. Cover tightly for a month. When ready to use, take one ounce of this garlic wine, add some honey or rock sugar and two ounces of water, and drink. Do this twice a day, once in the morning and once in the evening, for a month. This can relieve irregular menstruation and pain.

• For general menstrual dysfunction, make a porridge out of one bean curd, one ounce of gingko fruit, and two ounces of rice. Eat it for breakfast.

• To relieve uterus bleeding, grind the bones of a cuttlefish into powder. Swallow two spoonfuls of this powder with warm water. Do this twice a day.

• Stew one ounce of sliced *Polygomum multiflorium* (a Chinese herb), first soaked in water for two hours, with two eggs in water. Eat as a dish.

• Pound four ounces of peach seeds into a powder. Cook the pounded peach seeds in water for thirty minutes. Then add five ounces of honey. Continue to cook for fifteen minutes until it becomes creamy. Eat one spoonful of the cream at a time on an empty stomach. Do this twice a day, once in the morning and again in the evening.

• Soak three ounces of black beans overnight. Mix them with one ounce of dong quai and some sliced garlic cloves. Cook together for twenty minutes. Eat in two equal servings in one day. Do this continuously for three days after each menstrual cycle. This warms the blood, boosts energy, and relieves pain.

• Eat some fresh pork, beef, or chicken liver twice a week.

• Fry some fresh sheep liver with some fragrant-flowered garlic to make a dish. Eat it as part of a meal.

• Cut three ounces of chives and four ounces of lamb liver and fry them in peanut oil for a short while. Then add some soy sauce and cover for a few more moments. Eat the dish once a day for three successive days.

• Slice four ounces of fresh celery and an equal amount of lotus roots. Fry them in a hot pan with peanut oil for about five minutes. Add some salt for seasoning. Eat this once a day.

• For excessive or abnormal menstruation, bake some wake-robin (herb) and grind it into a powder. Cook some celery in water together with some brown sugar for fifteen minutes. Use this celery mix to make a tea of the powder. Drink the tea once a day.

• For deficient menstruation, cook a female chicken in water for forty-five minutes together with some moxa leaves, sesame seeds, pepper, bamboo roots, and green onion stalks. When done, add three spoonfuls of rice wine. Drink the soup and eat the chicken as a dish.

• The following vegetables and fruits are very helpful for menstruation dysfunction: spinach, carrots, sweet potatoes, oranges, grapes, and bananas.

• These sea foods are very good for menstruation: mussels, kelp, and seaweed.

To relieve menstrual pain

- Take two eggs, water, and some coriander to make a soup. Eat as part of a meal to relieve stomachaches.

- Combine one ounce of red dates, one ounce of fresh ginger, and half an ounce of red pepper. Cut the ginger and pepper into small pieces and then boil in water for thirty minutes. Drink the soup hot.

- Cook a few sweet basil leaves with an egg in water and add some rice wine.

- Cook a few sweet basil leaves with ginger, green onion, and fish in water and eat.

- Eat soft-shelled turtle once a week.

- Cook two eggs (whole) together with two ounces of black soybeans and four ounces of rice wine over low heat. Eat the eggs and drink the soup.

- Boil some hawthorn fruit and cinnamon twigs with brown sugar in two cups of water until there is only one cup of water left. Drink this twice a day.

- Boil one ounce of red dates, one ounce of dried ginger, and one ounce of brown sugar in water for about twenty minutes. Drink and eat everything.

- Take five ounces of dong quai root and twenty red dates. Boil them with two cups of water for twenty minutes. Eat everything. This dish is traditionally used in China as a women's supplement. It has the effect of nourishing the blood and female energy and regulating the menstrual cycle.

Other natural therapies

- Avoid cold water and swimming during menstruation. Chinese medicine holds that cold water is detrimental to the health of women during menstruation.

- Manage stress and maintain a light heart. Go to bed early in the evening and get up early in the morning.

- Learn some soft exercises and practice them regularly.

- Practice breathing exercises every day.

- For irregular menstruation, acupress the following acupoints: Qihai, Guanyuan, Sanyingjiao, and Xingjian.

- For painful menstruation, acupress the following acupoints: Zhongji, Hegu, Sanyingjiao, Xingjian, Qihai, Guanyuan, and Diji. (See appendix 7.)

- For absence of menstruation, acupress Guanyuan, Zhongji, Qihai, Zusanli, Sanyingjiao, Tianshu, and Zhongwan.

- For excess bleeding in menstruation, acupress Qihai, Zhongji, Sanyinjiao, Renzhong, and Baihui. (See appendix 7.)

Myopia (Nearsightedness)

Description

Myopia, or nearsightedness, is a defect in the vision where light entering the eye is brought to a focus in front of the retina instead of at the retina. Those afflicted with myopia have a hard time seeing far away objects clearly without the aid of glasses.

Causes

Myopia can be caused by genetic factors if there is a long family history of the disease. Modernization has added some strong triggers of myopia, mainly in the form of television sets and computers, which have become a way of life in this country. If this tendency continues, by the next century myopia will be the rule in our society and normal eyesight will become the exception.

Prevention and treatment

Natural therapies

- Eat plenty of fish oil, carrots, and animal liver, which are helpful to the eyes.

- Stop for a while every half an hour after reading or working at a computer. Look outside the office into the distance, or just close your eyes for a few minutes. This can go a long way toward maintaining good eyesight and treating bad eyesight.

- Avoid reading or working at a computer under a light that is too strong or too weak. Do not read on the bus, in bed, or while walking. Limit the length and time you watch television.

- Rotate your eyes seven times in each direction—clockwise and counterclockwise. Do this several times a day, especially in the morning after getting up. (See appendix 5.)

- Rub your hands until they are warm, and then cover the eyes for a while. Doing this several times a day can also help restore your eyesight.

- Eat plenty of kidney beans, carrots, grapes, and animal livers. You can cook the liver with the kidney beans and carrots to make a dish.

- Apply finger pressure to the following acupoints several times a day: Chuanzhu, Ganshu, Geshu, Yintang, Taiyang, Chengqi, Zhongshu, Sibai, Jingming, Jujiao, and Xinshu. (See appendix 7.)

Nausea

Description

Nausea is an unpleasant feeling in the stomach. Sufferers of nausea may feel weak and sweaty and produce lots of saliva. Vomiting is the result of intense nausea, which forces the stomach contents up the esophagus and out of the mouth. Dehydration is the greatest risk of vomiting, and is marked by increased thirst, infrequent urination, dry mouth, and dry skin.

Symptoms or signs

These include an upset stomach, vomiting, sweating, excess production of saliva, and feeling weak.

Causes

There are several causes of nausea: a virus (such as a viral stomach flu); food poisoning; stress or nervousness; diabetes; pregnancy; and head injuries. Persistent nausea without vomiting is most likely due to medication and occasionally to ulcers or cancer.

NOTE: It must be pointed out that the therapies listed below are tailored to temporarily relieve the condition. It is advised to get the condition diagnosed as soon as possible in order to find out the exact cause of the ailment. See a medical professional if you do not feel better.

Prevention and treatment

Dietary therapies

- Take nothing by mouth for three hours after vomiting.

- Drink only water, green tea, or diluted juice for the first twelve hours. Drink as much clean water as your stomach can take, but do not drink too much at any one time.

- Avoid solid foods. Eat only clear soups, mild foods and liquids the next day until all symptoms are gone.

- Chewing ginger or drinking ginger tea can bring relief. Do this as soon as the symptoms show up.

Nearsightedness

(See "Myopia.")

Neurasthenia

Description

This is the most common variety of neurosis. It is often associated with intellectuals who used a lot of their brain and did little physical exercise. Nowadays more and more people have fallen victims to it due to our modern way of life. While initially a problem with the nervous system, it can affect various parts of the body.

Symptoms or signs

These include headaches, dizziness, ear ringing, fatigue, indigestion, jaded appetite, constipation, insomnia, dream-laden sleep, palpitations, weak memory, depression, lassitude, frequent urination and/or bowel movements, night sweats, and menstrual disorders.

Causes

Neurasthenia is often caused by chronic nervous tension, an unbalanced lifestyle between mental and physical activities, chronic stress and depression, emotional upsets, and indulgence in sex. All of these can lead to functional disorders of the cerebral cortex with resultant disturbances of the autonomic nervous system.

NOTE: Be sure to see a medical professional if the condition doesn't improve.

Prevention and treatment

Dietary therapies

- Stop smoking and avoid alcohol.

- Regularly consume honey with milk for breakfast. The Chinese believe that this can nourish the brain system and therefore relieve the ailment.

- Steam a pork brain in water with some tuber of elevated gastrodia (*Gastrodia eleta*) and Chinese wolfberries (*Lycium chinese*). Eat the soup and the brain before going to bed at night. The Chinese believe this can nourish the brain system and therefore relieve the ailment.

- For night sweats, fry chives in vegetable oil together with some fresh sheep's liver, or with some fresh pork kidney. Eat it as a dish.

- Regularly eat peanuts, walnuts, mushrooms, and animal marrow and brain.

- Regularly drink chicken or beef soup.

- Cook together ten ounces of fresh green soybeans. Eat it as part of a meal.

- Soak two ounces of lotus seeds and some lily in water for two hours. Then add five ounces of sliced lean meat. Stew them together for thirty minutes, add a little bit salt, and eat it as a dish.

- Soak ten dates and one ounce of Chinese wolfberry in water for two hours. Break in two eggs, along with some rock sugar and salt. Stew for fifteen minutes and eat it as a dish at dinner time. Do this once a day for two weeks.

- Cook two ounces of red dates together with two ounces of dansheng (*Codonopsis pilosula*) in water for forty-five minutes. Drink the soup and eat the dates. This can relieve palpitations.

- Mix one spoonful of sesame oil and one spoonful of granulated sugar with boiled water to brew a tea. Drink it three times a day.

- Fry some fresh sheep's liver with some fragrant-flowered garlic to make a dish. Eat it as part of a meal.

- Fry one ounce of dried peaches until brown. Add some water immediately and then add one ounce of red dates. Boil together for a few moments and eat before going to bed.

- Cook clams with some chives. Eat it as a meal once a day for two weeks.

Other natural therapies

- Practice qigong, Dharma's internal exercises, and other soft exercises every day.

- Take a cold bath everyday.

- Be very abstinent in sex, especially ejaculation and even masturbation.

- Apply finger pressure to the following acupoints several times a day: Shenmen, Sanyinjiao, Baihui, Daling, Neiguan, Tianshu, Guanyuan, Yintang, Taiyang, and Zusanli. (See appendix 7.)

Night Blindness

Description
The medical term for this disease is retinitis pigmentosa. This ailment is characterized by the inability to see objects at night, and an inability to navigate in or adapt to the darkness. If the disease progresses, peripheral vision is also lost.

Symptoms or signs
Those afflicted can have difficulty seeing at night or in reduced light and have poor central vision.

Causes
Night blindness is due to a defect of the rods of the retina. It may be a hereditary defect or an early symptom of a deficiency of vitamin A. According to traditional Chinese theory, this is caused by a deficiency of liver energy.

Prevention and treatment
Natural therapies
- Regular consumption of animal livers, especially sheep liver, can greatly treat the disease.
- Regular consumption of fresh carrots or carrot juice can prevent and cure night blindness.
- Cook some pork liver with one ounce of Chinese wolfberries. Eat as a dish.
- Drink plenty of apple juice. The Chinese believe this can strengthen the eyesight and relieve the ailment.
- Eating fresh peanuts on a regular basis as well as fish oil can strengthen the eyesight and relieve the ailment.
- Cook two tomatoes with three ounces of pork liver. Eat it as a meal, once a day for two weeks.
- Regularly eat bitter gourd as a vegetable, or fry it with pork liver to make an appetizing dish. This is because bitter gourd, according to Chinese theory, can nourish the liver and therefore improve eyesight.
- Fry beef or lamb liver together with some chives to make a dish. Eat it once a day. Chicken liver has a similar effect. This can strengthen the eye function and relieve the disease.
- Apply finger pressure to the following acupoints several times a day: Sibai, Zanzhu, Jujiao, Jingming, and Chengqi. (See appendix 7.)

Nocturnal Emissions

Description
Alternatively known as "wet dreams," this is an exclusively male disease, characterized by involuntary ejaculation during sleep, without actual intercourse or masturbation. An occasional seminal emission without discomfort or other symptoms is a physiological phenomenon, usually when an adult male sleeps alone.

However, frequent seminal emissions are considered to be much more harmful to the health than most people think. It can lead to a number of ailments such as neurasthenia, dizziness, ringing in the ear, fatigue and weakness, insomnia, emaciation, loss of appetite and weight, loss of memory, impotence, and premature aging.

Symptoms or signs

These include involuntary discharge of semen during sleep, once a week or more often; feeling tired, weak, or sleepy; lack of strength in the limbs; loss of appetite; decrease in memory; ear ringing; heart palpitations; frequent colds, and night sweats.

Causes

This disease is diagnosed in traditional Chinese medicine as a looseness in the "sperm gate," which is caused by an imbalance of the heart qi and kidney qi (or lack of communication—so to speak—between the heart and the kidneys), leading to a deficiency in kidney qi energy. Such a deficiency can be caused by many different factors such as masturbation, indulgence in sex, excessive drinking, exposure to pornographic or sexually stimulating images, and wishful sexual thinking.

In the Chinese natural health care system, the kidneys stand for water, and the heart stands for fire. These two seemingly conflicting elements must be in balance for the body to function properly. Typically, when a fire is roaring, water evaporates. The overheating of fire (in one's body) can result from a mental preoccupation with sex, an excess eating of fried, spicy, and hot-natured foods, and a lowering of kidney qi energy as a con-

sequence of sexual indulgence. This is the case with nocturnal emissions and sexual dysfunction. Physical exertion and fatigue during the day can also loosen the "sperm gate" during the night, resulting in a nocturnal emission.

Prevention and treatment

Oddly enough, marriage has been shown to be an effective cure for nocturnal emissions. Many single men report the disappearance of this ailment once they marry.

To prevent wet dreams, avoid heavy meals in the evening, especially spicy foods and alcohol. Free the mind of encumbrances, and abstain from masturbation. Keep regular hours, going to bed and waking up early. Wear loose and comfortable clothes in bed. While asleep, lie on your side to avoid any pressure on the penis. Since emissions are most likely to occur when the bladder is full, make sure to urinate whenever you feel the need during the night.

Dietary therapies

- Avoid spicy, stimulating foods such as hot peppers, alcohol, and fried foods.

- Cook in water for half an hour one pound of fresh pork bones together with half a pound of fresh mussels. Drink the soup and eat the mussels. Do this once a day to make up for the loss of sexual essence.

- Eat pork or beef kidneys every day or every other day to strengthen the kidney qi energy.

- Stew one ounce of Chinese wolfberries with a cut beef penis and some ginger. Drink and eat everything. Do this every other day.

- Stew two ounces of walnuts and one ounce of silkworm cocoons in water for thirty minutes.

- Fry chives in vegetable oil together with some fresh, sliced sheep liver. Eat them as a dish.

- Lotus plumule, oyster, walnuts, and black fungus are good foods for the condition. They are good at either nourishing the kidneys or strengthening the Gate of Heaven so that nocturnal emissions can be stopped.

- Stew lotus seeds and lean pork meat together for an hour. Eat it as a dish on an empty stomach.

- Fry two eggs and some chives together and eat.

- Stew five ounces of lotus seeds in water for thirty minutes. Eat the lotus seeds and drink the soup. Do this twice a day, once in the morning and again in the evening, for two weeks.

- Cook three ounces of mussels and an egg together, seasoned with some salt and sesame oil. Eat everything and drink the soup. Take this once a day for two weeks.

- Mix five ounces of fresh oysters and two eggs. Fry them in peanut oil for three minutes together with some ginger and salt. Eat once a day for two weeks.

- Cook pork bones in water to make a cup of thick soup, by cooking it for a couple of hours. Use it to cook two pork kidneys, one ounce of peach seeds, some pepper, three green onion stalks, and a bit of salt. When done, eat the kidneys and drink the soup.

- Cook walnuts and silkworm chrysalis together. Eat them at dinner time.

- Fry some fresh sheep liver with some fragrant-flowered garlic to make a dish. Eat it as part of a meal.

- Cook in water for one hour a fresh beef penis (cleaned and cut) together with some pork feet, ginger, green onion stalks, and salt. Eat everything.

- Bake ten to fifteen silkworm cocoons in moderate heat. Put them in a glass, and add some lotus hair. Boil a cup of spring water and use it to soak the silkworm cocoons and lotus hair. Drink as a tea twice a day.

- Stew one ounce of sliced *Polygomum multiflorium* (first soaked in water for two hours), with two broken eggs in water. Eat the eggs as a dish.

- Fry one ounce of dried peaches until the surface is yellowish. Add some water and one ounce of red dates. Boil together for a few minutes. Eat before going to bed.

- Drink fresh raspberry juice before going to bed.

- Fry one ounce of walnuts, two sliced pork kidneys, and a little lard together. Eat it hot everyday at bedtime for one week.

- Bake one ounce of the seed of Chinese arborvitae. Put the baked seeds in a glass and brew the seeds with boiled spring water. Drink it as tea twice a day.

- Cook chives with an egg to relieve nocturnal emission and night sweating.

- Boil yams with some ginseng and eat at bedtime.

Other natural therapies

- Practice qigong. Lie on your back, cover your naval with your right palm, and press the acupoint of Huiyin with the middle finger of your left hand. (See appendix 7 for the location of the acupoint.) Breathe deeply and naturally, with your mind focusing on the acupoint. Huiyin and the navel are directly linked to the "sperm gate," according to the Chinese natural health care theory.

- Frequently accumulate and swallow saliva. (For methods of accumulating and swallowing the saliva, see appendix 1.)

- Each night at bedtime, rub your hands against each other until warm. Then cup the scrotum with a warm hand for a few minutes. Rub both hands against each other again until warm, and then cup the scrotum again for a few minutes with the other hand.

- Rub both hands against each other until warm. Use the warm hands to rub the soles of your feet, one sole at a time.

- Practice Dharma's internal exercises, especially "Rub the Neck," "Rub the Abdomen," and "Shake the Heavenly Pillar." (See appendix 5.)

- Practice sound qigong, making the sound of "Ha" while exhaling. (See appendix 3.)

- Drink the middle third of your midnight urination. In practice, pass away your urine until it is almost three-quarters done. Then use a cup to hold the rest of your urine and drink it right away.

- Frequently contract and release your anal muscle and toes alternately. These parts of the body are thought to be linked to the "sperm gate."

- Soak the feet in warm water for five minutes immediately before going to bed. Or, use a cold towel to rub the soles of your feet.

- Pressing the following acupoints several times a day can strengthen the kidney yin energy and help control nocturnal emissions: Sanyinjiao, Zusanli, Guanyuan, Xinshu, Shenshu, Zhishi, Neiguan, Qihai, Zhongji, and Zusanli. (See appendix 7.)

Nosebleed

Description

Just as the name implies, this ailment is characterized by blood coming out of the nose. It is inconvenient and messy, and can cause unnecessary panic when it's unexpected. Fortunately, it can be effectively tackled by natural means without knocking on a doctor's door.

Symptoms or signs

A nosebleed is sudden bleeding from one or both nostrils.

Causes

Low humidity (dryness in the nose) is a common cause of nosebleeds. Colds, allergies, high altitudes, and, according to Chinese theory, excess consumption of hot-natured foods, such as tropical foods, are all causes of nosebleeds.

A study done in England suggests that regular drinking of alcohol increases the risk of nosebleeds. Doctors surveyed the drinking habits of 140 hospital patients. They found that 45 percent of those with nosebleeds were regular drinkers. One explanation for this is that alcohol in the bloodstream makes clot-forming more difficult.

Prevention and treatment

Dietary therapies

- These foods are believed to be able to arrest bleeding: black fungus, chestnuts, chicken eggshell powder (grind the eggshell into power and take one small spoonful of it with warm water), spinach, and vinegar.

- Stew two to five ounces of peanuts in water with some garlic cloves for forty-five minutes. Eat everything as a dish.

- Crush a few garlic cloves and make a cake out of it. Place it on the sole of your foot.

- Squeeze the juice out of fresh chives. Drink a small cup of juice twice a day.

- Eat fresh peanuts to stop bleeding.

- Drink a cup of juice made of fresh lotus roots to stop bleeding.

- Cook peanuts with garlic cloves and eat them up as dish or meal.

- Boil corn silk with banana peel in water.

- Drink celery juice.

- Drink plenty of water to increase the internal humidity of the body.

Other natural therapies

- Humidify your house, especially your bedroom, and keep the temperature low in sleeping areas.

- Bend your head back to face the sky and cover your forehead with a towel soaked in cold water. Stay in that position and rest for fifteen minutes. Applying ice to the bridge of the nose works, too.

- Blow all the blood clots out of your nose. Pinch the nostrils between your thumb and forefinger for ten minutes. Resist the urge to peek after a few minutes to see if it has stopped bleeding.

- Apply finger pressure to the following acupoints: Fengfu, Ximen, and Hegu. (See appendix 7.)

Obesity

Description
Obesity is an excessive amount of fat in the body, largely located in the abdomen, buttocks, and thigh areas. Being 20 to 30 percent over your normal weight is considered obesity. According to a report by the American Heart Association, 65.7 million Americans were above the healthy range of weight in a 1988-1994 study.[30] The fact is that more Americans suffer from obesity than we would like to think.

A nasty consequence of excessive weight is that it adds an unnecessary burden to many parts of the body: the heart, lungs, pancreas, kidneys, gallbladder, joints, and even the genitals. This is why obesity often contributes to hypertension, diabetes, heart disease, and other health problems.

It is not a matter of how much you weigh, but a matter of how your body weight affects your life. If you are slowed down or unable to do normal daily activities as a result of the excess weight, then obesity is a problem. Measures should be taken to tackle it before it leads to more serious health problems.

Symptoms or signs
Obesity is being 20 to 30 percent above your normal weight, with low flexibility and low muscle tone.

Causes
An unhealthy diet and lifestyle are by far the two most important causes of obesity, although there may be hereditary factors involved. It is what you eat, how you eat, and how much you eat, as well as how much exercise you get that determine whether you are heading toward obesity or not.

Bad eating habits that can lead to obesity include eating between meals, eating close to bedtime, regularly eating a heavy dinner, drinking alcohol with meals, and eating protein foods together with starchy ones, or eating fruit together with protein or starchy foods. These are habits that hamper proper digestion of the foods you eat. Unless fully digested and used as energy, the food will turn into fat and be stored in the body.

Recent studies show that even moderate drinking can increase your waistline. This is because alcohol in the diet seems to protect the body's reserves of fat, since the body prefers to burn alcohol and store food as fat. For instance, drink two cans of beer a day and you will take in roughly 300 calories of the 2,300 to 2,900 calories you need each day if you are a moderately active man (1,900 to 2,200 calories if you are a woman). That is how beer gains its reputation as a "belly maker."[31]

The most effective means of turning food into energy and expending that energy is through daily exercise. The more you exercise, the harder it will be for you to become obese. Exercise effectively burns up the fat and calories one takes in. We may see some people who eat a lot of fat but remain slender throughout their lives. Their secret is regular exercise. Your occupation or lifestyle can determine how much food you can eat without gaining weight. My teacher is a typical example. Dr. Wan Laisheng enjoyed animal meat, fatty meat in particular, throughout his life. However, he remained very strong and slender to the very end. This is because his occupation as a martial arts master required him to exercise a lot every day. The animal fat he took in served only to provide the energy he needed for his daily activities and vitality.

Please do not misunderstand me. I am not advocating animal meat or fat, but rather showing how important exercise is to one's health. As not many of us have the time or ability to exercise as efficiently as Wan Laisheng, it is advisable to watch our diet carefully if we want to avoid obesity. This does not mean, however, that you cannot enjoy meals or eat what you like to. Actually, there are many foods that are both delicious and healthy.

Prevention and treatment

The latest research shows that popular and miraculous-sounding weight loss methods, such as the diet pill Fen-phen, can have serious side effects. These can range from frequent fatigue and diarrhea to serious heart trouble.[32] In the Chinese natural health care system, weight loss is treated quite differently. Since what really makes up the weight gain is fat and water, the focus of treatment should be on how to get rid of the excess fat and water in the body as well as reducing the number of calories consumed. This can be done by internally burning up or absorbing the fat and water, or externally taking out the excess fat and water through sweating and urination.

One of the best suggestions is to follow a diet that is rich in fresh fruits and vegetables. Such a diet provides the active enzymes, organic alkaline minerals, and fiber required for digestion, bowel movements, and metabolism. A diet high in protein but low in carbohydrates will better utilize fat and protein as energy. Seafood and fish are excellent sources of protein that are low in saturated fat, light on calories, and high in vitamins, minerals, and omega-3 fatty acids, which help reduce the risk of heart disease. Just as important, you should exercise regularly on a daily basis to burn up calories.

Dietary therapies

- Avoid all refined foods and high carbohydrates: candy, chocolate, pizza, fatty meats, chips, sodas, corn, carrots, junk foods, milk, beets, and potatoes.

- Avoid caffeinated products such as coffee and commercial soft drinks. Caffeine activates sugar into the system from glycogen stored in the liver, leading to weight gain.

- Avoid alcohol. Alcohol is high in calories, and it tends to work against your self-control when eating.

- Eat plenty of spinach, which is one of the most potent antidotes for lower bowel stagnation, a common cause of obesity.

- Regularly drink plenty of lemon juice to reduce weight and relieve obesity. My teacher told me that lemon juice can help carry away the fat in the body.

- Sniff food deeply before eating. Sniffing the odors of your favorite foods can help in weight reduction by diminishing your hunger. That is why cooks usually do not get fat because they are exposed to delicious odors too frequently to feel hungry.

- Chew thoroughly to give your brain time to warn you regarding how full your stomach is, thus avoiding overeating.

- Eat early during the day. As the saying goes: Eat breakfast like a king, but dinner like a pauper. If you eat most of your calories earlier in the day, you may actually burn fat faster. You have the entire day ahead of you to burn up the fat you have taken in, even just through normal activities. Studies show that obese people eat a big dinner, consuming more than 75 percent of their calories in the evening when the body is entering its resting stage.

- Cook small red beans until they are soft and eat them as a meal at least once a day. It is even better to cook them with red dates and a few garlic cloves.

- Boil some soybeans and garlic together as a meal to promote urination. Mung and hyacinth beans have a similar effect.

- Drink plenty of pure water between meals to rid the body of toxins and help with the elimination of undigested foods.

- Regular consumption of fresh ginger can promote perspiration and the burning of fat inside the body.

- Drink a cup of grapefruit juice one hour before a meal. Grapefruit contains the enzyme that promotes digestion.

- Eat plenty of bananas. Bananas are a healthy food with multiple nutrients. They help bowel movements, kill hunger without adding a lot of calories.

- Drink plenty of carrot juice and cabbage juice.

- Mixing apple cider vinegar with olive oil to dress a dish can help digestion.

- Boil dried ginger and dried orange peel together. Then add some brown sugar and boil for another minute. Drink as a tea.

Other natural therapies

- Practice soft exercises, such as Dharma's morning exercises, on a daily basis. Exercise is the best weapon we have in fighting obesity, because it helps fix what makes us fat in the first place: our metabolism. Exercise promotes the metabolic process, and makes our muscle cells better at utilizing the glucose by encouraging the growth of calorie-consuming enzymes.

- In addition to daytime exercise, it is highly advisable to exercise in the evening, too. This will help burn up the calories you consume at dinner, which will otherwise stay in the body and add to your weight.

- Practice sound qigong and make the sound of "High." (See appendix 3.)

- Move your bowels at least once a day, preferably right after you get up in the morning.

- Pressing the earlobes between the thumb and forefinger thirty times daily can stimulate the appetite, help digestion, and lose weight.

Osteoporosis

Description

Osteoporosis is a condition that affects a quarter of women over the age of sixty. It is much less common and severe in men than in women. Literally, osteoporosis means "holey bones," i.e., your skeletal structure has become demineralized, brittle, and riddled with holes, making your bones very susceptible to breakage.

Symptoms or signs

Osteoporosis is a silent disease so there may be no symptoms until a bone breaks. The first sign may be hip or low back pain, or painful swelling after a fall.

Causes

Osteoporosis is caused by loss of bone mass and strength. Estrogen withdrawal, malabsorption of calcium, and low calcium intake are other risk factors. The risk of developing osteoporosis is greater for women than for men, especially women who lose 3 percent of their bone mass every year after menopause as a result of estrogen withdrawal. That is why about 70 percent of women eventually develop some degree of osteoporosis.

Interestingly, fewer cases of osteoporosis are reported in obese women. This is because fat stored in the body increases the levels of estrogen in the blood, and estrogen can protect the bones from the breakdown of osteoporosis through two or more different hormonal mechanisms.

A sedentary lifestyle or lack of exercise is another major factor leading to the condition. Bones gain strength in response to use and exercise. It is not an exaggeration to say "use them or you lose them."

Yet another cause is caffeine which, in the form of tea or coffee, seems to interfere with the body's absorption of calcium. Scientists tell us that our bones are constantly going through metabolic cycles, in which the dissolution of destroying cells and the synthesis of replenishing cells interact and try to offset each other. After thirty-five years of age, the speed of dissolution exceeds that of synthesis, leading to the loss of calcium in the bones. Thus, the risk of osteoporosis increases in direct proportion to age.

Prevention and treatment

First, you need to dispel the myth that calcium deficiency is only of concern to women as they approach menopause. The truth is that it's never too early for women to increase their calcium intake. Even teenagers should start eating more foods rich in calcium (such as milk and seafood) to build bone strength. Bones that are strong at an early age are in a better position to avoid running out of calcium and developing osteoporosis later on. Even during middle age, it is important for women to strengthen their bones, for bone productivity is at its highest at this time. This means eating more calcium-rich foods to prepare for "rainy days." Meanwhile, regular exercise, a balanced diet, and weight control are also extremely important in preventing osteoporosis.

Dietary therapies

- Reduce the daily intake of coffee, soft drinks, sugar, salt, alcohol, meat, and fatty foods. These foods all promote loss of calcium from the body. Focus your diet instead on fruits, vegetables, fish, nuts, seeds, and dairy products.

- Eat plenty of soy products such as tofu, soybean sprouts, and soy beverages. Soy consumption can greatly increase the bone density.

- Eat plenty of salmon, which has been shown to have the best therapeutic effect on preventing and treating osteoporosis. The next best choice is eel.

- Spend one hour a day in the sunshine, if possible (for the vitamin D).

- Cook sesame seeds with rice, or mix it with bread, and eat it regularly as a meal. Sesame seeds contain a lot of vitamin D.

- Drink carrot, parsley, or celery juice. These natural juices are rich in organic sodium, iron, and calcium. They can facilitate oxygen metabolism, dissolve deposits of inorganic calcium in joints, and relieve the discomfort of osteoporosis.

- Cook some soybeans or red beans and sliced pig leg together. Eat this as part of a meal. The Chinese fathers hold that pork leg contains certain properties that are nourishing to human legs and joints.

- Drink apple cider vinegar each day since it aids calcium absorption.

- Black walnuts contain silica which can relieve the pain of osteoporosis. So also can towel gourd do the job.

Other natural therapies

- Strengthen your bones with exercise. Since the bones are already weak, Chinese soft exercises are the most suitable and helpful for patients of osteoporosis.

- Protect your joints by pacing yourself, positioning yourself properly, and using a walking aid such as a cane.

- Massage the afflicted joints.

- Press the acupoints of Chenfu and Kunlun several times a day. (See appendix 7.)

Parkinson's Disease

Description

This disease is characterized by the nervous system's loss of control over the muscles. It is estimated that about one and a half a million Americans are afflicted with this disease. Most of them are over seventy years old. Quite a few world leaders, including China's Mao Tse-tung and Deng Xiaoping, have died from Parkinson's disease.

Symptoms or signs

These include cramping, muscle rigidity, shaking, staring or a blank facial expression, speech impairment, drooling, shuffling gait, weight loss, memory loss, and slowness in overall physical and mental activity.

Causes

Exact causes of Parkinson's disease are not well known, but preliminary studies show that the disease has a lot to do with an imbalance of brain chemicals such as dopamine and acetylcholine. These two neurotransmitters act as message-transferring tools between the central nervous system and muscles. Another explanation is that heavy metal toxicity tends to slow the energy-producing area of the brain cells that control the muscles. The Chinese fathers also believe that an excessive use of the brain, as in the case of many thinkers and intellectuals, also contributes to the occurrence of the disease.

Prevention and treatment

To prevent Parkinson's disease, it is important to nourish and relax the brain cells regularly. This is achieved through a healthy diet, sufficient sleep, and regular relaxation of the brain. Regular exercise and breathing fresh air on a daily basis is also recommended. The following methods can help relieve the symptoms and treat the disease.

NOTE: See a medical professional if the condition does not improve.

Dietary therapies

- Follow a low-protein, high-complex carbohydrate diet that will supply a higher amount of glucose needed to nourish a brain deficient in energy.

- Eat whole grains such as oatmeal, whole wheat bread, millet, rice, and barley. These foods are rich in vitamin E, a very helpful nutrient for the brain, which can improve the brain cell function.

- Eat plenty of apples, pears, strawberries, and cherries. The Chinese believe that these are good for the brain.

- Eat tofu regularly, preferably two meals a day.

- Drink a lot of fruit and vegetable juices.

Other natural therapies

- Practice qigong regularly. Qigong is a very effective means of keeping the brain healthy and fit, because qigong can relax an overused brain, replenishing energy and restoring balance. To bring more blood flow to the brain, imagine yourself bringing the qi energy up to the brain while inhaling. (See appendix 1.)

- Practice Dharma's internal exercises every day, especially "Rub the Face," "Rub the Head," and "Beat the Heavenly Drum." (See appendix 5.) These exercises directly impact the brain cells, activating them and keeping them in healthy condition.

- Spend plenty of time outdoors every day. This serves two purposes: it ensures that your brain is provided with sufficient fresh air, and that your brain gets enough rest after working.

- Apply finger pressure to the following acupoints many times a day: Fengchi, Taiyang, Shangxing, and Baihui. (See appendix 7.)

Pneumonia

Description

This disease is characterized by severe inflammation or infection of the smallest air passages in the lungs called alveoli. When these passages are filled with mucus, oxygen cannot reach the blood. Ranked as the sixth greatest killer in this country, pneumonia claimed more than 80,000 lives in 1996.

Symptoms or signs

Symptoms include pain in the chest, especially when coughing or taking a deep breath, nagging cough, chills, high fever, labored and shallow breathing, loss of appetite or upset stomach, chronic fatigue, sweating, and a flushed appearance on the face around noontime each day. If you experience these symptoms regularly, most likely you have contracted pneumonia.

Causes

The main cause of pneumonia is the intrusion of infectious pneumonia bacteria into the body while the immune system is weak.

Prevention and treatment

Healthy diet, sufficient rest, and a clean living environment with fresh air and sufficient sunlight are the best defenses against this disease. Pneumonia is a great consumer of energy. Therefore, nutrition and rest are of primary importance for its treatment. Make sure that your house is well ventilated and well lighted. Regularly hang your clothes, bedding, and often-used materials in the sunlight to get rid of potential pneumonia bacteria. Try to avoid catching a cold or the flu. Also, avoid living in humid, windowless rooms (because of bacteria).

NOTE: See a medical professional if the condition does not improve.

Dietary therapies

- Avoid tobacco products and alcohol.

- Limit the consumption of shrimp, fish, and crabs, as well as eggs.

- Eat foods rich in vitamins A, C, and E, such as green vegetables, carrots, tomatoes, sweet potatoes, mango, papaya, apples, lemons, oranges, peanuts, persimmon, strawberries, milk, lean meat, and chicken.

- Apricots, tremella, sheep's milk, malt sugar, olives, pears, an edible bird's nests are strongly recommended for treating pneumonia. This is based on Chinese folk tradition.

- Soak ten dates and one ounce of Chinese wolfberries in water for two hours. Add two eggs, rock sugar, and salt. Stew for fifteen minutes and eat it as a dish at dinner time. Do this once a day for two weeks. This serves to strengthen the lung function and help treat the disease.

- Soak one ounce of tremella in water for an hour. Add some rock sugar and twenty red dates and stew it for another hour. Drink the soup and eat the tremella. Enjoy this once a day for two weeks. This serves to strengthen the lung function and help treating the disease.

- Eat three raw garlic cloves, three times a day before meals. This can help kill pneumonia bacteria.

- Cook freshwater mussels with lean pork and eat them as a dish. This serves to strengthen the lung function and help treat the disease.

- Cook enough millet in water to make a meal. When it is becomes a porridge, add some white sugar and eat it. Do this once a day. It is a Chinese folk belief that millet can strengthen the lung function and relieve the symptoms of pneumonia.

- Cook one to two ounces of tremella in water until it is fully soft. Add some rock candy and eat it, preferably for breakfast. This is especially helpful to patients with a burning sensation in the lungs.

- Cook sesame powder in water, add an egg and some rock candy. Eat it on an empty stomach.

- Clean a fresh pork lung and cook it in water for half an hour together with fifty apricots and one ounce of fresh ginger. When done, add some honey. Eat the soup on an empty stomach. Do this once a day or every other day.

- Each half of a duck everyday for a month. This will have obvious results.

- Combine sliced Chinese yams and kelp and cook them in water for half an hour. When done, add white sugar and eat either as a meal or before a meal.

- Eat ten walnuts on an empty stomach in the morning, every day for one month. Avoid coffee or tea for an hour so that the walnuts can be fully absorbed.

- Take one teaspoonful of garlic syrup every three hours. Or chew several garlic cloves three times a day.

- Cook some noodles in water until they are half done. Add eight ounces of oysters and one ounce of crushed fresh garlic. Boil them together for another ten minutes and eat as a meal. This can both strengthen the lungs and kill the bacteria.

- Boil together some seaweed, kelp, dried lichee (a fruit produced in south China and Southeastern Asian countries), and some wine in water. Eat this every day for a week. This can help relieve pneumonia.

- Grind into powder the bones of a cuttlefish. Swallow two spoonfuls of this powder with warm waterbefore breakfast each morning. This can stop bleeding and pain. This has no side effects and can be taken regularly over time.

- Fasting is an ancient way of treating pneumonia, and is one of the most effective treatments for some people.

Other natural therapies

- Get plenty of rest to restore and build up the body's energy level in order to fight the pneumonia bacteria.

- Practice qigong three times a day, imagining the qi entering your chest while exhaling. Qigong derives its healing power for pneumonia from its ability to influence the starch enzyme in the saliva. Clinical observation found that through qigong practice, pneumonia patients can increase the starch enzyme level in their saliva to that of a normal person. (See appendix 1.)

- Practice Dharma's morning exercises and breathing exercises every day. This series of exercises are especially beneficial because they can effectively strengthen the lungs' function and effect a healing internally. (See appendix 4.)

- Regularly expose your personal belongings to sunlight, especially bedding, clothes, books, and so on. Sunlight is the strongest killer of viruses and bacteria.

- Open the window of your bedroom or the door of your house every day for a while to let in fresh air and sunlight.

- Frequently accumulate saliva in the mouth and swallow it down to the lower abdomen.

- Drink your own urine, only when you have not been drinking, smoking, or using drugs for the past twenty-four hours. Do this twice a day, once in the morning and once late at night. When you get up in the morning, pass away the first half of your first morning urine, but save the second half in a glass. Drink it warm right away. Then at midnight, do the same thing again. It is a Chinese folk belief that urine can kill pneumonia bacteria.

- Practice sound qigong and make the sounds of "Sang" and "Shi." (See appendix 3.)

- Apply finger pressure to the following acupoints several times a day: Waiguan, Yutang, Kongzui, and Taiyuan. (See appendix 7.)

Poisoning

Description

Poison is anything that is not compatible with the human body. Poison can be ingested, breathed in, or exposed to the skin. Apparently, all pharmaceutical drugs fit into this category when not taken according to medical directions, i.e. overdosing. Chemicals, certain metals (lead), household cleaners, and contaminated air, food, or water also fit into this category.

Symptoms or signs

Poisoning symptoms include severe shock, diarrhea, vomiting, dizziness, pale face, shortness of breath, and even immediate death. It can also cause malignant boils on the body.

Causes

Poisoning can be the result of eating foods contaminated by poisonous chemicals or spoiled foods, drinking contaminated water or too much alcohol, breathing in poisonous gas, or exposure to radiation or lead. One source of contamination can come from the ocean. Seafood can be a major cause of food poisoning because the water in the ocean often gets polluted or contaminated. Animal meat is another potential source of contamination. Because of the bacteria that remain in it as a result of processing, meat can frequently contains poisonous elements in it. Since people vary in their immunity, some become ill more easily than others after eating these foods.

Prevention and treatment

To prevent chemical poisoning, avoid chemical contaminants such as air pollution resulting from the burning of coal or gas.

To avoid food poisoning, choose younger, smaller fish, since their capacity to accumulate contaminants is much lower than their larger and older counterparts. Before cooking fish, always trim the skin, belly flap, and dark meat along the top or center. Do not use the fatty part to make sauces.

Do not eat the green part in lobsters (found in the head), the hairy part in crabs (found in the soft tissue of crab when it is opened) because these parts are where the greatest potential concentration of chemical contaminants will be.

Avoid shellfish whose shells remain closed after cooking. Most likely such shellfish were already dead before cooking, therefore poisonous materials will remain inside the shell for a longer time. It cannot be cleaned by water as it can when the shellfish is alive, as it opens its shell from time to time. Wash and cook all fish, shellfish, and seafood thoroughly.

Other suggestions are to use a quality water filter at home to remove lead and other contaminants. Never buy meat that has been packed a week ago. Thoroughly clean vegetables before eating.

Natural therapies

- Cook half a pound of pork blood together with some salt. This can clean up the body by helping it to excrete the poisons.

- Clean and cut a bitter gourd as well as two chicken wings. Fry the bitter gourd in vegetable oil first. Then, take out the bitter gourd and cook the chicken wings. When done, add the bitter gourd back, along with some salt and green onions. Eat them as a dish. This can relieve some of the symptoms of poisoning.

- Alternatively, fry the bitter gourd and eat it alone as a dish.

- To relieve alcohol poisoning, drink a cup of sugar cane juice. This can relieve some of the symptoms of poisoning.

- Eat fresh radishes, or better still, drink a cup of fresh radish juice to relieve some of the symptoms.

- Drinking two teaspoonfuls of rice vinegar can relieve most symptoms of food, alcohol, and water poisoning.

- Clean up one pound of fresh kelp. Slice it and boil it in water. Eat the kelp and drink the soup once a day. Kelp can slow down the process of chemical radiation becoming an indissoluble substance in the body, ensuring it leaves the body in the urine and stool.

- Garlic and milk are good at preventing and curing poisoning caused by lead and other toxic metals.

- For alcohol poisoning, drink a cup of strong tea, or take two spoonfuls of rice vinegar.

- Boil in water two ounces of mung beans together with some licorice for twenty minutes. Add some salt and eat. You may prefer to simply boil the mung beans in water and eat them that way.

- Cook some bladderwrack in water after cleaning. Drink and eat everything.

- Drink your own urine in the morning, fresh and warm. The ancient Chinese believed that urine was an antidote to poisoning.

Pregnancy Ailments

Description
Though not a disease, pregnancy can cause a variety of health problems for both the mother and the unborn baby. For instance, pregnant women are likely to experience heartburn and indigestion, fatigue, sore breasts, nausea (morning sickness), constipation, and excess weight gain. These ailments should be addressed to ensure that mother and baby are healthy.

Symptoms or signs
Ailments can include nausea, swelling, lactation problems, and lumbago.

Causes
Pregnancy often brings about various forms of physical changes and ailments. For instance, pregnancy after the age of thirty-five can cause fibroid tumor problems. Morning sickness and kidney discomfort (frequent

urination) are the most common complaints of most pregnant women.

Other health problems include anemia, lack of milk, fainting, and chronic headaches. According to Chinese theory, a lack of milk is largely due to a weak physique, indigestion, or emotional upset. Chronic headaches can result from exposure to cold and wind during the month of confinement (refers to the month in which delivery happens).

Treatment

During this critical period, following the principles of natural health care can greatly improve the health of mothers and lay down a solid health foundation for their babies. This means adopting a healthy diet appropriate to the situation. To begin with, you should eliminate cigarettes, alcohol, and drugs. You should also control your stress level, maintain a happy mind, and have moderate but regular exercise. Ensure that you get enough sleep, read books that are healthy in content, listen to light melodies, and enjoy peaceful, beautiful views.

General therapies

- During pregnancy, the need for calories and nutrients, such as protein, iron, and multiple vitamins, is increased to meet the requirements of the fetus. Thus, it is important that pregnant women have a nutritious diet that includes fish, eggs, lean meat, fruits, green leafy vegetables, whole grain foods, and legumes. These foods are rich in protein, vitamins, and folic acid, which helps prevent certain birth defects.

- Drink a lot of water—at least twelve glasses of water every day. Although that may send you to the bathroom frequently, you will be handsomely rewarded. Drinking plenty of water helps the whole process of pregnancy, from effective elimination of waste products through the kidneys and intestines, to the ability to perspire, thus avoiding the common problems of constipation and indigestion.

- Stop smoking and drinking. Smoking is particularly hard on unborn babies and is one of the leading causes of low birth weights. It retards fetus growth.

- Reduce the caffeine intake significantly.

- Eat plenty of grapes or drink plenty of grape juice, both before and after delivery. This can enhance the immunity of the pregnant woman and the mother of a newborn baby.

- Regularly do moderate exercise—hard enough to create a light sweat but not so hard that you have trouble speaking.

- Qigong and Dharma's internal exercises are especially helpful. (See appendices 1 and 5.)

Therapies to relieve edema (swelling)

- Boil two ounces of mung beans in water with four ounces of pork liver and some rice. Eat it as a meal.

- Drink one glass of fresh sugar cane juice, three times a day.

- Simmer a cleaned chicken (with internal organs discarded) with one ounce of small red beans stuffed inside. Divide the chicken into smaller meals.

- Steam ten ounces of cleaned gold carp along with three ounces of small red beans until the beans are soft. Eat this every day for a week.

- Boil two ounces of small red beans and wax gourd peel in water. Drink it as a tea.

- Fry four ounces of fresh peanuts, ten red dates, and thirty thin-sliced garlic cloves in peanut oil for a while. Pour in some water and boil for fifteen minutes until the peanuts are soft. Eat this once a day for a week.

- Boil some water and then add three ounces of black soybeans, one ounce of sliced garlic cloves, and one ounce of brown sugar. Simmer over a low heat until the beans are soft. Eat this once a day for a week.

- Soak four ounces of small red beans overnight and then boil them in three cups of water until the beans are soft. Eat it as a soup.

Therapies to prevent miscarriage

- Eliminate coffee, alcohol, and cigarettes.

- Increase the intake of protein and calcium by eating foods such as eggs and dairy products.

- Avoid refined foods.

- Soak cleaned moxa leaves in water for one hour and then add two eggs. Stew them together for fifteen minutes. Eat the eggs and drink the soup.

- Chicken liver is a tonic to the liver and kidneys. Regular consumption of it can heal repeated miscarriages.

Therapies to relieve morning sickness

- Steam some ginseng with dried ginger and drink the soup.

- Boil one ounce of grapefruit peel in water. Drink it as a tea.

- To avoid an empty stomach, eat smaller but more frequent meals, such as five or six small meals a day. Make sure that the diet contains enough protein, calcium, and iron.

- Drink fresh ginger juice in the morning.

- Fry eight ounces of sweet rice with one ounce of fresh ginger juice until the rice breaks. Grind it into a powder. Take half an ounce of the powder with warm water each day.

- Bring two ounces of rice vinegar to a boil over low heat. Add some sugar and a whole egg. Eat it all when the egg is cooked. Take this once a day for a week.

- Cook rice for fifteen minutes and then put in two ounces of fresh apple peel. Boil them together for another five minutes. Drink the soup in the morning.

- Eat more whole grains and cereals, nuts, seeds, and legumes.

Therapies to relieve lumbago

- Cook two ounces of sword beans with a pork kidney. Eat as a meal once a day.

- Sometimes pregnant women may experience itching all over the body. In such cases, mix rice wine with honey and drink it twice a day.

- To get rid of fibroid tumors, avoid mental and emotional stimulation, eat apples, potatoes, and sesame seeds, and do some soft exercises.

- If feeling faint after delivery due to a loss of blood, drink a mixture of brown sugar and red wine.

- Apply finger pressure to the following acupoints: Guanyuan, Qihai, Zhongwan, Zusanli, Sanyinjiao, and Tianshu. (See appendix 7.)

Therapies to increase lactation after childbirth

- Stew a leg of pork and some peanuts together for an hour. Eat it as a dish.

- Stew a pig trotter and a bean curd together for an hour. Eat it as a dish.

- Fry one ounce of sesame seeds with some salt. Eat the fried sesame seeds once a day.

- Eat mutton regularly. This can greatly nourish the mother and help lactation.

- Eat towel gourd as a vegetable every day.

- Cook a fresh hairtail. This is a delicious fish found in the ocean. (It has a very slim and long body). Cook it with some papaya and eat as a dish.

- Boil two figs with half a pound of lean pork and three red dates. Eat once a day.

- Steam or boil fresh pork feet for an hour until they are very soft. Add some vinegar and salt. Drink the soup and eat the meat.

- Boil one pork foreleg together with three ounces of peanuts. Eat with a meal.

- Soak in water two ounces of small red beans for two hours. Stew it together with a fresh carp, adding some green onion stalks. Eat them as a dish and be sure to drink the soup.

- Boil four ounces of red beans in water and eat it as a meal.

- Soak one pound of shelled fresh shrimp in hot rice wine for ten minutes. Drink the wine. (In this special case, hot rice wine is used.) Cook the shrimp and eat it with a meal.

- Apply finger pressure to the following acupoints several times a day: Zusanli, Hegu, Quchi, and Sanyinjiao. (See appendix 7.)

Premature Aging

Description

This is diagnosed when certain biological conditions that normally pertain to elderly people happen in people who are not old. It is marked by the degenerative process of the breakdown of cellular matter, which starts with most people at around the age of thirty. The speed of this process varies.

There is no specific age of premature aging. Anyone who is below fifty years of age but is experiencing marked symptoms of old age can be considered prematurely aging.

Symptoms or signs

Symptoms include wrinkling in the face, rough skin, blurred eyesight, lack of flexibility, gray hair, loss of hair, decreased interest in sexual activity, fatigue, poor memory, high blood pressure, and hearing loss.

Causes

In the Chinese natural health care system, premature aging is diagnosed to be a kidney problem of qi deficiency which, in turn, is mainly driven by excessive sex, particularly generous ejaculation. In modern science, the deterioration of cellular structures is caused by a process known as free radical production. These free radicals penetrate into other molecules, causing an imbalance of their electrons. As a result, substances within the cell that are derived from basic vitamins and minerals are depleted.

What really triggers this deteriorating process is primarily an unhealthy lifestyle: lack of physical exercise, poor diet, nutrition deficiency, excessive use of alcohol and tobacco, low-quality sleep or insomnia, poor physical hygiene, stress, depression, emotional excess such as chronic worry and fear, and excessive ejaculation. Smoking has been shown to be closely associated with premature white hair or loss of hair, wrinkles, and brown teeth.

Prevention and treatment

Knowing the causes of premature aging is the first step toward its avoidance. If inactivity—both physical and mental—accelerates the aging progression, then we need to be active. Regular exercise is the logical answer. Life lies in exercise. If mental stress and depression contribute to aging, then we need to be optimistic and enthusiastic. If poor diet is another risk factor, then we need to keep a close eye on what we eat and ensure that we follow a healthy diet. We should also drink plenty of water each day.

Give up cigarettes if you are a smoker. Smoking constricts blood vessels and thus impairs blood circulation. Impaired blood circulation means premature wrinkling. That explains why the complexions of heavy, chronic smokers are of a yellow-gray pallor, and their skin is rough and wrinkled long before they reach sixty years of age. A survey found that the skin of smokers in their forties was as wrinkled as nonsmokers twenty years their senior.

Avoid excess drinking of alcohol. Drinking to excess can permanently dilate the facial blood vessels, making the person look prematurely old.

Conservation of essence (sperm) occupies an exceptionally important position in the Chinese system, for sperm is considered the material basis of vital life energy. The vitality of life, and indeed the length of life, depends primarily on the supply and storage of sperm turned vital energy. The greater the amount of sperm inside the body, the higher will be the person's spirit, the stronger his immunity, the more flexible and energetic he will be, and the more sanguine he will look. His skin will be smooth, he will look younger than his years, and the aging process will slow down. This, however, does not mean avoidance of sex. Chinese longevity theory encourages frequent sex, which is considered by ancient Chinese to be indispensable to health and longevity, but only under the guidance and regulation of the Taoist principles (discussed in chapters 11 and 12, "Secrets of Sexual Vitality" and "Secrets of Rejuvenation and Longevity").

Dietary therapies

To delay the aging process, people should eat wholesome, raw, fresh foods, such as whole grain, fresh fruit, and vegetables. Replace red meat with fish for protein and vitamin B. Eat foods that are warm but not hot, cool but not cold. Do not overcook foods. The heat used in cooking can destroy the enzymes contained in the food, which is an essential factor in keeping one feeling young and vital. Water is of special importance because older people are more prone to dehydration due to numerous factors. Consequently, older people should drink at least eight glasses of clean water or juice each day. Water is essential for the maintenance of the skin and proper functioning of the body.

- Sesame seeds are an excellent anti-aging food. You can cook them together with rice to make a porridge or use sesame oil. They will nourish your kidneys, help the hair grow, and generate saliva.

- Fresh sugar cane, especially the juice made from it, has been successfully used by the Chinese for centuries to delay the aging process.

- Daily consumption of soybeans and its products, such as tofu, can effectively prevent and treat premature aging.

- Stew one ounce of sliced *Polygomum multiflorium* (first soaked in water for two hours) with two broken eggs in water. Eat as a dish. This can prevent and relieve premature aging.

- Ginseng is a potent anti-aging healer. Drinking ginseng tea regularly can delay the aging process.

- Eat dove rice. Cook or steam cleaned, sliced fresh dove meat together with some rice, two red dates, three pieces of mushroom, and two slices of ginger in water for thirty to forty minutes. Eat this as a meal once a week. It can delay the process of aging.

- Take gingko every day because it helps increase peripheral circulation and improves mental sharpness.

- Heshouwu, literally "making any head (hair) black," has been used in China for centuries as an anti-aging material. Boiling the root of this plant and drinking it regularly will delay the aging process, turn gray hair black (or its natural color), and stimulate the regeneration of red blood cells.

- Cook one pound of mussels and three ounces of heshouwu together. Eat the mussels and drink the soup to keep your appearance young and your hair its natural color.

Other natural therapies

- Avoid stress. If you cannot avoid it completely, at least reduce the level of it. As the proverbs say, "To think of you makes me old," and "Worry can kill a cat." Indeed, it can kill a man. Stress disturbs the yin-yang balance of the body. It hinders the production of hormones, depresses the morale and spirit, and weakens the immune system, thus speeding up the aging process.

- Follow a regular schedule. This means having a relatively definite time for meals, sleeping, exercise, work, and bowel movements. In so doing, you set the internal biological clock to the right settings, which stimulates your metabolic function and delays the aging process.

- It is particularly important to get good quality sleep. Do everything you can to ensure the success of your sleep. Do not trade necessary sleep for something else, just for the sake of temporary pleasure or wealth.

- Follow the rules of nature. Remember: The Chinese system of health is an imitation of nature. Hence the highest rule and wisdom of the Chinese natural health care system is to learn from nature. Thus, go to bed after it is dark and wake up after the sun rises.

- Develop mental images for your affirmations. For example, imagine a cool and soothing fluid pouring over your hands, making them more and more flexible, and consequently free of pain.

- Become a "cheerleader" for your immune system. Encourage it and see it successfully defeating the aging process and other illnesses.

- Open yourself to humor, society, and love. These aspects of life have been proven to be conducive to a youthful look.

- Ban negative self-images and self-criticism. Instead, think of yourself as a young person who is capable of performing many activities. Never accept aging, never acknowledge defeat. It is part of the holistic health care typical of the Chinese natural healing system which recognizes the significant influence of the mind on the body.

- Massage your face five times a day, thirty-six rounds each time. Massage has the healing effect of stimulating the lymphatic system, the body's cleansing program, which promotes the blood and energy circulation, and makes the muscle cells of the massaged portions active and energetic. Many friends and colleagues ask me why I look so young for my age. According to them, I look at least ten years younger than I am. I told them the secret I have kept for many years, and that is . . . to frequently rub your face with warm hands.

- Use coconut oil to rub into the hair periodically, or use coconut milk for shampoo. This can give luster to the hair and keep it from becoming gray.

- Practice qigong every day, preferably twice a day. The tranquillity of mind, circulation of internal energy, and delicate massage of internal organs qigong provides magically reverse the aging process and make you look and feel younger.

- Follow the soft exercises described in the appendix of this book. Exercise can help delay the aging process. Besides the often-cited effect of promoting circulation, enhancing immunity, and boosting morale, it also promotes greater elasticity in your skin, thus preventing wrinkles from forming on your face as a result of aging. Skin reacts to exercise by strengthening its structure and increasing its elasticity, and turning over fresh supplies of oxygen and nutrients. Keep in mind the truth that life lies in exercise, so you need to be active. With regular exercise, your body will not grow old as rapidly.

- A fulfilling sex life can actual retard the process of aging. The willingness and ability to engage in sexual activity is a sign of longevity. Indeed, the very thought of sex can make many people feel young or forget their actual age. For one thing, sexually active people often refuse to submit to aging. They feel they are still capable of many things claimed by younger people. Here, the key lies in regulation and coordination. Sex should serve to enhance rather than reduce the vital energy of both partners if well regulated. Find a willing and healthy partner, and practice regulated sex (see chapter 8). You will be able to tell the difference.

Prostate Ailments

Description

The prostate is a doughnut-shaped cluster of glands located at the bottom of the bladder about halfway between the rectum and the base of the penis. It encircles the urethra, the tube that carries urine from the bladder out through the penis. This walnut-sized gland produces most of the fluid in semen. When enlarged, the prostate squeezes the urethra, hinders the flow of urine, and in some cases can completely stop the urine flow.

There are three types of common prostate ailments: prostatitis (infection) which is a deeply painful inflammation of the prostate, prostate enlargement (benign prostatic hypertrophy), and prostate cancer.

It is estimated that one man in five will develop prostate cancer in his lifetime, and three out of 100 men will die from prostate cancer. According to a report in *Men's Health*, in 1996, prostate cancer killed an estimated 41,000 American men, and more than 317,000 were diagnosed with the disease.[33] It is the second leading cancer killer among men, next only to lung cancer. Bob Samuels, president of the National Prostate Cancer Coalition, says that many patients of prostate cancer are reluctant to have the condition diagnosed. This is because of the side effects of conventional treatment such as impotence and incontinence, which strike at the very center of their manhood. Prostate cancer strikes men of all ages, but it is most common among men in their fifties and sixties. Indeed, its occurrence rate is in direct proportion to age, because the prostate tends to grow as one ages.

Another condition called benign prostate hyperplasia, such as the painful inflammation of prostatitis, or the nonpainful enlargement of the prostate, afflicts 30 percent of fifty-year-old men, 50 percent of sixty-year-olds, and 80 percent of men over seventy.[34]

Symptoms or signs

These are symptoms for prostate enlargement and prostatitis: difficulty in urination with dripping of urine, urgent and frequent urination, a weak urine stream, urination that starts and stops, a need to push or strain to start urination, painful urination, a whitish secretion at the end of urination or during bowel movements, incontinence, nocturnal emissions, premature ejaculation, chronic weakness, and fatigue.

As for prostate cancer, there are no specific symptoms. Most men have no symptoms at all. In some cases, it can cause urinary symptoms very similar to those of prostate enlargement.

Causes

Prostate ailments are caused by chronic congestion of bacterial infection, nutritional deficiency, indulgence in sex (Chinese wisdom holds sexual indulgence partly responsible for prostate ailments), and excessive drinking.

Researchers find that dihydrotestosterone is the key male hormone that is mainly responsible for prostate enlargement, and it may also be the key contributor to the risk of prostate cancer. The Chinese believe the following factors can lead to the increase of this hormone. First, clogged arteries slow circulation to the prostate, depriving it of the nutrients it needs. Therefore, it enlarges to make up for the lack of nutrients. Excess sexual intercourse weakens the immune system, lowers the level of vital energy that the body needs to fight against disease, and directly affects the prostate function because emissions bring about the excitement and prostate fluid with it, thus enlarging it. The arteries and capillaries feeding the prostate can also harden and crack, like a frozen garden hose, preventing the blood from reaching the prostate tissues to nourish them.

Prevention and treatment

Mainstream medicine employs prostatectomies and expensive drugs to tackle prostate ailment and cancer. The Agency for Health Care Policy and Research acknowledged in 1994 that these treatments may actually be harmful to patients' health. Thus, natural treatments such as diet and exercise are much preferred alternatives. Besides the lack of side effects, another big plus of natural methods lies in their preventive abilities in addition to their healing properties. For instance, maintaining a low-fat diet is a wonderful way to reduce the risk of prostate cancer. Another natural therapy is to increase your fluid intake to at least ten glasses per day. Extra fluids help clean the urinary tract. Also important is mental treatment, by which I mean keeping stress under control. Stress is also closely associated with prostate ailments.

Dietary therapies

- Avoid alcohol, caffeine, coffee, tea, and spicy or fried foods; steam foods instead.

- Avoid all shellfish because they are high in calcium, which is believed to store up in the bladder and aggravate the prostate.

- Avoid smoking cigarettes and cigars. Recent studies showed that men who smoke face a higher risk of prostate cancer.

- Follow a diet rich in nuts, seeds, tofu and soy products, and whole grains. Such a diet contains plant hormones and oils that can decrease swelling, congestion, and inflammation of the prostate. Pumpkin seeds and sunflower seeds contain oils that can reduce prostate pain and enlargement. Soy products, rice, and Chinese cabbage can relieve prostatitis.

- Chew two fresh chestnuts twice a day, one in the morning and the other in the evening. This can be very effective in reducing the frequency of urination, especially for older men.

- Eat plenty of tomatoes every day. Tomatoes are rich in lycophene, a carotenoid that can reduce the risk of prostate cancer (Edward Giovannucci). [35]

- Soak one ounce of dried mushrooms in water until they are soft; cook them with the white heads from fifteen green onions. Eat them in a meal to relieve prostate pain.

- Boil five ounces of string beans in water, and add a little salt as seasoning when the beans get soft. Eating this on an empty stomach can help reduce the urination frequency.

- Eat less meat and dairy products that are rich in fat. As with heart disease and other forms of cancer, prostate cancer is more common in men who enjoy a fatty diet or who are obese. Saturated fat found in red meat and dairy products are especially dangerous, because such fat is particularly effective in promoting tumor development.

- Significantly increase the zinc intake in your daily diet. Zinc is a potent nutrient that can reduce protein levels with no side effects. Zinc is crucial for the maturation of the sex gland and for their function, particularly the prostate, and can prevent enlargement of the prostate.[36] Under normal circumstances, the prostate gland contains ten times more zinc than any other organ of the body.

- One of the best natural sources of zinc is found in fresh oysters. Eat twenty to forty ounces of them each week.

- Sunflower seeds and pumpkin seeds are rich in iron, pangamic acid, and unsaturated fatty acids. They are good for the male prostate gland, and can relieve prostate ailments.

- Drink ginseng tea twice a day, once in the morning and again at bedtime. Ginseng is a potent prostate healer, and can shrink the prostate, improve vitality, and prolong sexual life.

- Put small red beans and fresh carp together to make a dish. First, soak one ounce of red beans in pure water for three hours. Wash and cut a fresh carp into small pieces. Put the sliced carp into the red beans, then steam or cook them for about thirty minutes, adding some ginger and salt. Eat it as a meal. If you prefer, you can divide the dish into two meals. Do this once a day for two weeks. This is one of the most important traditional Chinese dietary treatments for prostate disease because it has been found effective in many patients.

- Chew about three ounces of raw pumpkin seeds each day. The Chinese think that pumpkin seeds can prevent a man's prostate gland from developing cancer cells and enlarging, keeping it healthy and in good shape throughout life.

- Steam a pork stomach and gingko nuts together, and eat them as a meal. To prepare, clean the pork stomach and soak the gingko nuts in water for an hour. Then steam them together until done.

- Cook pineapple slices together with beef spareribs, adding some ginger slices, onions, and vinegar. Eat it as a meal.

- Eat red clover sprouts, beans, beets, fish, onions, parsley, asparagus, barley, carrots, Chinese wax gourds, coconut, corn, cucumbers, grapes, hops, kidney beans, lettuce, oranges, mangos, muskmelon, pineapple, plums, star fruit, water chestnuts, watermelon, and soy products. Soy products contain phytic acid, protease inhibitors, saponins, and isoflavones, which have been shown to be anticarcinogenic and may mimic the hormone occupying sites in cells, thus preventing estrogen from locking on.

- Dramatically reduce fat intake, especially animal fat. Fats, animal fat in particular, are conducive to the growth of tumors.

- Drink as much water as possible—at least twelve glasses a day—to help clean out the urinary tract.

Other natural therapies

- Practice qigong or Chinese breathing exercises on a regular basis. Qigong requires deep and rhythmic breathing, which will trigger rhythmic massage of the prostate in men, promoting prostate health and preventing/limiting enlargement or tumor development in that organ. That is why qigong masters are never known to be afflicted with this disease, despite their old age.

- Learn to control your stress level. Keep it to the minimum. This is because stress can cause and aggravate the condition of prostate ailments. Stress control can be achieved by practicing qigong, regularly involved in exercise, listening to music, go sightseeing, and other relaxing methods.

- Do not hold back ejaculating unless you are adept in the art of bedroom skills. Semen held back after it is already on its way out becomes stagnated in the prostate, adding more pressure to it.

- Take a warm sitz at least once a day. Sit in water as hot as you can stand, for thirty minutes each time. This will relieve the enlargement problem, soothe pain, and reduce stress. This is designed to promote local blood circulation for the treatment of the disease.

- Practice abstinence. Cool down your desire while under treatment.

- Regularly contract and relax the anal sphincter muscle, several times a day, together with breathing exercises.

- Apply finger pressure to the following acupoints several times a day: Gongsun, Zhongji, Guanyuan, Zhishi, Yinlingquan, and Sanyinjiao. (See appendix 7.)

Sexual Dysfunction

Description

Sexual dysfunction can be anything ranging from lack of sexual desire, inability to attain orgasm, ejaculation pain, premature ejaculation, to impotence. Since impotence is an extreme yet common form of sexual dysfunction, I purposely listed it separately (see listings for "Impotence").

Most people take the decline in sexual drive after the age of thirty for granted. They accept the conventional wisdom that human beings reach their sexual peak at around twenty, and that it steadily decreases after that. The fact of the matter is that normal people should be able to maintain their sexual ability well into their eighties. Any consistently decreased sexual drive in middle age (apart from relational causes) is considered a health problem, which may signal other related health problems. This is clear if we agree that a healthy body is a sexual body, and vice versa. The reason we accept sexual coolness and do not consider it to be a disease is mainly because it does not cause physical pain, although it does cause a great deal of psychological "pain" for many of us.

Symptoms or signs

These include decreased sexual drive, premature ejaculation, and impotence.

Causes

In Chinese medicine, sexual dysfunction is diagnosed to be a deficiency of yang-qi, the vital energy made up of sperm and spirit. This can be caused by different factors, including genetic factors. There is no denying the fact that genetics play a key role in determining our sexual vitality. Some people are born more sexually vital and capable than others. Of course, there are physical as well as mental, dietary as well as environmental, causes of sexual dysfunction. As the Chinese see it, a common cause of sexual dysfunction is found in masturbation. Another hidden but common cause lies in wishful sexual thinking. (The harm to health and sexual vitality of such wishful sexual thinking is explained in chapter 8.)

A recent study completed at the University of South Carolina School of Medicine shows that constant pressure on the groin as in the case of extreme, long-distance bicyclists may cause irreversible damage to people's sexual ability, even impotence, because such activity hurts the critical arteries and sexual nerves. In fact, continuous long-distance cycling affects the sexuality of both experienced cyclists and novices, due to peripheral nerve compression it creates. The

frequency of impotence as well as numbness of the penis in bicycle sport may be higher than hitherto recognized.[37]

In terms of diet, vegetarians usually have a lower sexual drive than those who eat meat and fish. This is because vegetables are low in zinc, a vital mineral for sexual drive. Moreover, one's physical condition has a lot to do with normal sexual functioning. Thus, if you are afflicted with diarrhea or ulcers, your sexual function will be decreased, partly because such medical conditions will interfere with the absorption of zinc.

Prevention and treatment

Since one's sexual vitality is a directly related to one's health status and, particularly, qi energy level of the kidneys, prevention and treatment of sexual dysfunction lies first and foremost in strengthening and conserving the kidney qi energy. Again, it requires a holistic approach toward the problem, which includes mental discipline, a healthy diet, regulated sex, proper exercise, and sufficient sleep and rest. From a dietary viewpoint, for instance, zinc and calcium are vital to sperm production, ejaculation, sexual drive, and potency. Each ejaculation costs about 0.7 milligrams of zinc.

Dietary therapies

- Eat oysters every day or every other day. The Chinese discovered long ago that oysters are an excellent natural aphrodisiac, and have been used for centuries in treating kidney deficiencies and impotence problems. Oysters are rich in zinc, a mineral that is essential for male potency and the production of testosterone.

- Lean meat, lean beef, and turkey are also rich in zinc.

- Soak ten dates and one ounce of Chinese wolfberries in water for two hours. Break in two eggs with some rock sugar and salt. Stew for fifteen minutes and eat it at dinner time. Do this once a day for two weeks to enhance sexual ability.

- Fish and green vegetables are rich in calcium, which is another vital mineral for sexual vitality.

- Eat walnuts regularly. Walnuts were considered by the ancient Chinese to be able to nourish the kidneys and boost sexual vitality.

- Cook walnuts and silkworm chrysalis together. Eat them at dinner time.

- Fry some Chinese chives and fresh shrimp to make a dish. Eat it once a day.

- Drink a cup of grape wine every day, preferably at bedtime.

- Drink two cups of beer every day..

Other natural therapies

- Frequently accumulate saliva by putting your tongue against the upper palate, and swallow saliva as it fills the mouth.

- Each night at bedtime, rub your hands against each other until warm. Then use a warm hand to cradle the scrotum for a few minutes. Rub both hands against each other once more until warm, and use the other hand to cradle the scrotum for a few minutes.

- Rub both hands against each other until warm. Use the warm hands to rub the soles of the feet, one sole at a time.

- Practice Dharma's internal exercises, especially "Rub the Neck," "Rub the Abdomen," and "Shake the Heavenly Pillar." (See appendix 5.)

- Practice qigong on daily basis and focus your mind on the acupoint of Yongquan, located at the center of both soles.

- Practice sound qigong and make the sounds of "Hay" and "Ha" while exhaling. (See appendix 3.)

- Clench your teeth several times a day. Also contract your toes and anus frequently. This can enhance your sexual function.

- Pull your ear tips and earlobes several times a day. This can enhance your sexual function.

- Apply finger pressure to the following acupoints several times a day: Earlobes, Fengmen, Guanyuan, Juque, Mingmen, Qihai, Sanyinjiao, Shenshu, Yaoyangguan, Yinlingquan, Zhishi, Zhongji, Yongquan, and Zusanli. (See appendix 7.)

Sinusitis

Description

Sinusitis is an inflammation or infection of the sinuses, which are cavities, or hollow spaces in the head that are lined with mucous membranes. This is a disease that affects 32 million Americans.[38] It has become endemic in this country. If untreated or mistreated, sinusitis can develop into a chronic problem which defies any effective, quick cure.

Symptoms or signs

Symptoms can include headaches, facial pain in the cheekbones, over the eyebrows, or around the eyes, head congestion, fatigue, discharge of yellow mucus from the nose, fever, insomnia, and a weakened memory.

Causes

There are many causes for sinusitis: a repeated cold, asthma, smoking, long-term cold air exposure, air pollution, allergies, occupational hazards, and emotional stress.

Prevention and treatment

If the symptoms of a common cold last longer than two weeks, seek treatment promptly. The best prevention against sinusitis is a healthy lifestyle that sees to it you eat good food, exercise regularly, and stay away from polluted air as well as cigarettes and secondhand smoke. That way, you will most likely remove the causes for the ailment, such as common cold, asthma, and allergies. In terms of treatment, the following provides some solid alternatives.

Dietary therapies

- Drink plenty of water to help keep the mucus thin and draining.

- Eat a lot of fresh vegetables and fruit. This will enhance your immunity and maintain your health.

- Frequently drink the combination of carrot and ginger juices.

- Avoid sugary, spicy foods and dairy products, as well as caffeine and alcohol.

- Chew garlic cloves and eat them with some water. Do this twice a day to enhance your immunity and maintain your health so as to keep sinusitis at bay.

- Eat plenty of pineapples. Pineapple contains an enzyme that is beneficial to sinusitis treatment.

- Eating grapefruit can help also.

- Use sesame oil (white sesame oil is best) as nose drops and apply it three times a day, two drops in each nostril. Repeat for a week.

- Break two eggs and cook them in water together with twenty flower buds of a lily magnolia. Eat the eggs and drink the soup. Do this once a day for two weeks.

Other natural therapies

- Exercise regularly. The Chinese breathing exercises, Dharma's internal as well as morning exercises are especially helpful. (See appendices 4 and 5.)

- Regularly rub the bridge of your nose, and apply finger pressure on the acupoints beside the nostrils, Yingxiang.

- Slice several garlic cloves and put them on a spoon. Place it close to the nose and deeply inhale the garlic odor for several minutes a day.

- Ensure that the house in which you live is moist enough.

- Soak some sliced mint and dried ginger in pure water for fifteen minutes and then bring to a boil. As the water boils, deeply inhale the steam. Do this three times a day, and you will find your sinus passages open up, mucus will be discharged, and breathing will become easier.

- Keep your own urine in a glass. Sniff it forcefully many times a day. This can help relieve sinusitis and other nose problems.

- Soak a towel in hot water, wring it, and apply the towel right on your nose, especially your nostrils. Heavily inhale the warm steam from the towel while massaging your nostrils. Alternatively, breathe moist air from a hot shower, a basin filled with hot water, or from a humidifier.

- Apply finger pressure to the following acupoints several times a day: Yintang, Hegu, Yingxiang, Lieque, Baihui, Shangxing, Fengfu, Sibai, Jujiao, Taiyang, and Fengchi. (See appendix 7.)

Skin Cancer

Description

As the name states clearly, it is a form of cancer that develops on the skin. Usually, it starts with a portion of the skin and spreads to a greater area, potentially the entire body. Skin cancer itself has various types. The most dangerous is malignant melanoma. Other types of skin cancer are less threatening but are nonetheless worrisome. This kind of cancer deserves special treatment if only because it is becoming more widespread these days, largely due to widespread environmental pollution around the world. An estimated 800,000 skin cancer cases are diagnosed each year.[39]

Symptoms and signs

These can include an open sore that persists for three weeks or more, an irritated red area on the skin that may be painful or itchy, a smooth growth with an elevated border, a pearly or translucent nodule that resembles a mole, a white or yellow lesion that is similar to scar tissue, and changes in the shape, size, or surface texture of a mole.

Causes

Causes of skin cancer can be genetic, dietary, or environmental. Genetically, some people are born with a greater vulnerability to skin cancer than others. These people include those with fair skin that burns or blisters easily, those with red or blond hair, those born with many moles, blue, green, or gray-colored eyes, and those with a family history of skin cancer. Environmentally, it is the body's long exposure to the dangerous ultraviolet rays of the sun or tanning devices that is the greatest cause of most skin cancer cases. There are many harmful effects of sun exposure, with malignant melanoma being the most dangerous.

Skin cancer as a disease is a relatively new phenomenon, at least in terms of the large number of cases. In olden times, farmers worked day in and day out in the fields, constantly exposing themselves to the sun with no protection. They never heard of skin cancer. On the contrary, they enjoyed a very healthy life, and their skin color resulting from long exposure to sun had been taken as a symbol of robust health. What has happened since then?

What has happened is due to us humans. It is our industrialization and the resulting massive release into the air of industrial smog and fumes that have greatly damaged the ozone layer, creating holes that let in an unprecedented amount of dangerous ultraviolet rays into the earth, which had been so well protected by the ozone layer until recently.

Only in this sense can we understand why the cases of skin cancer have increased to an astronomical figure, and why that figure is still on the increase. It is beyond our foreseeable ability to mend the sky, or shoot down the sun. Interestingly, those feats were performed successfully according to the Chinese legends of Empress Nyuwa and warrior Yi 20,000 years ago. The Chinese legend says that a long time ago, there were ten suns. Holes suddenly appeared in the sky, making

the sunlight too much to bear. Volunteering to save the earth and its inhabitants, the master shooter Yi used his arrows to successfully shoot down nine of the ten suns, saving the last one to give humans light and warmth. Because of the big hole in the sky, the remaining sun was still too much for the humans. So Empress Nyuwa flew up to the sky and successfully mended the hole. We could definitely use Empress Nyuwa now.

Prevention and treatment

The good news is that all types of skin cancer including malignant melanoma are curable, if detected in their early stages. But if left alone undiscovered or untreated, they may quickly spread throughout the body and lead to death. While we have no choice at all over our genetic background, there are several things that we can do to prevent or lessen the possibility, of skin cancer.

NOTE: It is advised that you see a medical professional if you suspect you may have skin cancer.

Natural therapies

- Cook fresh snake meat in water for one hour. When done, add some ginger and salt, and drink the soup twice a day for one week. This can relieve and treat skin cancer because snake is considered in Chinese tradition as a potent antipoisonous substance.

- Limit the amount of sun exposure, especially between 10 A.M. and 4 P.M. every day. The ultraviolet rays of the sun are strongest during these hours. If you have to be out, take an umbrella or a broad-brimmed hat and wear sunglasses and protective clothing, such as long shirts and pants, preferably white in color. (White reflects the sunlight and reduces the absorption of ultraviolet rays significantly.) This is also true if you are swimming outside in the sun. Water can absorb ultraviolet rays and increase their intensity.

- If you are outside, find a big tree or man-made shelter to give protective shade.

- Stay away from tanning machines. These devices supposedly give you health and beauty, but in reality give you skin cancer.

- Eat whole-wheat products such as whole-wheat bread as a staple food, just as the northern Chinese do. Whole-wheat products contain rich selenium, a mineral which has proven to be a potent fighter against cancer, skin cancer in particular.

- Drink sugar cane juice, or use it to rub the diseased part of the skin.

- Drink plenty of carrot juice or eat plenty of carrots, or a combination of carrot juice and apple juice. This is because the Chinese think that carrots and apples are very beneficial to the health of skin. Therefore, they think of them when they have skin problems.

- Rub coconut oil on the skin once a day.

- Apply your own urine to the affected part of your body by rubbing it with a urine-soaked towel. This natural product has an antiseptic effect, and a magical healing effect on all kinds of skin ailments.

Stomach Ailments

Description

Stomach disorders are fairly common. When the stomach is in trouble, the foods you take in cannot be well digested and absorbed by the body, leading to malnutrition and many other medical problems. In severe cases, you may feel your stomach burning or gnawing, and may vomit food or—worse still—vomit blood. If this is the case, it is clear sign that you have stomach ulcers, which are nothing but holes in the inner lining of your stomach or duodenum. The types of stomach ailments covered here include excess stomach acid, indigestion, stomachaches, abnormal swelling of the stomach, intestinal rumbling, but not stomach cancer.

The stomach is regarded as the factory of postnatal qi energy, which is needed to supplement the primordial qi energy. As such, it is of vital importance to our health and life itself, at least until you have mastered the art of bigu, or avoidance of foods, as some Chinese immortals can do.

Symptoms or signs

These can include stomachaches, abnormal swelling, stomach prolapse, intestinal rumbling, excess stomach acid, gas, indigestion, nausea, mild pain, or heartburn.

Causes

Obviously, the biggest cause of stomach ailments is unhealthy dietary habits in terms of the foods we eat, the amount we take in, and the time we take them. All of the following could cause stomach problems: excessive eating and drinking, especially of fried foods; coffee and alcohol; irregular mealtimes, especially not eating when one is hungry or eating between meals; being in a depressed mood at mealtimes or thinking while eating; not thoroughly chewing before swallowing; and exercising or working right after a meal.

Prevention and treatment

Follow a diet that is composed mainly of fresh vegetables, fruits, and whole grain products. Change your diet from time to time instead of eating the same foods over and over. Chew thoroughly before swallowing. Try not to mix foods and juices, for fear that you will not chew the foods thoroughly enough before swallowing them. That is one sure way to invite stomach trouble.

Do not eat between meals and eat only until your stomach is 70 percent full. Do not eat food that is too hot or too cold; warm food is best for the health of the stomach. Wait at least half an hour after a meal before exercising. Try not going to bed right after a meal, but instead sit down or slowly walk for ten minutes afterward, before you engage in other activities.

In terms of healing, try the following. Those therapies that are not specified for a specific type of stomach ailment are considered good for all stomach ailments.

NOTE: See a doctor if symptoms do not get better.

Dietary therapies

- Avoid late dinners, particularly large ones. An early dinner releases less stomach acid than a late one.

- Avoid alcohol, coffee, soft drinks, and other sources of caffeine. Instead, drink green tea. (While green tea does contain some caffeine, its health benefits far outweigh the limited caffeine it contains.)

- Avoid honey, soy sauce, garlic, red meat, bitter gourd, apples, pears, and wine. These foods either will produce more stomach acid or will irritate the stomach.

- Eat small and frequent meals, chewing your food thoroughly.

- These foods are considered by the ancient Chinese to be beneficial to the stomach and have therapeutic effects: crucian carp, pork or beef stomach, soup made of pork bones or mutton, persimmons, eggplant, oatmeal porridge or porridge made of burned rice, cabbage, and carrots.

- Add some pepper to the dishes. This hot-natured food can greatly relieve a stomachache. It is the Chinese belief that the stomach likes warmth and hates coldness in terms of diet.

- To relieve a stomachache, stomach bleeding, and excessive stomach acid, grind into powder the bone of a cuttlefish. Before breakfast each morning, swallow two spoonfuls of the powder with warm water.

• To stop stomach bleeding, drink a cup of juice made of lotus roots every day.

• To relieve stomach lowering, stew two ounces of walnuts and one ounce of silkworm cocoon in water for about thirty minutes.

• To relieve excess stomach acid, frequently drink warm red tea and avoid acidic foods such as lemons, apples, and pineapple.

• To relieve ptosis of the stomach, stew ginseng and ginger together to make a tea and drink it.

• Use two eggs and some coriander to make a soup. Eat it as part of a meal to relieve a stomachache.

• Cut a papaya and throw away the seed. Cook the papaya together with some ginger slices. Add three spoonfuls of rice vinegar when done. Eat this once every other day to strengthen the functioning of the stomach.

• Use some dried rose to brew a tea and drink it twice a day. This can strengthen the function of the stomach and help relieve stomach ailments.

• Cook Gorgon fruit together with rice until done. Add in some rock candy and eat as a meal. Do this once a day. This can strengthen the function of the stomach.

• Mix ginger juice, milk, and some sugar. Drink the mixed juice.

• Clean a seedless watermelon and cut it into small pieces. Cook it over moderate heat for two hours until it is creamy. Eat two spoonfuls of this watermelon cream twice a day, once in the morning and once at bedtime.

• Cook half a pound of rice in water for fifteen minutes. Reserve one cup of the boiled rice water. Mix two ounces of honey and one ounce of sesame oil in a bowl. Use chopsticks to stir them for a minute, then pour into the bowl of boiled rice water. Drink this mixture warm on an empty stomach. Eat the rice later. This can strengthen the function of the stomach.

• Fry some cooked taro in peanut oil and sesame oil. Add some water, soy sauce, and garlic cloves and eat it as a dish. This can strengthen the function of the stomach and help relieve stomach ailments.

• Drink potato juice mixed with some honey on an empty stomach, preferably early in the morning before breakfast. Do this every day for two weeks. This can relieve stomach prolapse.

• Clean and cut in two halves a yellow croaker (fish) for cooking. Stew the fish together with some ginger, green onion stalks, pepper, and a little bit of salt. When the fish is done, add some sesame oil. Eat and drink everything. This can nourish and strengthen the stomach.

- Stew a crucian carp and some radishes together, seasoned with some salt and sesame oil. Eat it as a meal. This can nourish and strengthen the stomach.

- Drink plenty of raw cabbage juice. It is a good source of the potent anti-ulcer compound known as S-methylmethioine.

- Clean and cut a fresh crucian carp and a radish into small pieces. Cook them in water together with some green onion roots and fresh ginger. Add in some sesame oil and salt when done. Eat the fish and the radish as dinner. This can nourish and strengthen the stomach.

- Eat a lot of bananas. They also contain a potent anti-ulcer compound.

- Contrary to popular belief, milk does not help cure ulcers. Milk actually generates more acid in the stomach.

- Peppermint tea can promote digestive enzymes, which in turn relieves intestinal gas, soothes upset stomachs, and relieves heartburn.

- Use five red seeded dates, twelve raw black peppercorns, and six apricot seeds and immerse in warm water for one day. Then boil them into a thick soup and drink it with water, twice a day. This can nourish and strengthen the stomach.

- Drinking plenty of potato juice, apple juice, and carrot juice can reduce the level of stomach acid.

- Drinking a lot of vegetable juice made of spinach, celery, and carrots can help relieve stomach disorders. These can be taken separately or mixed.

- Soak some ground cinnamon in a cup of warm water for twenty minutes and drink. This can relieve stomachaches.

- Drinking a glass of beer each day can relieve stomach ailments and promote digestion.

- To relieve a stomachache, boil eight dried kumquats in water for half an hour and drink the juice, three times a day.

- Cook five ounces of bean curd, adding some brown sugar into it. Eat it as a dish or a meal to stop stomach bleeding due to an ulcer.

Other natural therapies

- Practice Dharma's internal exercises, especially "Rub the Abdomen," three times a day. (See appendix 5.)

- Practice sound qigong making the sounds of "Gong," "Huu," or "High." (See appendix 3.)

- Practice qigong every day, imaginatively guiding your qi to the stomach while exhaling. (See appendix 1.)

- Apply finger pressure to the following acupoints several times a day: Taichong, Tianshu, Xiawan, Qihai, Daling, Daheng, Zhongwan, Guanyuan, Hukou, Zusanli, Dazhui, Fengmen, and Neiguan. (See appendix 7.)

Stroke

Description

Strokes cause damage to the brain, resulting in mental and physical impairment. A common stroke is a cerebral thrombosis, caused by a blockage of an artery in the brain. When blood flow to the brain is interrupted, vital supplies of oxygen and nutrients are cut off and brain cells in the affected area begin to die immediately. A complete shutoff of blood to the brain can lead to permanent damage in just five minutes. It can sometimes lead to death in a matter of minutes. There are two kinds of strokes. One is hemorrhagic stroke, and the other is ischemic stroke which is by far the more common type of stroke, making up about 80 percent of all strokes. Stroke is the third largest killer of Americans, claiming 162,000 lives every year. It is one of the top causes of disability in the U.S.

Symptoms or signs

A stroke may be accompanied by a sudden, unexpected vision loss, sudden weakness and numbness or paralysis in your face, arm, or leg, loss of speech or trouble talking or understanding, loss of balance or coordination, confusion, or rapid onset of a severe headache.

NOTE: If you are experiencing symptoms, see a medical professional immediately. These are preventive and healing therapies—not first aid.

Causes

Hemorrhagic stroke occurs when blood vessels burst, causing bleeding within the brain, often as a consequence of high blood pressure. Ischemic strokes are caused by reduced blood flow to the brain when blood vessels are blocked by a clot or become too narrow for blood to get through. Reasons for the formation of such a clot in the blood vessels include hardening of the arteries, inflammation or trauma of the blood vessels, migraines, and drug use.

Prevention and treatment

Contrary to popular belief, you do not have to sit around waiting for a stroke to happen. There are many steps to take beforehand to keep a stroke at bay. To prevent a stroke, you have to keep a close watch on your blood pressure. High blood pressure is a clear warning sign that you are at risk for a stroke. High blood pressure is highly conducive to strokes because it accelerates clogging of the arteries and it can cause one of the tiny blood vessels in the brain to "explode." Therefore, it is very important that you reduce elevated blood pressure to within normal limits (under 140/90) to dramatically lower the risk of a stroke.

To prevent hypertension or to lower high blood pressure, you need to control your diet, limiting the saturated fat intake, and eating high-fiber, complex carbohydrate foods such as whole grains, vegetables, and fruits, especially bananas, oranges, cantaloupe, potatoes, yams, figs, and spinach.

It is also important to stop smoking completely. Smoking dramatically increases the risk of a stroke by speeding up the clogging of the carotid arteries, the large vessels found on each side of your neck. Clogging these vital arteries means blood can't get to your brain. In fact, blockage of these main vessels to the brain accounts for nearly two-thirds of all stroke deaths. So it is important to check your neck regularly to see if there is any thick buildup in the neck. Surgery may be needed if there is a serious plaque buildup.

At the same time, exercise regularly, but moderately. It is well proven that exercise can dramatically reduce the risk of strokes. The best exercises are soft Chinese exercises, which consciously train not just the body, but the mind as well, thus ensuring a smooth flow of blood to all parts of the body, including the brain.

Natural therapies

- Eat at least one banana a day. The ancient Chinese recommended this fruit for prevention and treatment of many diseases, including strokes. One study suggests that eating just one banana a day is enough to protect you. This is because bananas are rich in potassium, a substance that can prevent plaque buildup on artery walls.

- Eat plenty of potatoes. Potatoes are rich in potassium, which can effectively lower your blood pressure and prevent plaque buildup.

- Eat more carrots. Carrots have been a favorite vegetable in China for a long time. It often appeared in the palace feast either as a decoration or as a dish in itself. Chinese people living in the countryside who eat plenty of carrots rarely have hypertension or a stroke. A recent study found that a diet high in carrots was responsible for a substantially lower risk of strokes. This is because carrots contain rich beta-carotene, a vitamin that can attack damaging oxygen molecules in the blood, preventing plaque from forming in the artery walls.

- Mix one spoonful of sesame oil and one spoonful of granulated sugar together. Use boiled water to brew a tea out of them. Drink it three times a day.

- Fry one ounce of sesame seeds with some granulated sugar in a pan. Eat the fried sesame seeds once a day. This can prevent and treat a stroke.

- Stew a small cup of fresh tortoise blood with some rock sugar for fifteen minutes and eat. This is a popular Chinese treatment.

- Eat a lot of pineapple. It contains bromeliad, an enzyme which can decrease the risk of blood clots.

- Cook half a pound of finless eels and eat. To relieve the palsied face that can occur as a result of a stroke, use the blood of finless eels to rub the face. You have to rub with care. If the face is aslant toward the right side, rub the left part of the face. If the face is aslant toward the left, rub the right part of the face. The Chinese believe that the blood of the finless eel can contract the facial muscles. If the muscle of the right side of the face is contracted, the face askew to the left can be corrected, and vice versa.

- Apply finger pressure to some or all of the following acupoints several times a day: Zhongwan, Shousanli, Dazhui, Fenglong, Laogong, Yingxiang, Shenque, Qihai, Renzhong, Neiguan, Baihui, Fengchi, Fengfu, Fengmen, Chengjiang, Zusanli, Taichong, Lieque, Qihai, Hegu, Yongquan, and Saoshang. (See appendix 7.)

Tooth Ailments

Description

Under this category, I refer to specific tooth ailments such as toothaches, tooth decay, and bleeding gums. These ailments can be marked by pain in the teeth and gums, change of teeth color, as well as bad breath. The pain can occur when eating or drinking hot or cold foods, or even when inhaling cool air. It can also be accompanied by a headache and swelling of the gums. If persistent, tooth ailments can cause a lot of discomfort and lead to indigestion, insomnia, depression, and other health problems.

Symptoms or signs

These include gum inflammation, bad breath, pain when eating cold or hot foods, headaches, fever, swelling, redness around the tooth, or bleeding of the gums.

Causes

From the standpoint of Western medicine, a toothache is caused by bacteria growing within the mouth cavity, leading to plaque, tooth decay, and gum inflammation. However, the real cause is an unhealthy lifestyle including negligence of oral hygiene, eating foods rich in refined sugars, and smoking. Sugary foods are the favorite of bacteria, and they directly contribute to the development and aggravation of the problem.

Another reason people develop tooth ailments is because they do not brush their teeth consistently and correctly. Using a hard toothbrush and brushing teeth horizontally from side to side can wear away the protective surface of the teeth. Brushing the teeth forcefully can be as harmful as not brushing them at all. Bleeding gums are usually the result of poor oral hygiene, such as negligence of brushing the teeth, or brushing them in a wrong way. (Refer to the chapter on "Natural Health through Hygiene" for the correct way to take care of your teeth.)

Yet another hidden reason is stress. This is because stress weakens the immune system. Researchers at the State University of New York at Buffalo studied 1,400 people and found that those who were stressed and highly emotional had more severe gum disease than those who were more easy-going.

From a Chinese medical viewpoint, excessively eating fried foods and foods of a hot-nature such as goat, wild animals, and fruits grown in the southern part of the country such as longon, lichee, and mangos, can also lead to toothaches and swollen and bleeding gums.

Prevention and treatment

To prevent tooth ailments, follow a healthy diet that consists mainly of wholesome grains, fresh fruits, and vegetables. Such a diet contains plenty of fiber that can help scrape away bacteria and plaque in the mouth. It is found that people who eat a lot of carrots, apples, and other hard or juicy foods enjoy healthy teeth in their old age. Part of the reason is because these are hard foods and need to be bitten and chewed, which strengthens the teeth and scrapes away plaque. These foods are also rich in beta-carotene, a nutrient conducive to strong teeth.

Make sure you do not snack between meals and avoid smoking, coffee, and sugary foods. A survey conducted in Japan showed that children who snack between meals have a much higher rate of tooth decay than those who do not.

Another thing to keep in mind is that teeth are for chewing foods. Teeth that are out of use are out of order. Chewing exercises the gums and ligaments around the teeth, stimulating blood flow to the area and discouraging bacteria growth. This is another illustration of the principle Hua Tuo established 2,000 years ago—running water is never stale and a door hinge is never worm-eaten. Modern diets composed of soft, processed foods have a tendency to not need the teeth, because they contain less and less raw food. To make up for this loss of "exercise" resulting from eating overprocessed foods, frequently yet gently bite or clench your teeth together.

It is important to follow good oral hygiene, which includes rinsing the mouth after each meal and brushing the teeth at least once a day, preferably at bedtime. As far as brushing the teeth is concerned, there is much to talk about. First, the toothbrush should be made of soft materials. Second, the water should be warm. Third, the movement of the toothbrush should be up and down, not from side to side. Fourth, brushing should be slow, gentle, and rhythmic, rather than vigorous.

Natural therapies

- Avoid foods that are rich in sugar, especially refined sugar.

- Avoid fatty, fried, and hot-natured yang foods, such as French fries and barbecued foods.

- To relieve a toothache, use three to five *Sterculia scaphigera* (a Chinese herb) and two ounces of rock sugar to brew a cup of tea to drink.

- Stew two to five ounces of peanuts in water together with some garlic cloves for forty-five minutes. Eating the peanuts can stop gum bleeding.

- Drinking a cup of fresh celery juice can also stop gum bleeding.

- Clean and slice some leaf mustard, then soak it in pure water for several hours. Drink the soup to stop gum bleeding.

- Make juice out of fresh star fruits. Drink it three times a day to relieve a toothache.

- Eat plenty of green vegetables such as spinach, cauliflower, and carrots. These natural foods contain a lot of vitamins which are thought to be beneficial to the health of teeth.

- Drink a lot of carrot, apple, pineapple, and vegetable juices.

- To relieve gum bleeding, drink a cup of juice made of lotus roots.

- Gargle several times a day with your own urine, fresh and warm. This can relieve toothaches and prevent tooth decay. Afterward, gargle with pure water to get rid of any smell or aftertaste.

- To relieve toothaches, drink a mixed tea made of green tea and mint powder.

- Soak some soybeans in water for two hours and then boil them for thirty minutes. Pour out the soup and let it cool before adding some honey. Drink the soup twice a day and eat the beans. This can relieve tooth ailments.

- Be sure to brush your teeth each day, at least once at bedtime, but preferably after every meal. Use only warm water to brush the teeth, and soak the toothbrush in the water for a while to soften it first.

- Young children should be helped to make sure they maintain their own dental health.

- If it is too troublesome to brush the teeth after each meal, be sure to rinse the mouth with warm water or salt water after each meal.

- Apply finger pressure to the following acupoints several times a day: Hegu, Shousanli, Baixie (Yemen), Xinjian, Shaohai, Nuxi, Chengjiang, Fengchi, Jiache, Renzhong, Taixi, Shousanli, and Xiaguan. Pressing Hegu is helpful in relieving a toothache in the lower jaw, while pressing Xinjian is especially helpful to toothaches in the upper jaw. The effect of acupressure will be further enhanced if you soak your finger in your own urine first before pressing the acupoints. (See appendix 7.)

Ulcers

Description

An ulcer is an inflamed and worn-down patch of tissue in the lining of the stomach or small intestine. Ulcers develop when something damages the protective lining and allows stomach acid to eat away at it. This severe inflammatory condition causes pain and a sense of burning when the stomach is empty or while food is being digested.

Every time food drops in, the lining is awash in acid-rich digestive juices. Normally the lining rebounds fairly well from activity. Excess stomach acid or other irritants in the stomach or intestine can result in the formation of ulcer craters. These craters are often as large as a thumb. A breakdown of the protective mucous barrier of the stomach accelerates the damage. Ulcers may develop in the stomach or in the upper part of the small intestine. It often bleeds, and the blood will show up as a dark color in the stool.

While all of us form small ulcers every now and then, large and severely progressive ones can lead to pain and hemorrhaging. They can even make holes all the way through the wall of the stomach or small bowel. If not properly treated, ulcers can lead to the point where a person will die of excessive bleeding.

Most patients are young males who enjoy stimulation from food, rush through meals instead of spending time chewing before swallowing, and who tend to experience more stress and emotional upheavals.

Symptoms or signs

Usually, it is a burning or sharp pain in the abdomen, most often occurring in the fall and winter seasons (because the stomach is afraid of cold). It is generally felt between meals and may wake the person during the night. The occurrence of pain is periodic and somewhat rhythmic. Each occurrence will last anywhere from one to two hours before disappearing by itself. Also, patients may suffer from vomiting, insomnia, and emotional upheaval and disruptive temper.

Causes

An unhealthy diet is one of the major causes of ulcers. This includes unhealthy foods, improper food combinations, irregular meal times, overeating, use of alcohol and tobacco, constant consumption of spicy foods that irritate the stomach lining, and insufficient chewing of food before swallowing it, as well as chronic use of drugs such as aspirin and aspirin-containing medicines as well as drugs used to treat arthritis.

According to traditional Chinese medicine, stress is a major contributing factor of ulcers. This is because stress triggers liver fire, which will attack the stomach, causing an imbalance in the stomach and improper functioning. Stress weakens the immune, central nervous, and digestion systems. As a result, the body loses its power to check the development of ulcer craters.

In a five-year study involving more than 8,000 men, scientists found that the quality of a man's marriage can influence his risk of developing an ulcer. Men who felt they got love and support from their wives were only half as likely to get ulcers as men who felt their marriage was a mess.

While not a direct cause, smoking causes the constriction of small vessels, preventing adequate nourishment to the wall of the stomach and increasing your risk of ulcers. Smoking can also slow the healing process, encourage repeated occurrences, and increase the risk of bleeding or the need for surgery to remove ulcerated tissue.

Alcohol, particularly strong liquor, can stimulate acid flow and damage your stomach, thus increasing the chance of developing an ulcer. Irregular eating habits can also be a factor by preventing the buffering of the acid by food. Studies also found that overproduction of hydrochloric acid from the stomach may erode the stomach lining, leading to ulcers over time. In addition, regular use of aspirin and other anti-inflammatory drugs is another major cause of ulcers.

Prevention and treatment

As the risk factors of ulcers clearly show, this problem can be prevented and controlled by ourselves. Since it is by-and-large a matter of lifestyle, we are the best doctors if we can stay away from the bad habits mentioned above.

To start, avoid foods that are too hot or too cold, fried, or spicy such as hot peppers. Stop smoking and drinking alcohol. Avoid coffee, commercial soft drinks, and illegal drugs. Be very regulated in sexual intercourse. This is because ejaculation will further lower the immunity and qi energy level of the person who is in need of such energy and immunity to fight the disease.

Dietary therapies

- Avoid foods that increase the stomach acid such as vinegar, dairy products, wheat products, tomatoes, coffee, sugar, pineapple, citrus fruits, strawberries, grapes, peaches, and plums.

- Eat smaller, but more frequent meals (five to seven meals instead of three big ones).

- Chew food thoroughly before swallowing.

- Eat more of these foods: pork bone soup, chicken soup, mutton soup, pork stomach, beef stomach, and carrots. These foods are good for the stomach and can relieve ulcers.

- Cook five ounces of bean curd, adding some brown sugar into it. Eat it as a dish or meal.

- Grind into powder the bone of a cuttlefish. Before breakfast each morning, swallow two spoonfuls of this powder with warm water. This can stop bleeding and pains, and has no side effects. The bones of a cuttlefish contain rich calcium phosphate and sodium chloride, which stop the bleeding and decrease inflammation.

- Eat plenty of raw cabbage or drink plenty of raw cabbage juice each day.

- Eat high-fiber foods and foods that are warm in temperature.

- Burn a pork stomach into ashes. Take one spoonful of the ashes with warm water each morning on an empty stomach.

- Regularly eating pork lung can relieve bleeding from ulcers.

- To relieve bleeding, drink a cup of lotus root juice every day.

- Regularly drinking potato juice and cabbage juice can relieve the ulcer.

- Eat one kind of food at a time. Try not to mix different foods at the same meal. (Don't eat a meal that consists of a salad and meat and potato at the same time.) This is the safe way to go for ulcer patients.

Other natural therapies

- Practice breathing exercises regularly, thinking of the stomach. Once the saliva fills the mouth, rinse it and swallow it in three small mouthfuls, guiding it down to the stomach with your mind.

- Practice sound qigong and make the sounds of "High," "Huu," and "Xu" while exhaling. (See appendix 3.)

- Massage the stomach and abdomen several times a day.

- Reduce your stress level. Stress may slow the healing process.

- Apply finger pressure to these acupoints several times a day: Neiguan, Zusanli, Tianshu, Qihai, Taiyi, Shenshu, Juque, and Sanyinjiao. (See appendix 7.)

Urination Problems

Description

Urination problems assume many forms. These ailments affect women more often than men. One common type of problem are urinary tract infections. They occur more commonly in women than in men, because women's shorter urethras make it easier for bacteria to migrate from outside the body into the bladder.

Symptoms or signs

These can include pain or burning during urination, a sense of pelvic fullness, pain during intercourse, cloudy or bloody urine, frequent urination, or lower abdomen pain.

Causes

Causes of urination problems include infection of the bladder or prostate gland, unhealthy sexual habits, illegal drug use, and excess consumption of caffeinated products such as coffee and soft drinks. Cystitis, often known as a urinary tract infection, is caused by fecal bacteria that migrate to the urethra and then into the bladder. These bacteria stay on the walls of the bladder, where they grow and cause damage.

In traditional Chinese medicine, urination problems are diagnosed to be a deficiency in kidney energy, and an imbalance in the kidney function, which in turn can be caused by a number of factors, such as sexual indulgence. It is believed that chronic nocturnal emission and neurasthenia often lead to urination ailments such as frequent urination, pain during sexual intercourse, and even muddy urination.

Prevention and treatment

To prevent urination ailments, take good care of your physical hygiene. For one thing, clean your genitals each and every day with soap, especially after sexual intercourse, using your own towel. Make sure to wear clean underwear every day. Do not indulge in sex merely to seek carnal pleasure and conserve your sexual essence to maintain a high level of immunity.

Natural therapies

- Avoid coffee, soft drinks, tea, alcohol, and fried foods.

- Eat less animal protein.

- Drink at least three cups of cranberry juice each day. Cranberry juice can help stop the bacteria from sticking to the bladder.

- Urinate and wash the genital organs with clean water as soon after sexual intercourse as possible. Limit the frequency of sexual activity.

- Stew one ounce of Chinese wolfberries with a cut beef penis and some ginger. Drink the soup and eat the penis. Do this once every other day. This can clean up the urine and relieve pain during urination.

- Make a porridge out of one bean curd, one ounce of gingko fruit, and two ounces of rice. Eat it for breakfast every day for a week. This can relieve pain during urination.

- Stew two ounces of walnuts and one ounce of silkworm cocoons in water for thirty minutes. Eat tand drink everything.

- Drink more fluids such as water and juice—at least ten glasses of water each day—to put more acid into the urine and help flush bacteria from your system.

- Cranberry juice, orange juice, and apple juice are good choices because they are contain natural antibiotics. Treatment of urinary tract infections relies mainly on antibiotics.

- Eat a lot of watermelon and asparagus, which can stimulate kidney function.

- Boil two ounces of dried pear peels in water. Drink it as a tea three times a day to relieve pain when urinating.

- Cook rice soup (water and rice) and add two persimmon cakes. Cook them together and eat it once a day for a week to stop bleeding during urination.

- Add some cold water to strawberry juice and drink it three times a day to relieve pain during urination and red-colored urine.

- Soak ten dates and one ounce of Chinese wolfberries in water for two hours. Crack in two eggs with some rock sugar and salt. Stew for fifteen minutes and eat it as a dish at dinner time. Do this once a day for two weeks. This can relieve the pain during urination and clean up the urine.

- Stew some maize corn hair together with some freshwater mussels and water. Eat the mussels and drink the soup. Do this once a day for two weeks to relieve the urinary infection.

- Cook sliced pork liver in rock sugar and eat it as a dish. This can stop bleeding in urination.

- Drink fresh raspberry juice or plenty of cherry juice to stop frequent urination.

- Bake one ounce of dried chestnuts and eat them twice a day, once in the morning and again in the evening, to cure frequent urination.

- Eat plenty of watermelon to relieve urination pain and red urine.

- Eat half a pound of ripe loquats. Loquats are a very delicious fruit grown in the southern part of China. They taste very sweet when ripe. Eat them in the morning and again in the evening to relieve urination difficulty.

- Eat half a pound of muskmelon twice a day to relieve painful urination.

- Boil bamboo leaves for twenty-five minutes and add some honey. Drink the soup to relieve urination difficulties.

- Boil dried corn silk in water and drink the soup as tea, three times a day. This can promote urination, and reduce urinary albumin—a type of simple protein.

- Boil four ounces of barley in water for thirty minutes. Mix the soup with some fresh ginger juice. Drink it before your meal to relieve painful urination.

- Boil barley leaves and drink it as a tea. This can relieve pain during urination and stop bleeding during urination.

Therapies to relieve frequent urination

- Cook walnuts and silkworm chrysalises together. Eat them at dinner time.

- Chew a few fresh chestnuts twice a day, once in the morning and again in the evening. This can be very effective in reducing the frequency of urination, especially for older people.

- Soak one ounce of dried mushrooms in water until they are soft; cook them with the white heads of fifteen green onions. Eat as a meal.

- Boil five ounces of string beans in water, and add a little salt as seasoning when the beans get soft. Drinking the soup on an empty stomach can help reduce urination frequency. Eat the beans, too, but half an hour later, not at the same time. This is meant to let the essence of the food, which is thought to be contained in the soup, to work out its medical effects first.

- Apply finger pressure to the following acupoints several times a day: Hegu, Qihai, Sanyinjiao, Zhishi, Zhongji, Shenshu, and Yinlingquan. (See appendix 7.)

Vaginitis

Description

Vaginitis is any vaginal infection, inflammation, or irritation that causes a change in the normal vaginal discharge. Common types of vaginitis include yeast infection and nonspecific infection. Women who are pregnant or diabetic are known to be more vulnerable to this disease.

Symptoms or signs

These can include burning, itching, or redness around the vagina; a whitish vaginal discharge; and change in the color, odor, or amount of discharge.

Causes

Vaginitis is usually caused by an upset in the normal balance of the vagina. For instance, irritation caused by excessive douching, strong soaps or perfumed feminine hygiene products, tight pants or jeans, bicycling, or sexual intercourse. Stress, pregnancy, diabetes, hormonal changes, a compromised immune system, birth control pills, and medical conditions that can damage the body's normal defenses against yeast infections are listed as common causes, too.

Prevention and treatment

Avoid intercourse until you are completely healed. Avoid douching—a healthy vagina will clean itself. Wash the genital area once a day with plain water mixed with a little salt. Avoid tight pants and jeans and perfumed feminine hygiene products, which can irritate tender skin. Take a cold sitz bath twice a day to help relieve vaginal discharge and inflammation. Make sure to change your underwear every day or even twice a day.

NOTE: See a medical professional if the condition does not improve.

Dietary therapies

*   Take apple cider vinegar, alfalfa, parsley, soya beans, and red clover.

*   Boil black fungus in water and add some brown sugar. Drink the soup and eat the fungus to relieve vaginal bleeding.

*   Eat garlic cloves alone or boil them in water and drink as a tea twice a day.

*   Boil half an ounce of dried radish leaves in three glasses of water and add some salt. Drink the soup hot twice a day for one month.

*   Boil two cuttlefish with eight ounces of lean pork in water, adding a little salt. Eat it twice a day for a week to relieve abnormal vaginal discharge.

*   Combine half an ounce of hyacinth beans, one ounce of yams, and two ounces of sweet rice, and boil them together in three cups of water over a low heat. Drink it hot as a soup. This can relieve vaginitis and reduce abnormal vaginal discharge.

*   Boil two ounces of hyacinth beans in water, adding some sugar and drink it hot as a tea. This can reduce abnormal vaginal discharge.

Vomiting

Description

This ailment is marked by the contents of the stomach being forced back up the esophogas and out the mouth.

Causes

Vomiting can have many causes including, but not limited to, poisoning, drug use, indigestion, motion sickness, gastroenteritis or other infections, uremia, stomach disorders, ulcer, or allergy to certain foods. A woman vomiting in the morning could be in the early stages of pregnancy.

NOTE: Vomiting could be a sign of a more serious illness. You should see a medical professional if it keeps occurring and does not improve.

Prevention and treatment

Dietary therapies

- Mix ginger juice and milk, add some sugar and drink.

- Chew a few plums slowly.

- Make a cup of warm tea mixed with some fresh ginger and dried orange peel.

- Drink lemon juice with some salt added to it.

- Mix some fresh ginger juice with some honey. Drink it with a little warm water.

- Steam two teaspoonfuls of fresh chive juice with one teaspoonful of fresh ginger juice plus eight ounces of fresh milk. Drink it warm on an empty stomach.

- Radish juice can relieve vomiting.

- Boil a bit of cloves with some persimmon calyx (this is the cake made of fresh persimmon) and fresh ginger in water. Drink half of a cup three times a day.

- Boil black dates and a few whole cloves in water. Eat the dates and drink the soup on an empty stomach. Do this once a day.

- Boil fresh ginger slices together with some pieces of dried orange peel in water. Drink it as a tea.

- Slowly chew two ounces of honeyed grapefruit peel to relieve vomiting.

- Swallow two egg yolks to relieve vomiting.

Other natural therapies

- Apply finger pressure to the following acupoints several times a day: Zhongwan, Burong, Yutang, Zusanli, Tianshu, Youmen, Juque, Quchi, Shangwan, Jiuwei, Xiawan, and Qihai. (See appendix 7.)

- Gently pat the upper part of the back of the patient with your fists or palms for five to ten minutes.

Endnotes

1. Allan R. Cook, *Environmentally Induced Disorders Sourcebook* (Detroit, MI: Omnigraphics, Inc., 1997), 17.

2. *USA Today* (April 29, 1997).

3. Kate Lorig and James Fries, *The Arthritis Helpbook* (Massachusetts: Addison-Wesley Publishing Co., 1995).

4. Linda M. Ross, *Allergies Sourcebook* (Detroit, MI: Omnigraphics, Inc., 1997), 77–78.

5. Donald Vickery & James Fries, *Take Care of Yourself* (Addison-Wesley Publishing Company, Inc., 1990), 7.

6. Allan R. Cook, *The New Cancer Sourcebook* (Detroit, MI: Omnigraphics, Inc.,1996), 4–5.

7. David Frahm and Anne Frahm, *Reclaim Your Health* (Colorado: Pinon Press, 1995), 69.

8. Donald Vickery, *Take Care of Yourself* (1990), 8.

9. "Prevention's New Encyclopedia of Common Diseases," *Prevention Magazine* (Emmaus, PA: Rodale Press, 1984), 184–6.

10. K. Yamaoka, et al., "Health-related quality of life varies with personality types," *Quality of Life Research* 7, no. 6 (August 1998): 535–44.

11. A. Panzer, "Depression or Cancer: the choice between serotonin or melatonin," *Medical Hypotheses* 50, no. 5 (May 1998): 385–7.

12. *Men's Health,* May 1997, 76.

13. Allan R. Cook, *Men's Health Concerns Sourcebook* (Detroit, MI: Omnigraphics, Inc., 1998), 129.

14. *Journal of Longevity* 4, no. 1 (1998): 6.

15. *Journal of the American Medical Association* (February 10, 1997).

16. Karen Bellenir, *Diabetes Sourcebook*, (Detroit, MI: Omnigraphics, Inc., 1999), 596.

17. *Men's Health,* January/February 1997.

18. *Men's Health,* January/February 1998.

19. "Prevention's New Encyclopedia of Common Diseases," *Prevention Magazine* (1984): 221–22.

20. Frahm, *Reclaim Your Health*, 18.

21. *Journal of Longevity* 3, no. 2 (1997).

22. Mary Kane et al., *Sound Decisions* (Boston, MA: Mosby Consumer Health, 1995).

23. K. V. Andersen et al., "Impotence and nerve entrapment in long distance amateur cyclists," *Acta Neurologica Scandinavica* 95, no. 4 (April 1997): 233–40.

24. Joseph Pizzorno, *Total Wellness* (Rocklin, CA: Prima Publishing, 1996), 242.

25. *Consumer Issues in Health Care Sourcebook* (Detroit, MI: Omnigraphics, Inc., 1999), 179.

26. Heather E. Aldred, *Women's Health Concerns Sourcebook* (Detroit, MI: Omnigraphics, Inc., 1997), 239.

27. Rosalind Cartwright, *Crisis Dreaming: Using Your Dreams to Help Solve Your Problems* (New York, NY: Harper Collins Publishers, 1993).

28. Linda M. Ross, *Kidney and Urinary Tract Diseases and Disorders Sourcebook* (Detroit, MI: Omnigraphics, Inc., 1997), 45, 76.

29. Ross, *Kidney and Urinary Tract Diseases and Disorders Sourcebook*, 87.

30. *Investor's Business Daily*, 3 January 1998.

31. Peter Jeret, "The Burden of Beer," *Health*, September 1992, 22–5.

32. R. Li et al., "Dose-effect of Fenfluramine On the Severity of Valvular Heart Disease Among Fen-phen Patients with Valvulopathy," *International Journal of Obesity Related Metabolistic Disorders* 23, no. 9 (September 1999): 926-8.

33. Scott Martin, *Men's Health,* January/ February 1997.

34. *Natural Health*, April 1999, 50.

35. Edward Giovannucci is a well-known American expert on prostate ailments. He is widely published in medical magazines of national and international reputation, such as *Prostate, Cancer Epidemiol Biomarkers Preview, Cancer Causes Control, Cancer Research, American Journal of Clinical Nutrition*, and *Journal of National Cancer Institute*.

36. Michael Sharon, "*Nutrients A to Z* (London: Prion Books Limited, 1998), 271.

37. K. V. Andersen, *Acta Neurologica Scandinavica*, 233–40.

38. Linda M. Shin, *Ear, Nose and Throat Disorders Sourcebook* (Detroit, MI: Omnigraphics, Inc., 1998), 299.

39. Allan R. Cook, *The New Cancer Sourcebook*, (Detroit, MI: Omnigraphics, Inc., 1996), 4–5).

Epilogue

Much has been said about the Chinese natural health care system. Contained in this system is a genuine, healthy life philosophy, and numerous precious techniques and methods designed and discovered by the ancient Chinese for life to function optimally. The principles and methods of this unique health care system are derived from and based on the observation of the laws of nature. Obey these laws and you will be healthy and live a long life. Break them and you will find yourself in trouble and eventually broken by nature.

Emerson once said something to the effect that health is the greatest wealth over the long run. This conviction was confirmed by Elbert Hubbard who declared: "If you have health, you probably will be happy, and if you have health and happiness, you will have all the wealth you need." Indeed, good health is a blessing, and the most important key to a happy life. However, in the hubbub of modern life deluged with materialistic objectives and vain glory, people often forget about this power-ful truth until they lose their health. In light of this reality, it becomes all the more important for us to cultivate a healthy life-style as early in life as possible so that it will become our second nature and health will take care of itself. Practice makes perfect. As long as the mind is willing, the flesh will become strong.

I wish all of you good luck and success in your pursuit of optimal health and longevity.

Appendix 1

Qigong:
The Chinese
Breathing Exercise

It may sound strange to Westerners to consider breathing an exercise, all the more so as a skill or an art. To them, breathing is a biological function that comes naturally so why bother to learn the skill of breathing. After all, we all breathe all the time. But the fact is that breathing is an art of a healthy life, a supreme art at that. The way we breathe can have a significant impact on our health and the healing process. For one thing, the way we breathe determines how much oxygen we take in and how efficiently we utilize it, and nothing is more vital to life than oxygen.

I purposely put qigong, the Chinese breathing exercise, before all the other Chinese fitness exercises because I believe this is the logical starting point. Indeed, breathing is to natural health and the healing process as air is to life. In fact, all Chinese fitness exercises uniformly incorporate into them the art of qigong, and require that practitioners coordinate their actions and movements with the rhythm of respiration. It is no exaggeration to say that qigong is a "red thread," a link, running through all other forms of Chinese fitness exercise. In fact, it is central to the Chinese methods of natural health and healing, and constitutes the cornerstone of all fitness exercises that have existed in China over the past 5,000 years. Therefore, a clear understanding of the principles of qigong and a solid foundation in qigong skills are prerequisites for gaining the greatest benefit from other forms of Chinese exercises.

It is stated in *The Yellow Emperor's Classic of Internal Medicine*: "Inhale and exhale the essential air, sit alone guarding one's spirit. . . . If you have kidney disease, get up at around 3 A.M. and practice qigong facing the south." Clearly, the Yellow Emperor and his medical advisors regarded breathing as a skill to be learned and a method of healing. Today, qigong is increasing in popularity around the world. In China alone it is estimated that 200 to 250 million people practice qigong on a daily basis.

The term "qigong" in Chinese is made up of two separate words: qi and gong. Literally, qi means "air" or "the breath one inhales and exhales," while gong means "exercise, skill, and mastery." Qigong aims at empowering, regulating, and controlling the qi of human beings, with the purpose of maintaining and restoring the yin-yang balance in the body, strengthening immunity, healing diseases, improving sexuality, prolonging life, and ultimately, merging into the universe and becoming one with nature. Thus, qigong is more than an exercise; it is a philosophy, an ancient Chinese philosophy that lies at the very center of the Chinese natural health care system. Since qigong combines meditation and regulated breathing to promote the circulation of vital energy in the body, it is preventative and therapeutic at the same time, and therefore can be used by the healthy as well as the sick.

Qigong is a special exercise aimed at promoting the flow of vital qi energy in our body in order to increase our immunity and self-healing power. To a large extent, all Chinese natural health and natural healing methods, as well as martial arts, rely on the mastery of qigong techniques for the achievement of their therapeutic effects.

Qigong exercise has multiple dimensions: delicate movement, right postures, regulated breathing, concentrated meditation, as well as a guided energy flow inside the body. Indeed, it is about the essence of life itself. It is required that all these aspects work in good harmony to produce the best therapeutic results. Of course, the effectiveness of qigong will be greatly enhanced if it is combined with other forms of natural health exercises that are outlined below. As a matter of fact, all the forms of natural health exercises I am going to describe utilize breathing exercise as an integral part of their performance. Indeed, qigong has become so important a part of Chinese life that Chinese sages declare that qigong should be practiced no matter if one is sitting, walking, or lying in bed.

Qi Energy

Not surprisingly, such an important exercise is backed up by rich theories. First and foremost is the theory of qi. The Chinese are so preoccupied with qi because they hold that qi is the origin of all life forms. Indeed, it is the origin of the universe. In the Chinese natural health care system, qi is considered a basic material and driving force for the development and maintenance of life. As we know, the body and mind are undergoing constant changes throughout life. This process of constant change is called metabolism, and the metabolic process includes respiration of air, digestion of foods, circulation of blood, secretion of wastes, distribution of saliva, and modulation of emotions. From the Chinese point of view, this entire process is driven and controlled by qi energy in the body. In this sense, the whole purpose of qigong is to strengthen the qi energy so as to promote the metabolic process, and with it, the overall health of the body.

However, qi is a much broader concept than breath or air; it is also used to describe the vital life energy of the human being. Although invisible and intangible, qi is the key substance linking the body and the mind, and is considered to be closely associated with blood and saliva. Indeed, they are interdependent upon one another. The ancient Chinese held that qi is the commander of blood. As such, smooth circulation of blood depends on smooth circulation of qi. If the qi is interrupted, the blood will clot as a con-

sequence. If the qi stops circulating, blood circulation will cease. Therefore, to promote blood circulation we must first promote qi circulation. To nourish, strengthen, and warm blood, one must first nourish, strengthen, and warm one's qi energy.

On the other hand, blood is the material basis of qi energy. In the absence of blood, there will be no qi energy. If the blood is clotted, the flow of qi will be obstructed as a consequence. Obstructed qi and clotted blood signify the imbalance of body energy, and cause dysfunction to the internal organs and various diseases. For instance, if lung qi is blocked, coughing usually follows. In very much the same way, if heart qi is deficient, one feels tired and low in spirit. If stomach qi is out of balance, vomiting and stomach acid will follow. If kidney qi is deficient, one will experience sexual dysfunction and incontinence.

Many factors can disturb the proper circulation of qi inside the body. These include an unhealthy diet or food combinations, excess emotions, stress, fatigue, and unpleasant weather. Therefore, it is vitally important that qi circulation in the body remains strong and smooth.

This vital qi energy in the body originates from the Gate of Life, located between the kidneys, and was considered the root of life by the ancient Chinese. Vital qi can be accumulated, stored, controlled, concentrated, regulated, guided, and even released through qigong training. It is the key link between sexual essence and spirit. In fact, the ultimate goal of qigong practice is to bring sexual essence, qi, and spirit together into a harmonious balance. Modern scientific experiments show that qi energy generated by qigong exercise can assume various physical properties—electricity, magnetism, light, and sound. It can be static electricity, electromagnetic waves, infrasonic waves, and particle currents. This shows that the human body is a powerful field that generates heat, light, electricity, and sound. The human body is a highly complex system full of mysteries and potentials. It challenges modern science to further explore and understand these marvelous properties latent in the human being. In this regard, qigong holds great promise, especially when combined with modern equipment and technology.

Broadly speaking, there are two major types of qi energy. One is prenatal qi, which comes with life as a heritage from the parents and is stored in the kidneys. The other is postnatal qi, which is derived from the nourishment gained from eating, drinking and breathing. It is stated in *The Yellow Emperor's Classic of Internal Medicine*: "True qi is a combination of what is received from heavens and the qi of diets. Qi permeates the whole body." The same concept is repeated in a slightly different way in Zhang's *Internal Classics*: "True qi is the original qi. Qi from heavens is received through the nose; qi from diets enters the stomach. What nourishes the unborn is the prenatal qi; what nourishes the born is the postnatal qi." Since the prenatal qi energy, or the primordial qi reserve, is limit-

ed and only comes once in life, it needs to be complemented by postnatal qi so that our body to function properly. Theoretically, if one does not spend any prenatal qi energy in life, one does not need much replenishment to survive, either. In this sense, prenatal qi functions in a way that is similar to a battery in an automobile. The less you use it, the longer it lasts. If you do not drive the car at all, you do not need to replace or replenish the battery.

In addition to the two broad categories of qi described above, the ancient Chinese have further classified qi energy inside the body into six more types: primordial or original qi, the essence qi, the blood qi, the organic qi, the circulatory qi, and the defensive qi. The primordial qi is also known as the genuine qi, which comes with life as an inheritance from the parents, and is stored between the kidneys in the Gate of Life. Primordial qi is the most basic qi of life, or the source of life, which can be transformed into essence qi. Primordial qi very much determines the hereditary characteristics of a person, and has a great influence on the person's health throughout life.

The essence qi governs and determines one's sexual vitality. Besides its source of primordial qi, it is also derived from diet, nutrition, and sexual activity, and is stored in the kidneys. The blood qi is derived from diet and is carried by the blood to various parts of the body. It determines our strength, courage, and the functioning of our organs. The organic qi exists in the body as a harmonizing factor among bodily organs. The circulatory qi is the qi that goes together with the blood in the vessels that can be stimulated by means of acupuncture or acupressure. The defensive qi, as the name implies, determines the immunity power of the body. It is the body's defense against diseases. Under normal conditions, the defensive qi is latent in bodily organs, but is called into action when the body is threatened by external viruses.

It is important to note that the different kinds of qi are intimately related to each other, although their functions may be different. In a broad sense, they are one entity. Only in its totality can we get a full picture of qi and understand its all around importance. Qi energy circulates throughout the body, nourishing and maintaining life, restoring yin-yang balance, and healing disease. More amazingly, it can be called into action for various purposes: diagnosis or healing, detection or combat, as shown by Chinese qigong masters and martial artists.

The biophysical functions of qi energy can be summarized by the following five words: promotion, regulation, preservation, prevention, and restoration. The promotional function of qi manifests itself in promoting the growth of energy, spirit, strength, blood, sexual essence, and saliva. Its regulatory function is manifested in its role in circulating the blood and nutrients throughout the body wherever it is needed. Its preservation function is shown in its ability to preserve the energy and essence of the body. Its preventive function works to boost the immunity of the body and to keep diseases at bay. Its restorative function lies in its ability to restore the proper balance between mind and body, yin and yang energies in the body, and eventually the health. This means correcting the disruption of such balances due to disease, fatigue, lack of sleep, nutritional deficiency, or excessive expression of emotions.

The therapeutic application of qigong falls into three areas. First, qigong is a health promoter and healer for its practitioners themselves. Second, it can diagnose diseases in others. Third, it is a healer for others.

Health Promoter and Self-Healer

Qigong is a highly powerful natural means of preventing and curing diseases. Numerous clinical surveys and thousands of years of Chinese experience bear witness to this truth. Qigong manifests its health promoting effects in several ways.

First, it can improve the regulatory ability of the central nervous system over the heart, strengthening the heart muscle, improving blood circulation, lowering blood pressure and heart rate, and promoting internal metabolism.

Second, it can also promote the movement of the stomach and colon, and increase the secretion of digestive enzymes, and raise the endocrine system's capabilities. Modern scientific experiments in China also find that qigong can regulate the substances cyclic adenosine monophosphate and cyclic guanosine monophosphate. These substances play vital roles in the respiration process and the provision of oxygen to the body's cells. In short, qigong can greatly enhance the immune system of the body, making us more resistant to disease and speeding up the recovery process.

In clinical experiments, qigong has also proven its abilities in treating degenerative and chronic diseases such as diabetes, asthma, chronic bronchitis, obesity, chronic kidney disease, peripheral vascular disease, rheumatism, cancer, hypertension, habitual constipation, stomach disorder, stress and depression, gastric and duodenal ulcers, heart disease, premature aging, insomnia, multiple sclerosis, menopause syndrome, post-stroke syndrome, and Parkinson's disease. Indeed, it is a cure-all in the arsenal of the Chinese natural health care system, which can help you fight virtually any disease. It is particularly effective in treating chronic dysfunction of the digestive, nervous, respiratory, and cardiovascular systems. In fact, many Chinese patients with diseases dismissed as incurable by Western medicine, such as cancer and heart disease, have been successfully treated by means of qigong.

Qigong benefits everybody, be they Chinese or not, young or old, male or female, sick or healthy. It is really a universal healer and health promoter. To understand how qigong works, we need to look closer into its underlying principles and premises.

One such premise is the ancient Chinese belief of yin and yang. These two aspects of life—yin and yang—must be kept in good balance and work in harmony in order to enjoy good health and longevity. For instance, the mind stands for yin, the invisible and intangible, whereas the body stands for yang, the visible and the tangible. One's mental health is inseparably linked to one's physical health. That is why in qigong practice, meditation goes hand-in-hand with regulated breathing, and quietness of mind with delicate movement of the energy inside the body. Thus, it is a holistic exercise and therapeutic tool that trains the body and the mind at the same time. It regulates the body through correct posture, relaxes the mind through focusing on dantian, and trains respiration through gentle, prolonged, and thread-like breathing—breathing that is very slow, delicate, and prolonged, as if it were a long thread. It influences one's physiological state and rectifies pathological conditions. It brings out the enormous power latent in the human body for healing and immunity uses.

Qigong derives its great powers from two basic requirements: tranquillity of mind and regulation of breathing. As the Chinese see it, all diseases are caused by the blockage of qi energy inside the body and the imbalance between the mind and body, which lowers the immunity of the body. The fundamental way to prevent and treat disease lies, therefore, in keeping the qi circulation smooth and uninterrupted inside the body, and boosting the immune system. A scientific clinical research study in China reported that patients increased their immune proteins by two to three times after practicing qigong. Clinical experiments also show that during a qigong exercise, the efficiency of white blood cells in the body to kill diseases increases. All these point to the conclusion that qigong can strengthen our immunity.

Qigong is a powerful means of maintaining or restoring the mind-body or yin-yang balance and harmony. It effectively relaxes the body and tranquilizes the mind. By regulating the function of the central nervous system, it leads to a serene mind, which comes partly from the increased body temperature and rate of oxygen absorption and a decreased heart rate. Researchers have proven that we are most susceptible to diseases when we are tired, physically and mentally, because fatigue weakens our immune system. As life is short and temptations of all kinds are so numerous, we all have a tendency to work or play too hard, and neglect the rest and relaxation that is indispensable to good health. Qigong, especially when it becomes a regular part of life, reminds us on regular basis that enough is enough and it is time to take a mental as well as physical break. Unlike other forms of rest, qigong relaxes not just the body, but the mind as well. The practice of qigong creates a state of tranquility for the mind and thus enhances the quality of rest, be it sleep or relaxation. Indeed, qigong itself is an excellent form of rest.

By inducing a state of tranquility and mental quietness, qigong stabilizes cerebral cortex activity, protects the cerebral cortex, stimulates blood circulation, lowers blood pressure, relieves insomnia and chronic pain, promotes the buildup and conservation of vital qi energy, restores the proper functions of the body, alleviates internal organ disorders, and enhances immunity.

Mental serenity means that the cerebral cortex is in a state of tranquility. Physiological experiments show that when a person is in a tranquil state induced by breathing exercises, the cerebral cortex is in an regulated state. This allays the overexcitation and fatigue of cortical cells that too often result in functional disorders and degenerative diseases. All this results in the mind and the body reinforcing and complementing each other in a harmonious state of dynamic equilibrium, improving overall health and assuring a longer life. Modern theories show that consciousness can implicitly and delicately affect our nervous system. This helps explain why qigong is so helpful and effective in treating diseases such as hypertension, gastric ulcers, aging, and neurasthenia, which are all closely connected with the cerebral cortex.

Equally significant is qigong's great ability to relieve mental stress and depression, which is wonderful news for many people. Modern surveys show that about 60 percent of all diseases are stress related. The mind and body are an inseparable entity; it is simply wrong to separate the two. Stress and emotional stimulation disturb the normal functioning of the nervous system, weakening our immunity, and aggravating medical conditions. Thus, tension, grief, fear, worries, and anxieties can lead to hypertension, insomnia, gastrointestinal disorders, peptic ulcers, palpitations, constipation, thoracic suffocation, incontinence, and mental disorders. Cancer, too, is found to be closely related to a person's mental and emotional condition. Typically, one whose mind is chronically depressed is doubly susceptible to an attack of cancer. Qigong, induces the mind to forget about external things and concentrate on the movement of qi inside the body. It also eliminates stress and brings about a healthy state of mind. Such a mental state is very helpful to recovery from disease and overall health.

As mentioned earlier, qigong promotes the circulation of blood. The ancient Chinese held that qi is the commander of blood and can generate, circulate, and regulate the blood. As such, smooth circulation of blood depends on the smooth circulation of qi. Clinical experiments show that during qigong exercise, arteries expand, showing that blood circulation is increased plus a lowered heart rate. Clearly, these effects are perfect for patients of hypertension and heart disease.

Qigong also makes one sensitive to the internal operations of the body through a process called "internal vision." By consciously guiding the mind's eye to look inward into one's own body and internal organs, rather than on external objects, one brings attention to oneself and consciously assists in the functioning of internal organs.

This practice improves the overall functions of the internal organs, and guards the body from external interferences.

The Chinese sages told us repeatedly: "Being tranquil and peaceful in mind will generate and conserve the vital energy. By guarding and saving your spirit and essence you can shy away disease." According to the theory of Chinese medicine, no disease can affect us if we have vital energy permeating the body and if the spirit stays quietly inside the body. Obviously, vital energy is viewed in Chinese medicine as the foundation of the immune system. The more you possess it, the healthier you are, and the more invulnerable you are to disease.

On a more active level, qigong exercise consciously guides the qi energy down to a small area in the lower abdomen known as dantian, which is the reservoir of qi energy. This practice directly increases the qi reserve in dantian. All consistent qigong practitioners will experience the qi flow and accumulation in the dantian area after several months of practice. As a result, their spirit is given a boost, work efficiency is enhanced, sexual vitality promoted, and immunity to disease strengthened. Experimental findings also indicate that, in the course of, and as a result of, qigong exercise, the number of rounds of respiration can be reduced from the ordinary fifteen to twenty per minute to an extraordinary four to five per minute. As well, the heart rate is obviously lowered, oxygen consumption is reduced by 30 percent and energy metabolism by 20 percent. All these demonstrate that qigong is a great energy saver. That explains why qigong masters have much less need for food and sleep, and yet possess greater energy and vitality than ordinary people.

Qigong exercise also massages the abdominal cavity. It produces this massaging effect through the regulated process of breathing, enabling the diaphragm to move up and down over a much larger range than usual. X-rays show that the magnitude of diaphragm movement of qigong masters is larger than ordinary people by as much as four or five times. Such active massage promotes gastrointestinal peristalsis, and aids digestion and absorption of dietary nutrients. This is turn promotes the functions of the heart, kidneys, liver, and lungs, thus greatly increasing one's digestion power, preventing and curing digestion and stomach related diseases. It is shown that after qigong practice, the digestive enzymes increase in the body. This is why qigong can boost one's appetite, and cure indigestion, habitual constipation, and stomach ulcers. At the same time, it effectively increases the capacity of the lungs, and the body's ability to clear the internal organs of wastes and obstructions.

Moreover, by combining meditation with regulated breathing, qigong strikes an optimum balance between the yin and the yang energies in the body, normalizes the level of sexual hormones, improves sexuality, and heals sexual dysfunction, including impotence. As has been discussed before, qigong training is fundamental to the practice of regulated sex, which in turn boosts one's sexual vitality and immunity, which is conducive to longevity and immortality.

Qigong, through chronic deep breathing, effectively helps cleanse our body and blood of the pollutants we take in. This is especially important in the modern world where pollution of various kinds has become a way of life. In this case, if one does not take in enough fresh air, or if one is a shallow breather, the intake of oxygen will be much lower than the outflow of carbon dioxide, encouraging the accumulation of poisonous carbon dioxide inside the body. Oxygen is a detoxifier that removes poisons from the body. Carbon dioxide is, by contrast, poisonous and its accumulation in the body can lower your level of vital energy, and cause pains and premature aging. By emphasizing deep breathing, qigong ensures that you take in the greatest possible amount of oxygen while getting rid of the greatest possible amount of carbon dioxide, thus keeping the body clean and potential problems at bay. Qigong is also excellent training for the lung function. Experience and observation tell us that the deeper one breathes, the longer one lives. The same rule holds for the animal world, too. The tortoise is a slow and deep-breathing animal. Its life span is much longer than most other animals. Accordingly, rabbits and pigs are fast-breathing animals, thus their lives are short.

Perhaps the most direct effect of qigong in natural healing is the potential ability of everyone to consciously induce their vital energy to flow to areas or organs afflicted by disease. Through qigong, you can direct the powerful qi thus built up to any portion of the body where a blockage or dysfunction occurs. Once the vital energy is directed and concentrated in the diseased area, it starts its healing and repair work in a very subtle, painless, and natural way. If you are well trained in qigong, you will be able to feel for yourself how it works inside your body—an alternating feeling of warmth and coolness in the area, perhaps accompanied by a light feeling of electricity running through the area, and the opening up of the qi channels throughout the body. It is in qigong that one realizes and experiences most clearly the great potentials of a human being, the incredible self-healing power, and the ability to merge into the universe. A survey performed by Beijing Qigong Institute several years ago, based on more than 5,000 patients of various chronic diseases who had received qigong therapy in the institute shows that after practicing qigong for three years, 25 percent of them had recovered completely, 44 percent had improved remarkably, and 22 percent had improved slightly. Apparently, the therapeutic effect of qigong varies with individual cases and depends on the individual's level of mastery of the art of qigong.

Last but not least, qigong puts us in closer contact with the universe, enabling its practitioners to take the live energy that abundantly exists in the universe and use it to supplement their own vital energy. The universe in which we live is full of live energy from various sources—the sunlight, the moonlight, the morning dew, even the odor emitted from the trees. It challenges us humans to take advantage of it in a natural way without disturbing the man-nature equilibrium, or the macrosystem of the universe. In ancient times, Taoist adepts used to live in the mountains and practice qigong all the time. They ate very little, and yet they outlived all of those people who were well fed. The mystery lies in the capacity of qigong to benefit its practitioners with the abundant supply of life energy in the universe.

In fact, Taoist adepts absorbed a great portion of their nutrition and life energy from nonfood sources in nature, by dint of qigong and other fitness exercises. This explains why people practicing qigong usually have lesser need for food than ordinary people. As has been mentioned in chapter 13, "The Road to Immortality," this reduced reliance on, and eventually independence of, food nutrients for physical existence. It is the royal road toward immortality, a practice known in Taoist literature as *bi-gu*, or avoidance of food.

This unique capacity of qigong tends to enhance your self-confidence and change your outlook toward life. It is little wonder that qigong masters normally have a very weak sense of competition, because they understand that life's purpose is to eventually merge with nature; that life's values are realized through working on one's inner self rather than competing with the outside world, and that there are unlimited resources existing in the universe that cost us nothing. This mentality greatly reduces the chance of stress and depression, improving immunity and overall health as well as the chance of happiness. Thus, the benefits of qigong go far beyond improving health. It allows us to tap into the potentials of life to self-actualize, to be the best doctors of ourselves. It awakens our sense of being a most intuitive member of the macrocosm, and puts us in closer contact with the infinity of the universe.

In practice, qigong stresses the significance of conscious concentration, which is required for qi circulation, and therefore contributes to preventing and treating diseases and prolonging life. Qigong therapy is, therefore, self-health care and self-therapy in that it uses your own hidden energy force to restore balance and kill diseased cells in the body. In fact, you do not need to become a qigong master to experience many of its health and therapeutic benefits. You just have to be persistent, consistent, and confident in what you are doing. Of course, to derive the full benefit of qigong takes time and patience, and sometimes even painstaking effort. Intelligence and genetic background also have a role to play in determining how successful one will be in mastering the art of qigong. Some people are born with stronger primordial qi energy, and smoother meridians and channels through which qi energy circulates, than others. That explains why not everybody who practices qigong with equal persistence for many years becomes a master. In fact, many people who have practiced qigong for decades cannot emit qi outside their body. This is not of primary importance. The really important truth to remember is this: the more you practice qigong—in terms of both frequency and length—the more you benefit from it, as long as your practice is guided by the correct principles (which I will illustrate step by step later).

Many highly sophisticated scientific experiments have been conducted in China to identify the nature of qi. It is now clear that qi is one kind of electric energy that can form a strong field around the lower abdomen or source of emission in any part of the body, as is the case with qigong masters. Also, qi can be defined as an informational message and a complex energy form vital to life itself. This finding opens up a whole new world of excitement in the diagnosis and treatment of diseases.

In recent years the therapeutic effects of qigong has aroused increasingly strong interest and enthusiasm from people all over the world. For instance, much attention has been drawn to the treatment of cancer by means of qigong, and the results are very encouraging. One of the well-cited examples is the case of Guo Lin. Since she was diagnosed with uterus cancer in 1985 at the age of forty, Guo continues to practice qigong every day, and her cancer has never recurred after two years of exercise. Guo Lin has summarized her intensive studies of qigong theories and her own clinical experience in her book *Qigong: A New Method for Combating Cancer*. The curative effect of qigong on cancer can be explained by the fact that qigong promotes circulation and clears obstruction inside the body, and in the eyes of Chinese medicine, cancer is exactly a problem of qi blockage and circulation.

A Tool for Medical Diagnosis

Using qigong as a means of diagnosis is another unique aspect of traditional Chinese medicine. Qigong as a diagnosis tool has been used for thousands of years in China. In the classical *Chronicles of History*, it is reported that the greatest doctor in the Han dynasty (206 B.C.–220 A.D.), Bian Que, could see the insides of his patients. He derived his diagnosis by means of his powerful sense of vision. He could not only tell what kind of disease a patient had, but also what kind of disease his patient had suffered before. The famous doctor Sun Shimiao also said in his *Secrets of Qigong Regimens* that a master of qigong could diagnose his patients 100 miles away. It goes without saying that this therapeutic application of qigong requires a higher degree of mastery than if it is used for the purpose of mere health promotion. In the latter case, the effect of qigong is almost immediate. The moment you sit down and devote yourself to qigong exercise, you gain some of its benefits, if not all. However, it takes a master of qigong to use it for clinical diagnosis. Only when one has achieved a high level of mastery over the art of qigong, can one project an electronic wave into the patient and get feedback from the body.

The great Chinese doctor Hua Tuo, whom we have mentioned before, is one such master. Hua Tuo was one of the first qigong masters who successfully applied the art of qigong to accurately diagnose his patients. Historical records tell us that one of his female patients suffered from a severe abdominal ache after a miscarriage. She came to see Hua Tuo for treatment. By dint of the incredible power of qigong, Hua was able to feel with his hands that there was another stillborn fetus inside the woman's body. He told her so, but she simply could not believe what Hua said. "I just had a miscarriage a week ago," she said. "Now are you telling me that I have another one? How can it be possible!" Hua Tuo told her that unless this second dead fetus was taken out of the body, her pains would only get worse. Helpless and desperate, the woman let Hua work on her, and after a two-hour surgery, Hua was successful.

There are quite a few modern examples of successful qigong diagnosis in China. For instance, Mr. Yan Xin of China—"the modern sage" as former president George Bush called him—is one such qigong master who often diagnoses for others. In late 1984, Yan demonstrated his qigong diagnosis ability to people in Chongqing, Sichuan province, of China. One of his patients was an old doctor. They had never met before. Yan asked the doctor to sit down in front of him. Shortly after Yan released his inner qi energy toward the old doctor, he told him: "Your right lung has been taken away by surgery. And the surgery is very unique; it cuts your right lung horizontally." The old doctor was astonished by Yan's diagnosis. He told Yan that his skill will shake the entire medical world some day.

Yan Xin provided an even more amazing example of qigong diagnosis. One day in late 1985 while Yan Xin was still in Sichuan, the general manager of *Canton's Economic Daily* newspaper came to see him and asked him to diagnose for his wife and daughter who were living in Canton, more than 1,200 miles away. Moved by the manager's sincerity, Yan accepted the request. Sitting on sofa in a quiet hotel room, Yan mobilized his inner qi energy while gazing at the carpet on the floor. A few minutes later, Yan raised his head with a smile as if he had just returned from Canton. He told the manager in an unambiguous manner: "Three days ago, your daughter caught a cold. She is now in red leather shoes, with one leg on the bed and the other on the ground. Your wife is lying in bed at this moment. Her bedding is made of three colors: black, green and blue. . . ." Upon hearing this, the manager cried out in amazement: "Marvelous! Marvelous! You are absolutely right, sir. I just received a phone call from my wife. She told me that my daughter is suffering from a bad cold."

Two years later, in 1987, Yan Xin was still in Sichuan. One day, a woman came to see him, telling him that her brother was very sick but did not know exactly what the problem was. The patient lived about thirty miles

away and had never met Yan. Employing the same skill, Yan was able to tell his sister that the patient was afflicted with a bladder ulcer. Moreover, Yan immediately made an effort to treat the patient with qigong even though he was many miles away. This, together with the prescription Yan made, finally cured the patient of his disease without the doctor and patient ever meeting each other.

Incidentally, Chongqing, Sichuan and Seattle, Washington are sister cities. In 1990, a native of Chongqing returned home from Seattle and brought a recent photograph of her old Seattle friend, Ms. Anna, to Yan Xin for diagnosis. Anna had been in ill-health for a long time. Gazing at the photo of Anna for about an hour, Yan Xin told the visitor that Anna was afflicted with otitis media, heart and lung diseases, gastric ulcer, twelve stones in her gallbladder, colon ailment, and had only eighteen teeth in her mouth. According to the visitor who had been living with Anna for many years, Yan's diagnosis was absolutely accurate.

What has given the above-mentioned Chinese masters the ability to diagnose without any tools, to see things clearly thousands of miles away? The secret lies in qigong, or more specifically, in something known as waiqi, or out-flowing qi energy in the world of qigong and Chinese martial arts. Waiqi is the inner qi released through the eyes, fingers, or palms and intensively projected onto others, which some seasoned qigong masters are able to perform. Inner qi released and projected onto other people can get a feedback, because both the human body and qi generate fields of electricity, magnetism, and heat. Fields are invisible substances and materials. Since similar fields possess the properties of mutual response, penetration, transmission, and field-induced light, qigong masters release their own qi energy to get feedback from their patients, in the same way that modern technology uses heat and radar to locate enemy planes and missiles. The changes in human health will be reflected in the field around the body. Normally, such fields and related changes are invisible to the naked eye, partly because their vibration is too weak. Only eyes sharpened by qigong practice can see them through highly condensed qi energy projected onto the field. The stronger the waiqi or outflowing qi, the more accurate and faster will be the diagnosis.

This unique ability to "see through" other people's bodies and discover objects hundreds of miles away is known in qigong literature as "the heavenly eyes opening up." Qigong exercise is the primary key to opening up the heavenly eyes. Qigong exercise calms the mind, reduces desires, conserves vital energy, nourishes the internal organs, sharpens the five senses, and eventually enables one to see things far away, in the past and in the future. The longer one practices qigong, the stronger the inner qi energy, the sharper will be the heavenly eyes. To facilitate the opening-up of the heavenly eyes, the ancient Chinese recommended that we practice qigong while gazing at the sun early in the morning. The idea is to take advantage of the beneficial solar energy to strengthen our vision power. Of course, the application of opened heavenly eyes is not limited to medical diagnosis. In fact, it has been successfully employed in areas where secret and hidden information is wanted, such as military espionage and criminal investigation.

A Healer for Others

Besides diagnosis, waiqi can and has been very successfully employed for active healing for others. My teacher Dr. Wan Laisheng was one such qigong master. The perfect combination of Chinese martial arts and qigong gave him the special ability to project qi out of his body to heal or to kill. He had successfully employed this ability to both defend himself and treat patients. He could do this by releasing the built-up energy against an object either through his fingers or through an acupoint in his palms known as Laogunxie. While waving or pushing his palms from a distance of about two feet from the patient's diseased part, Wan emitted waiqi through his right palm. The patient immediately felt a sense of warmth or electricity in the affected spot of his or her body, and then a feeling of numbness similar to that felt when one is undergoing a successful acupuncture.

One patient whom Dr. Wan had successfully treated suffered from arthritis in his right knee for more than ten years. When Wan released his qi energy toward the patient's knee, the patient sensed a warm current running through his knee. Several minutes later, there was sweat coming out of his forehead and a rhythmic beat in the surrounding muscles. After one month of qigong treatment, the arthritis had disappeared from the patient, never to return. Another patient who was cured by Dr. Wan had cancer in his thyroid gland for two years. Knowing that Dr. Wan could treat troublesome diseases with qigong, he came to seek help. Using the same method—waiqi treatment together with dietary and acupressure therapy—Dr. Wan cured the patient of his cancer in about five months.

Waiqi has been identified by Chinese scientists to be a low frequency current of modulated infrared radiation. It is a highly concentrated form of body energy, and has been shown in clinical experience to be able to kill cancer cells and to enhance one's immunity against such disease. In recent years, Russian psychic researchers have acknowledged the existence of qi energy and recognized it to be a kind of "bioplasmic energy." Chinese sages hold that every one of us has an energy field, which represents a largely untapped reserve of energy source for most people. The consciously directed emission of energy toward patients is a clear manifestation and demonstration of this energy field. The primary functions of such energy emitted toward a patient are to stimulate the energy system within the patient, trigger the self-healing potentials of the patient, and restore the patient's inherent healing ability that has become dormant or diminished due to illness.

Research is being carried out to treat patients of AIDS with waiqi. I have good reason to believe that this might be a promising approach toward the problem.

If most people have such a marvelous energy field, why can only a few "privileged" masters be able to manifest it while others can only stand by in amazement? Only the theory of qigong can answer that question. The fact is that man is a highly capable being, full of incredible, potential abilities. It remains a gigantic challenge to modern science to tap deeper into this huge reserve of human potential and reveal the true picture of human beings. As Dr. Qian Xueshen, the internationally famous Chinese rocket scientist and father of China's missile and system engineering, puts it: "The science of the human body is a high-tech area. It is the high-tech of high-techs."

It is now clear that qigong is the primary key that can open up all the energy potentials inherent in all people, Easterners or Westerners, who are supposed to be born equal, not only in human rights, but also in biological ability. It is through qigong that one starts to realize the existence of meridians and acupoints which are the keys to the energy field. The more you practice qigong in the right way, the more you will be able to tap into your own inherent potentials and build up your energy reserve. All these are guided and controlled by the mind. This is very well described by a famous motto in the qigong world which says: "Wherever the mind goes, qi follows; wherever qi goes, strength follows." This process of revelation and reservation is gradual and accumulative. Only when you have accumulated strong qi energy and are able to push it through its channels inside the body at will, will you be in a position to release the same qi towards external objects. While physical makeup and primordial qi heritage vary with individuals, I believe all of us are able to achieve this if we are willing to take the persistent effort under correct guidance.

Of course, there is no obligation that one should release such energy. In fact, one should be very cautious and conservative in releasing his qi energy. Projecting waiqi means releasing vital qi energy in huge quantity. That is why qigong masters feel tired after releasing waiqi and need time for rest and replenishment. Unreleased, qi is stored in the body for self-enhancement, benefiting its holder in many ways—restoring internal balance, improving resistance against diseases, healing one's own ailments, giving one a sanguine complexion, strong immunity, strong sexual vitality, and even supernatural physical strength.

To appreciate how wonderful and supernatural such strength is, let us see some of the feats that sophisticated Chinese qigong masters and martial artists can perform: chop through a stack of bricks or tiles with a single blow from the side of his hand, smash concrete blocks placed upon an exponent's chest with a large hammer, break free from a pair of steel handcuffs or from a tightly fastened rope around the body, take a sword or spear blow and emerge unscathed, walk through or lie on a board full of pointed nails and emerge unscathed, eradicate a tree from the ground or bend an iron bar with bare hands, drive a nail into the wooden wall with bare fingers, or easily lift an object weighing 1,000 pounds. When you see these miracles happen, you can be sure that qigong is at work.

The feats described above are known in Chinese martial arts as "hard qigong," which involves the direction of vital qi energy to the hands or fingers to accomplish such marvelous acts. Apparently, this ability can be effectively used to heal as well as kill. Strange to say, so hard and brutal force results, and can only result, from very delicate and gentle meditation and breathing. Here we see a classical example of appearance versus reality. Actually, the supreme achievement of Chinese martial arts comes from qigong practice. That is characteristic of the Nature School of martial arts which my teacher Dr. Wan Laisheng advocates and represents. Or, they are merged into one. Through qigong, one finds a perfect combination between force and delicacy, between action and nonaction, and in the final stage of cultivating immortality, between being and nonbeing.

Quite obviously, such skill on the part of a few qigong masters can be employed equally effectively to kill as well as to heal. Its killing ability makes it one of the most fearful weapons in the arsenal of Chinese martial arts, not only because it can kill, but more importantly because it can kill without your knowing it. Referred to in China as dianxue, or literally "pushing the acupoints," this is one of the supreme skills and highest attainments in Chinese martial arts. The attainment of this skill takes many years of persistent and arduous training in the area of hard qigong, aimed at being able to apply tremendous qi strength through the fingers to specific points in the body, coupled with the accurate knowledge of the timing of blood circulation to these acupoints. The ancient Chinese knew that each human body has a biological clock which marks the timing of blood coming to specific points—acupoints—in the body. Armed with this knowledge, one can apply the right finger strength to the right location at the right time to stop the blood circulation, resulting in physical death of the person applied.

Amazingly, the person on whom dianxue is applied will feel no pain at all. This is the supreme art, known as "cotton fingers" in Chinese martial arts. What cotton fingers means is that when such a finger touches you, you feel as if it is a piece of cotton falling on you. But its effect is delayed, penetrating, and fatal. Through decades of arduous training in hard qigong, a dianxue master such as my teacher Wan Laisheng can penetrate his force deep into his enemy's body without the latter feeling pain for the time being. Even more amazing is the fact that the exact time of the enemy's death can be programmed, so to speak, by the martial artist who applies the art of dianxue. The secret lies in the relation

of blood circulation to different acupoints. The lap in timing of death depends on how far a specific acupoint is ahead of time in terms of blood circulation at the time dianxue happens. The further an acupoint is ahead of the blood at the time of dianxue, the longer will the person survive. But eventually he or she is going to die, within twenty-four hours, because a full day is the cycle by which blood circulates throughout the body. It will stop where the master finger had touched, as also will the life itself.

Personally, I had seen one such thing happen during the turbulent years of the Cultural Revolution in China. A group of Red Guards stormed a Buddhist temple in my hometown at the urge of Mao. They smashed the Buddha images, broke the windows, put meat into the diet of monks, and physically humiliated and beat the monks. Still not satisfied with what they had accomplished, the leader of the group then threatened to kidnap the head monk of the temple if he refused to reveal where he had hidden the rest of the Buddhist classics. Driven to the limit of his forbearance and desperate, the elderly monk told the Guard leader: "Help me up, and I will show you where those classics are hidden." In response, the latter extended his hand over to help the monk up. Holding his left hand with the right hand of the Red Guard, the elderly monk gently put his right hand on the shoulder of the latter in an effort to stand up. That very night, the Guard leader mysteriously felt great difficulty in breathing.

Asked by his father, who was a high ranking official, where he had been, what he had done and eaten during the day, the young Guard related the scene at the temple. Having had some experience in martial arts himself, the father could roughly sense what might have happened to his son. He immediately sent for the elderly monk, and petitioned to the monk that if the latter could restore his son's life, he would forget everything and save the temple. Unfortunately, the answer he drew from the monk is "It is too late," an answer as gentle and quiet as his touch on the shoulder of his oppressor. The guard leader died shortly afterwards, about five hours after he left the temple.

In addition to hard qigong, there is another application of inner power known as "light qigong." My teacher Wan Laisheng, for instance, is a master of this special skill. He sometimes manifested his light qigong skill by walking along the brim of an empty bamboo basket dozens of times without falling down from the basket or destroying it. In one instance, using the power of light qigong, Wan Laisheng easily climbed up a perpendicular wall eight meters in height with bare hands and feet, approaching the agility and flexibility of a cat or a monkey.

Qigong Postures

The art of Chinese breathing exercise is composed of three pillars, or three regulations: regulating the body, regulating the mind, and regulating the breath. These three pillars must stand up together at the same time to achieve the optimum results. Regulating the body means assuming a proper posture in practicing qigong. Regulating the mind means controlling the mental activity during the exercise. Regulating the breath means keeping the breathing gentle, natural, and deep to the point that it seems as if no breath was coming in and going out of the nose. Let us first talk about regulating the body.

In its long history of development qigong has been developed into many forms, all of which involve the following three mutually dependent processes: regulation of posture, regulation of respiration, and regulation of the mind. Let us discuss the posture of qigong first. There are three postures commonly used in qigong: the lying posture, the standing posture, and the sitting posture.

Lying Posture

Many people, particularly weak and sick people, prefer to practice qigong while lying down in bed, facing the roof. Obviously, this is the least demanding posture of qigong exercise in terms of physical requirements. It makes you completely relaxed. While lying is a posture to assume in qigong, I would recommend that you lie on your side and put one hand on the pillow beside your head and rest the other hand on your hip. Your head should lean slightly forward. Bend your right arm (if you turn to the right side) and rest it on a pillow about half a foot away from the head, in a slightly fisted manner, while the left arm extends naturally and rests on the hip, palm downward. Rest the left leg on the right leg, with both legs bent slightly forward. If you choose to turn to the left side, just reverse the above positions.

While being the easiest posture to assume, the lying posture has its drawbacks. In fact, it is the hardest one in all three postures for the promotion of qi circulation and the attainment of serenity of mind. This is because while lying in bed, one has a much greater chance of falling asleep and thus completely losing one's consciousness and with it, all control over breathing and the mind. This situation is undesirable in qigong practice, otherwise qigong would be no different to ordinary sleep. Besides, qi has a harder time circulating throughout the body in a lying position than in a sitting or standing position. It seems that the principle "No pain, no gain" is working here, too. For this reason, the lying position should be the last resort reserved for those who have difficult sitting or standing.

Standing Posture

In contrast to lying, which is the most relaxed posture, standing is the most physically demanding posture of qigong in that it makes one tired the fastest. But it has its own rewards. With a standing posture, one's mind is more clear and regulated. Also, a standing posture seems to have the greatest power in promoting the circulation of qi energy in the body.

The correct standing posture is to stand with feet shoulder-width apart and slightly turned inward against each other, with arms raised to the level of shoulder in front of the breast as if encircling a column, and fingers forming a circle as if clutching a large ball, with shoulders slightly lowered.

Sitting Posture

This is by far the most popular posture for practicing qigong. Its popularity lies in the fact that it lies between standing and lying postures in terms of physical demand. As such, it prevents one from getting tired too easily, while at the same time avoiding losing one's concentration of mind. Thus, the sitting posture reaps the benefits of the other two postures while avoiding their pitfalls. Since qigong requires a certain length of time to take effect, the posture which will allow you to considerably extend the length of practice without losing your concentration of mind will naturally yield the greatest result. That is why the sitting posture becomes the most recommended position of qigong.

Sitting posture itself consists of three different variations. The first variation is the normal sitting form that everyone is used to, i.e., sitting on a hard chair (not a sofa) as you would normally do for a meal or work. To assume this posture, you must sit with your trunk erect on a square stool with feet flat on the ground, legs shoulder-width apart, knees bent at a 90-degree angle, thighs perpendicular to the trunk, palms resting in a relaxed manner on knees, or placed in front of dantian, elbows naturally bent, shoulders down, chin slightly withdrawn, chest in, and shoulders lowered slightly.

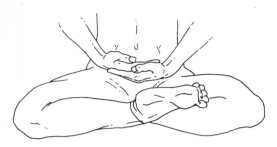

Figure 1-1
Half-lotus sitting position.

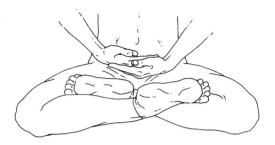

Figure 1-2
Full-lotus sitting position.

The second variation of the sitting posture is the single cross-legged position, or half-lotus posture. With this position, you sit on a cushion or on the ground, with one leg folded over the other. Keep the feet flat on the floor. Buttocks should protrude slightly, head erect, back straight, shoulders sunk, chin slightly withdrawn and chest slightly held in. With thumbs locked and the right hand holding the left hand, you place your hands just below the navel, with palms crossed and turned facing upwards. (See Figure 1-1.)

Yet another variation is the double cross-legged position, or the full-lotus position. This position is very similar to the half-lotus position. The only difference between them lies in the fact that rather than having one leg folded over the other, you tuck both feet under your legs and both knees are off the cushion. All other details remain the same. (See Figure 1-2.)

As you can easily tell, this is the most difficult of all postures. It takes good flexibility to perform it. Age is a big factor in determining whether you should adopt this posture or not. Those people who are used to this posture invariably start at an early age. This is because the younger you are, the more flexible your body is, and the easier it is for you to practice qigong in this form. For instance, Dr. Wan Laisheng always assumed a full-lotus posture while practicing qigong, even in his late eighties.

The trouble it takes to assume this position is worthwhile, because there are extra credits from the full-lotus posture. The unique benefit of the full-lotus position is its ability to keep one in good balance, leaning neither to the right nor to the left.

Naturalness is the principle of qigong to be followed in any posture one assumes. If you have trouble sitting in the full-lotus position, try the half-lotus position. If you have trouble sitting in the half-lotus position, just sit as you normally would. Otherwise, the cons will outweigh the pros. After all, postures are just a means to an end, and the end is the concentration of mind and construction of qi energy. The principle of naturalness dictates that one selects a posture that is most suitable to oneself based on one's physical condition. Do not throw the baby out with the bath water, so to speak.

There are some special suggestions in regard to posture based on one's special conditions. Patients with hypertension, heart disease, or neurosis are recommended to assume a sitting position when practicing qigong because this position induces the blood to move downward through the body, releasing the pressure on the head and heart. On the other hand, patients with gastrointestinal diseases are encouraged to take a lying position to promote gastrointestinal peristalsis.

Generally speaking, the sitting position is suitable for most people, sick or healthy, old or young, male or female. To prevent fatigue and prolong the time of practice, one may want to alternate positions during the session if it is going to be a lengthy one. For instance, one can sit for half an hour, and lie down for another fifteen minutes before resuming the sitting position. Assume whichever form suits you the best.

Guiding Principles of Qigong

Relax and remain at ease

This is the first principle of qigong. Unless you can manage to be relaxed and at ease with qigong, all the efforts you spend will be to no avail. In order to relax, you should keep in mind the following points. First, don't use force either in prolonging your breathing or in regulating your muscles; let everything go naturally. Second, don't strain yourself to maintain your posture; always stay comfortable. All muscles must be relaxed, especially those of the lower abdomen. Third, wear loose-fitting clothes. Fourth, set your mind at ease and adopt a cheerful and easy-going attitude, free from all cares and worries. Peace of mind is attained by focusing your attention on the exercise itself, banishing all other thoughts from your mind. Of great help to tranquillity of mind is to practice qigong in a place with tender light and free of all external interferences, such as noise, traffic, or movements. You will find yourself in a state of perfect calm wherein you will be unconscious of your own body weight. You may feel irritated at being unable to concentrate your mind in the beginning. This is quite natural and understandable. Just tell yourself repeatedly to calm down and be confident and patient. Persistent practice will bring steady progress.

Coordinate meditation with respiration

After initial tranquillity is attained, you can start to regulate your breathing. As the name of the breathing exercise implies, this is the central topic of qigong. The key difference between normal breathing and breathing in qigong lies in this: while the breathing process is purely natural in the normal case, the breathing process in qigong is regulated and deliberately prolonged. In other words, conscious efforts must be made to regulate the rhythm and speed of breathing, and to guide the flow of qi throughout the body. The regulation of respiration is achieved partly through meditation, i.e., you use your mind to guide the flow of qi energy as well as your respiration along certain prescribed routes within your body. While regulating your respiration with your consciousness, meditation serves two essential purposes of qigong at the same time: it guides your vital energy to flow along certain bodily routes, and helps your mind to concentrate on qigong exclusively to the negligence of all other things.

Progress gradually

Go slowly but steadily. Qigong is an art that can be perfected only through persistent and prolonged practice. Like any other art, practice makes perfect. Adjust the posture, the length of each practice and the speed of breathing to your own comfort level. Breathe naturally and rhythmically. Remember that in qigong as in any other forms of art, the result is cumulative. The more haste, the less

speed. It is advisable to just sow the seed and forget about the harvest for the time being. Don't worry about the harvest. When the harvesting time comes, qigong will let you know. For beginners, the length of each training can be anywhere from fifteen to twenty minutes. After three months of continuous training, one should be able to progress to thirty to forty-five minutes at a time. One year later, one will be able to do qigong for one to one-and-a-half hours at a time. Qigong masters like Dr. Wan Laisheng could sit for five hours in full-lotus posture without a stop. Experience points to the fact that the longer you practice qigong each time, the faster you will be able to accumulate enough vital energy in order to effect both the Minor Heavenly Cycle and the Major Heavenly Cycle, the ultimate attainments of qigong to be discussed later. This is because you have warmed up your body, or built up the momentum, as a natural consequence of prolonged practice, in very much the same way you drive a car. Each time you stop the car, you have to restart it the next time in order to assume the original speed, which costs time and energy. But it is important to remember that you should proceed in a natural way. Do not overextend yourself. After all, the way of nature lies in naturalness and persistency.

Constantly accumulate your saliva

Regularly swallow it down to dantian. Saliva was considered by the ancient Chinese to be of great value in promoting health and healing disease. The very character of "alive" in

Chinese speaks for its significance. In Chinese, the word "alive" is made of two components—the tongue and the water. Obviously, ancient Chinese regard saliva—the water of the tongue—as the symbol of life itself. There is an apparent reason for this, since only living people have saliva. Dead people don't have it. Moreover, it is an easy observation that the healthier you are, the more saliva you can generate in the mouth, and the easier it is to produce. This is demonstrated by the time length and strength in which one can speak continuously. Both the length and strength of speech one can sustain have a lot to do with the quantity of saliva one has. When one can only speak in a low voice or only for a short while before one is out of breath, he is said to be deficient in inner qi energy. Quite the contrary, Dr. Wan Laisheng could speak in a sonorous voice continuously for eight hours at a time without drinking even a mouthful of water. He can be said to be a manifestation of the Chinese natural health care system.

In this system, there is a profound set of theory governing the value of saliva. In the Chinese natural health care system saliva has been called "the water of the flowery pond," "the jade juice," and "the golden liquid." It is regarded as a vital life material intimately associated with sexual essence, blood, and qi energy. It is the key link between the heart and the kidney, and is an essential aid in the pilgrimage towards immortality. Recently, scientists have shown that saliva is closely related to one's immune system which, in the eyes of the ancient Chinese, is made up of nothing but the qi, the blood, and the sexual essence. Thus, frequently swallowing saliva down to dantian can nourish the vital qi, the sexual essence, and the blood, and greatly improve one's immunity and sexual vitality. The way to accomplish this in qigong is to put the tongue slightly against the upper hard palate while meditating. As the mouth is full of saliva, jiggle it in the mouth for a while, then swallow it down to dantian (using your mind to guide it) in three small mouthfuls through three rounds of exhalation. As time goes by, you will find your ability to generate saliva increases, and with it your immunity and overall health.

Suggestions for Practicing Qigong

About five minutes before practicing qigong, stop all mental and physical work. Go to the bathroom and get rid of the waste. Prepare yourself physically and mentally for the exercise. Tell yourself that you are going to be committed to qigong for the next thirty or sixty minutes; that qigong will be your sole occupation during that period of time and that nothing else should interfere with it.

Assume a south/north direction while practicing qigong. In other words, either face the south or face the north in qigong practice. A south/north orientation is known as *zi-wu* in Chinese philosophy, and is in line with the earth's magnetic field. Assuming this direction allows you to best promote your qi circulation and accumulation in the body, as well as to absorb the maximum amount of live energy in the universe.

Do not answer any calls during the exercise or stand up abruptly afterward. Otherwise, it will seriously damage your heart and kidneys over time. Another negative effect of violating this rule is the destruction of all the vital energy accumulated so far. No matter who calls or knocks at your door during your qigong practice, affect ignorance and continue with your exercise. If it is really something important and urgent, prepare yourself mentally that you have to stop the exercise for the time being. But do this slowly and leisurely, giving it at least two minutes' grace. During this short period of preparation, slowly withdraw your mind and consciousness from the mysterious world of qigong and return to the temporary reality. Loosen your body, stretch your limbs and body before you actually open your eyes and stand up in response. In a normal situation when you have finished the exercise and try to call a stop, retreat mentally from the qigong world first, and massage your face with both hands. Then gently stretch your arms and feet, gradually open your eyes and rotate them seven times before you get up to do some other things.

Other suggestions to follow include:

- Do not practice qigong immediately after a meal. Nor should you practice it while you feel hungry or are under the influence of alcohol.

- Do not practice qigong within one hour of sexual intercourse, before or after. The only exception is when you have mastered the art of regulated sex.

- Do not practice qigong while you have a bad cold, fever, coughing, diarrhea, or severe bodily pain. Nor should you do it while you are pregnant.

- Since qigong increases blood circulation, women should not practice it during menstruation. Nor should someone with bleeding problems practice it. Wait until the bleeding symptoms disappear.

- Do not exercise qigong under too high or too low a temperature, or in a noisy environment.

The Art of Breathing

It sounds ridiculous to people who know nothing of qigong to talk about breathing as an art. To them, breathing is a biological function that naturally. In other words, everybody can breathe without learning. This, however, is only partially true. The fact is that there is a lot to be learned about breathing, and it is an integral part of, and occupies a central position in, the Chinese natural health care system. Indeed, the ancient Chinese literally left no stone unturned in their search for means that would lead to better health, longevity, and immortality. They were especially careful in discovering the powerful effects of everyday, ordinary activities. Breathing is one of these activities that occupied their attention for centuries.

We all know that breathing is one of the most essential requirements of life. Without it, nobody can last more than five minutes. Since air costs us nothing, and the right and ability to breathe come with each one of us, we tend to neglect their significance and take air and breathing for granted. Not many of us ever think that the air we breathe is a precious resource, still less of us think of breathing as an art. When I talk about the art of breathing, it must sound odd to most people. But the fact is that for all its spontaneity, breathing remains a profound and supreme art of promoting health and healing.

Today, more and more people around the world are aware of the importance of clean air. This is a major progress towards environmental hygiene. However, not many people think of the very biological action of respiration as an art in itself. Indeed, the art of breathing remains a big enigma to most people. It was the ancient Chinese who elevated this biological function to the level of art. Qigong, the traditional Chinese breathing exercise, represents the earliest and most comprehensive accomplishment on the part of mankind to explore the potentials of the human body through regulated breathing and meditation.

The ancient Chinese were fully aware of the importance of fresh, clean air. That is one of the important reasons why all temples and monasteries in China are built in the midst of high mountains where the air is pure and fresh. Not surprisingly, most long-lived Chinese have been found in these places. But this is only part of their efforts to strive for better health and longevity. To them, the process of respiration is not just a matter of passively taking in the fresh air and getting rid of the stale air. It also involves the active participation of humans to prolong the respiratory process and to promote the accumulation and circulation of vital qi energy throughout the body. As essential supportive evidence of their theory, they observed that most long-lived animals are gentle, lengthy breathers, such as the tortoise. It stands to logic that if we humans can make our respiration cycle gentler and longer, we will enjoy better health and a longer life, too.

First, the Chinese sages discovered that breathing is the key link between man and superman, natural and supernatural, the mortal world and the immortal universe. In other words, longevity and immortality are attained through properly regulated breathing. The ancient Chinese regarded life as temporary and even external; they looked forward to an immortal world where the body and spirit hovered around nature and lasted hundreds, if not thousands, of years. To them, immortality is not something unthinkable. Rather, it is an attainable goal for humans. When your respiration is habitually tender, delicate, and prolonged like that of a tortoise, it is conducive to your longevity and immortality. If you keep the momentum and let the trend continue uninterrupted for decades, there is a good chance of having your spirit elevated to the supernatural immortal world, leaving your physical body behind. This is why many ancient Chinese were totally absorbed with qigong to the neglect of all worldly fame and wealth.

Second, through the persistent practice of qigong they discovered that there is an enormous energy potential inherent in everybody. This potential is so great that they came to believe the incredible similarities between man and god. Indeed, some of them even claimed that the distance between man and god is only one step. Might this be the reason why all gods are cast in the image of man? However, it takes long, persistent effort in the practice of qigong under the right guidance to bring man that close to god. This is why only a "privileged" few masters are able to manifest the amazing potentials which everybody has.

To appreciate how enormous that potential is, just look at the following facts. When someone pushes down a wall with his bare palms, it is human potential at work. When someone can see things hundreds of miles away, it is that same human potential at work. When someone can break a pile of bricks with his bare hands, or lie on nails and emerge unscathed, it is that same human potential at work. When you see someone causing the water in a well to surge by a mere wave of his hands, it is that same human potential at work.

Qigong is the key to opening up all these potentials. The nucleus of qigong lies in regulating qi (the vital energy) through the body with consciousness, and the purpose of this training is to set up a link in our body among essence, energy and spirit, known in the literature of the Chinese natural health care system as the "three treasures of life."

To master the art of breathing, however, we must first understand some essential concepts used in qigong practice. These are purely Chinese concepts, and may sound strange and even ridiculous to a Western mind that is absorbed with the tools and methods of scientific verification. By contrast, the Chinese culture emphasizes intuition and experience rather than experimentation and equipment. If you feel better by doing or eating something, that something is good for you. You do not need scientific verification for that. You yourself know it by heart, just as a fish knows best the temperature of the water. The Chinese ancients did not really bother about verifying the results, and still less do they rely on expensive equipment. So long as they felt better because of doing something, that something must be good for them. Nor did they worry about whether or not people believe them. In fact, many of them simply did not want to reveal the secrets. They kept such secrets of life to themselves, to their dear ones and trusted disciples. You may say that they were selfish. Again, who is not? But selfishness is not the sole reason why many secrets of qigong are not even known by the majority of Chinese. There are just too many secrets of life that can only be felt, but not adequately expressed in words. Here is another major point of departure between the Chinese and Western cultures.

One of the important concepts stressed over and over again in the theory of qigong is the that of dantian. What is dantian? In the Chinese natural health care system, dantian refers to that physical area in the lower abdomen about three inches below the navel. Also known as the Gate of Life and the "sea of qi," dantian is considered the origin and reservoir of the vital qi energy, the command of the twelve channels in the body, the point of convergence of all meridians and collaterals. It is dantian that determines the yin-yang balance, the respiratory efficiency, and the warmth and nourishment of the body. The importance of dantian to overall health is described by Zhao Xianke, a famous doctor in the Ming Dynasty, as follows:

Without the support of dantian, the kidneys become weak and there will be no sexual vitality to talk about. Without the support of dantian, the bladder will be out of function and urination problems occur. Without the support of dantian, the spleen and stomach will be dysfunctional and digestion problems arise. Without the support of dantian, the colon becomes stagnant and constipation happens. Without the support of dantian, the heart becomes dull and unable to think clearly. . . .

Since our energy level, our strength, our immunity, and ultimately our overall health and life expectancy are primarily determined by the strength of qi energy in our dantian, it makes sense to strengthen and improve this "sea of qi." The Chinese believe that by focusing one's attention on dantian from time to time, one can not only eliminate all distracting thoughts, but promote yang qi energy as well. By focusing our mind on the dantian area while practicing qigong, we will be able to concentrate our three treasures—essence, qi, and spirit—in dantian. In time, a sacred embryo will be formed there. To my understanding, dantian is also the center of gravity for the entire human body. My experience tells me that merely thinking about it can greatly increase our ability to maintain equilibrium and balance in exercise, a skill highly desirable for gymnastics, acrobatics, and all sorts of other sports.

From the standpoint of natural health and healing, the biological and therapeutic functions of dantian can be summarized as follows:

- It serves as the source and warehouse of vital qi.

- It reinforces the primordial qi.

- It strengthens the internal organs.

- It promotes blood circulation.

- It keeps breathing calm and smooth.

- It increases one's physical stamina.

- It keeps the body in balance while performing dramatic movements.

As has been mentioned before in many places, the Chinese fathers held that the very function of life itself depends ultimately on the supply of qi energy, since qi is the prime life force in the universe. Therefore, the more affluent qi supply one has or is capable of producing, the healthier one will be and the longer will be one's life. In terms of natural healing, the stronger the qi energy source, the shorter will be the healing process and faster will be the recovery from disease. More specifically, the self-healing power of qigong manifests itself when one induces one's own internal qi to flow to a diseased area in the body. This invisible but sensible energy flow will work wonders. However, before this can happen, one needs a strong bioelectrical source to propel it. Dantian is exactly such a source. Therefore, the strength of dantian very much determines our physical as well as mental health, and natural healing ability. This is why qigong exercise aims first and foremost at strengthening and enlarging the power base of dantian.

The way qigong accomplishes this end is two-fold: regulated meditation and regulated respiration. The first thing you need to learn is to focus your mind on dantian, i.e., to think of dantian as often as possible, even when you are not practicing qigong. Another thing you need to learn is to guide your qi, or the breath, down to dantian to the best of your ability. This may sound funny to many as dantian cannot be anatomically verified. All the more so when I talk about guiding breath with your mind. How can air be artificially guided to certain parts of the body? This is something that modern science finds hard to accept. Nevertheless, it is a powerful truth, a truth which points to the close connection of mind and body, and the supremacy of mind over body. It has worked wonders in many qigong masters and, believe me, it will work wonders on you if you take the effort to practice qigong. Focusing one's mind on dantian while guiding one's breath down to this area is at once a mental and physical exercise, which serves the following essential purposes at the same time: It brings about serenity and tranquillity of the mind; it builds up vital energy reserves; and it massages the internal organs and triggers abdominal movement.

Another important concept in qigong theory has to do with the routes along which qi energy travels and circulates inside the body. The Chinese sages identify two full cycles as basic routes for qi circulation. One full cycle is called the Minor Heavenly Cycle, and the other is called the Major Heavenly Cycle. Significantly, both are termed "heavenly," a fact which reflects the ancient Chinese view of humans as microcosms of heaven. Let us see how these two cycles work in our body.

The Minor Heavenly Cycle is composed of two semicycles. One is called the Functioning or Ren channel, which goes along the middle line of the front of the body from the acupoint Baihui (located at the apex of the head) to the acupoint Huiyin (found on the perineum). (See Figure 7-1, page 459.) The other is called Governing or Du channel, which travels from Huiyin to Baihui up the spine along the middle line of the back of the body, thus completing a full cycle. (See Figure 7-2, page 459.) The Functioning channel is regarded as the head of all yin channels, while the Governing channel is the head of all yang channels. Altogether, there are fourteen channels in each human body.

The Minor Heavenly Cycle works in this way: as you inhale, the qi begins to rise from Huiyin along the Governing channel until it finally reaches Baihui on top of the head. This coincides with the whole process of inhalation. When you exhale, the qi starts to descend from Baihui along the Functioning channel, through dantian, all the way to Huiyin, completing the Minor Heavenly Cycle in one round of respiration.

The Major Heavenly Cycle consists of four channels. In addition to the Functioning and Governing channels just described, we add the stomach channel and gallbladder channel to it. The stomach channel runs along the right leg, from the acupoint of Huiyin to that of Yonchuan on the right sole. This is an important acupoint at the middle of the sole. The gallbladder channel runs along the left leg, from Huiyin to the left Yonchuan. The whole cycle works like this: as you inhale, the qi begins to climb up from the two Yonchuan acupoints along the stomach and gallbladder channels simultaneously until they merge at Huiyin. There the two courses of qi join force and then continue their ascent along the Governing channel until it finally reaches Baihui at the very top of the head, thus completing the inhaling process of the cycle. After that, as the exhaling process starts, the qi begins to descend along the Functioning channel through dantian until it reaches Huiyin. At that juncture, the qi energy divides into two flows—one travels along the stomach channel and goes down the right leg to the right Yonchuan, the other along the gallbladder channel and travels down the left leg to the left Yonchuan, thus completing the major heavenly cycle in one round of respiration.

The opening up of the two heavenly cycles represent two higher stages of attainment in qigong practice. As a matter of normal procedure, one should not attempt the Major Heavenly Cycle until one has been successful and feels at home with the Minor Heavenly Cycle, just as one should not attempt the Minor Heavenly Cycle until one has accumulated strong qi in the dantian.

To begin with, one should practice the manipulation of qi along the Functioning channel only, which is half of the Minor Heavenly Cycle. Then one can proceed to the Minor Heavenly Cycle. Finally, one can embark on the adventure of the Major Heavenly Cycle. This is a logical order in terms of degree of demand and difficulty. The more haste, the less speed. This is the principle governing all arts. Qigong is no exception.

Beginners of qigong should first try to manipulate qi down the Functioning channel. This is how the semicycle works. As you inhale, you temporarily forget everything. When you exhale, you consciously guide your breath down your body along the Functioning channel all the way to dantian and stop there. Let your mind, together with qi, stay in dantian for a while until you have completed the exhaling process. Then you start another round of respiration, and repeat it again and again. The purpose of this training in the semicycle is to strengthen dantian and to accumulate as much vital qi energy as you can in preparation for greater cycles of qi manipulation.

Usually, this preparatory stage will take anywhere from three to eighteen months. Exactly how long it takes depends on many factors including the health status of the practitioner, how frequently qigong is practiced, how long each session lasts, what posture is assumed during the exercise, and how concentrated one is during each qigong session. Generally speaking, the more regularly and frequently one practices qigong, the sooner one will find sufficient qi built up in dantian. In the same way, the longer one practices qigong, the sooner one will accumulate qi in the body. Besides, as mentioned before, the sitting position is more effective in conducing the qi to the lower abdomen as compared with other postures. Another significant factor in determining the length of time it takes to build up qi around dantian is the health status of the practitioner. Believe

it or not, the healthier one is, the easier it is to accumulate vital qi around dantian. For one thing, a healthy person can practice longer each time, and the length of each practice does count in the mastery of qigong skills. For another thing, a healthy person already has more qi reserve in the body than a sick person. That gives the former a head start in the adventure of qigong.

One relevant question is: How can one tell whether the qi cumulated in dantian is powerful enough to proceed to the next stage, which in this case means the Minor Heavenly Cycle? This is a very individual question, which only the individual practitioner can answer. The thing to note is that for everybody, there is a stumbling block lying somewhere between the upper abdomen and the lower abdomen, which prevents the qi from flowing directly, uninterrupted into the dantian area. This stumbling block is the diaphragm. The diaphragm prevents most people from physically guiding their qi or air down to the dantian area. One of the major tasks of qigong in its first stage of training is to physically open up the diaphragm along the Functioning channel to allow the qi energy to flow uninterrupted to dantian. Your success with the heavenly cycles depends first and foremost on the opening up of the Functioning channel, or the removal of the diaphragm.

In this regard, there are no shortcuts. Anybody who wants to open up a route through the diaphragm to experience the magic and wonder of qigong must achieve this goal by persistent, consciously guided breathing exercises. This effort can take months, or even years, before the invisible route is opened up. The effect is cumulative. The more intensively, attentively, and frequently you practice regulated breathing, the sooner you will be able to open the Functioning channel and allow yourself to physically send your qi down to dantian and store it there for multiple uses later. Many qigong practitioners stumbled at this point, either because they were too lazy to devote enough time to the training, or because they did not focus on the project while training, or even because they were so eager for success that they unnaturally overexerted themselves. Overexertion in breathing is counterproductive in that it can lead to mental and physical ailments. The end result: the more haste, the less speed. Therefore, it is vital to keep in mind that success in qigong does not come overnight. It takes long and consistent effort. It is the cumulative effect of long time practice that will eventually work wonders for you. As a matter of principle, absolutely no force or exertion should be employed in the process. Everything should come naturally. This is one reason why longevity counts so much for those serious about qigong and immortality. To them, time is not money, but life.

Generally speaking, the longer you practice qigong, the stronger your dantian becomes. Then all of a sudden comes the exciting moment. You experience some strange sensations inside the body: a current of cool

or warm air flowing uninterrupted all the way down to dantian each time you exhale during qigong practice, a series of rolling sounds keep coming out of the lower abdomen, and sometimes you can even feel the vibration of your body and the rotation of qi around dantian for thirty-six rounds in each direction, clockwise and counterclockwise. At the same time, all your organs feel a sensation of pleasant warmth, comfortable coolness, and a feeling that all your internal organs are cleansed of pollutants. These are not fictions. They are truths experienced and confirmed by many qigong practitioners. It is a sure sign that the stumbling block in the abdomen has been penetrated. It is a green light inviting you to move on to the next stage in qigong practice. Your biological clock is ringing. This is a really exciting moment, a moment in which you experience how you heal yourself internally, a moment in which you realize the immense potentials latent in your body, and a moment you begin to notice a marked difference in your health status. If you are sick, your health will start to improve with each passing day. If you are healthy, you become even more healthy and energetic, catching a glimpse of the "supernatural."

Before I embark on the wonderland of the Minor Heavenly Cycle, I would like to say a few words that can be very helpful to you. That is: you do not have to experience the Minor Heavenly Cycle if you cannot attain it. Do not exert yourself; take it easily and naturally. The healing effect will certainly happen as long as you can practice qigong on a regular basis, and its effect and momentum will keep on growing just by continuing the experiment of the semicycle around the Functioning channel. As a matter of fact, many qigong practitioners have never experienced any heavenly cycle, although they have practiced qigong throughout their lives. Nonetheless, they gain health benefits from the very practice of qigong.

It would be better and more desirable, of course, to be able to carry the adventure of the qigong world into the stage of the Minor Heavenly Cycle. Once qi can automatically circulate around the upper trunk of the body, which is the portion of the body where the majority of diseases, and most of the fatal diseases, are found and located, the preventative and therapeutic effects of qigong will be further enhanced. Again, the principle is to regulate respiration with consciousness. Just imagine that the vital qi rises along the Governing channel from the acupoint Huiyin to Baihui as you inhale, and flows down along the Functioning channel as you exhale. Some day you will experience the circulation of air in the cycle, around and around, even after you stop thinking about it. This is one way in which qigong heals and cleanses the body. Here the key is the strength of qi, the primary healing materials of qigong. The stronger the qi energy, the faster and greater the healing. No qi, no cure.

The completion of the Minor Heavenly Cycle means success in opening up and connecting the Functioning and Governing channels. At this stage, there are some clear biophysical changes indicating the opening up of these vital channels. When you inhale, you will feel your qi energy descend all the way down to dantian. When you exhale, you will feel the qi energy ascend all the way up to the brain. Thus, each round of regulated inhalation and exhalation causes the inner qi energy to circulate along the Functioning and Governing channels.

You are to be congratulated on reaching this stage. It marks a major achievement in qigong practice, of which not many can boast. At this stage, some strange physical phenomena may happen. For instance, some practitioners may lift themselves up slightly as if about to fly, while others may experience a short pause in breathing as if life has ceased to exist. Strange and frightening as these phenomena may sound, they are quite natural from the standpoint of qigong. It is important that you do not get scared. Stay calm and composed in case these happen to you. Sometimes, at the higher stage of qigong exercise, one may even experience a brief pause between the end of exhalation and the beginning of inhalation as if life has stopped. This is a normal phenomenon, and there is no reason for panic. It help build up the qi in dantian. However, if it bothers you, you can slowly round up the exercise and do something else.

Now it is time to embark on the Major Heavenly Cycle, which represents the highest attainment in the skill of guiding qi energy inside the body. During this stage, one consciously guides the circulation of qi along the route of the major heavenly cycle described before. In a sense, the Major Heavenly Cycle can be thought of as an extension of the Minor Heavenly Cycle. Since the route of the Major Heavenly Cycle is much longer than that of the Minor Heavenly Cycle, with the addition of the length of the stomach and gallbladder channels, this apparently puts a higher demand on the qigong practitioner in terms of length of breathing. It takes time to attain this status, and it is logical to go from the Minor Heavenly Cycle to the Major Heavenly Cycle, because length of breathing is generally in proportion to the length of practice. This demand on the ability to breathe slowly and deeply alone explains why only a very small portion of qigong practitioners have the chance to experience the Major Heavenly Cycle.

Once successful in landing on the Major Heavenly Cycle, one can feel the same sensations experienced in the stage of the Minor Heavenly Cycle, only now these sensations have been extended to the entire body. As such, the opening up of the Major Heavenly Cycle gives its practitioner an added healing power for diseases located in the lower part of the body, such as arthritis in the knee. While not essential for the purposes of health, success in the Major Heavenly Cycle seems to be a prerequisite for the pursuit of immortality in the Taoist context.

Above all, the principles of qigong require that the mind be concentrated, while the breathing remains slow, smooth, deep, long, quiet, and natural. The two reinforce each other in a positive cycle. A concentrated mind helps prolong the respiration, and gentle, prolonged respiration further calms down the mind, eases the disturbed emotions, and helps bring about the internal balance of yin and yang in the body. Clinical experiments prove that regulated long and deep breathing can help bring the central nervous system to a state of dynamic equilibrium, thus improving and curing many stress-related diseases, including cancer.

The Art of Meditation

It would be incomplete to talk about the art of breathing without also discussing the art of meditation. For without adequate meditation going side by side with respiration, it would be hard to achieve the desired results in breathing, be it the Minor Heavenly Cycle or Major Heavenly Cycle. In fact, meditation and respiration are twins in qigong. Contrary to the Western concept which describes meditation as a process of deep thinking, meditation in qigong is concerned about the achievement of inner tranquillity of mind to the exclusion of all thinking and reflection, especially deep thinking. It is a process by which the mind becomes cleansed, purified, and elevated, rather than deep and complicated. In fact, the first and foremost principle of qigong exercise is to have the mind "entering a state of tranquillity," a semiconscious mental state free from all distracting thoughts and worry. Unless one can attain such a state, there is no point going further, because most of the efforts spent on qigong will be wasted.

In the Chinese natural health care system, this state of mind is described as *ruo-cun-ruo-wang* (as if existing, as if nonexisting), or *wu-zhu-wu-wang* (neither exerting nor forgetting). The famous Taoist immortal Zhang Shanfeng describes this mental state as follows: "Keeping your mind quiet and natural all the time is *wu-wan* (never forgetting); going with qigong naturally is *wu-zhu* (never exerting)." That is to say, one is only vaguely aware of the ongoing qigong exercise, but totally unaware of all other things going around. In other words, one is fully relaxed but not in a trance. In such a mental state, all cares and worries are laid aside for the time being. In their place, a peaceful, tranquil mind comes into being, with an enhanced self-confidence and a proud sense of spiritual detachment from this troublesome, competitive, dirty, and violent world. This is a special state of mind, the third state of mind which lies between sleep and full awareness. It is the ideal state of qigong, which seeks to control and regulate not just the breathing process, but also the mental process. Once one is fast asleep, one loses all control over one's mental state. That is why a sitting and standing posture are superior to a lying posture in qigong practice, because lying on a bed makes one sleepy, which is something qigong wants to avoid. Otherwise, there would be no difference between qigong and sleep.

Why should qigong seek such a mental state of tranquillity? It is because such a mental state is very helpful to overall health, stronger immunity, and the healing process. For one thing, clinical experiments show that in a mental state of quietness and tranquillity, one consumes 16 to 34 percent less oxygen than in a state of full awareness. This finding explains why qigong masters have much less need for food and sleep than ordinary people. For another thing, a tranquil mind promotes the orderliness of mental activity, thus greatly increasing the efficiency of the brain cells. This fact shows that regular qigong exercise can prevent and relieve Alzheimer's and Parkinson's diseases. A tranquil state of mind also promotes the connection and balance between mind and body, enhancing one's immunity against diseases. In addition, it brings about the following biological changes in favor of overall health:

- The rate of brain wave activities in the cerebral cortex diminishes, while the amplitude of alpha waves increases.

- Adrenaline decreases to about 60 percent of normal.

- The rate of protein renewal slows down.

- Vascular tension reduces.

- The secretion of hormones diminishes.

- The lactate concentration in the blood markedly reduces.

All these phenomena point to the fact that the metabolism is reduced or slowed down;

and that energy consumption decreases as a result of qigong exercise.

To attain this mental state, qigong requires its practitioners to concentrate their mind on dantian as the first step. This concentration of mind on dantian serves to kill two birds with one stone. If the goal is to solely forget worldly affairs, then concentrating on any part of the body will serve this purpose. Concentration of mind on dantian, however, has a dual effect of achieving a tranquil state of mind while building up the strategic reserve of qi. This is because dantian is the "sea of qi," the origin and warehouse of vital qi energy. This is especially important for beginners. For one thing, they normally find it hard to concentrate on the qigong practice itself. In the initial stages of training, their mind typically goes woolgathering, so to speak. Trying to think of dantian for a period of time is the best way for them to enter the tranquil state of mind.

Besides trying to focus your mind on dantian, the following points have been found helpful to the realization of a quiet state of mind:

- Find a peaceful and secluded environment to practice qigong. Such an environment is conducive to a peaceful mind. This is especially important for beginners. There is a rippling effect between the mind and the environment. That is why many Chinese spend years meditating in deep mountains.

- Find an easy, carefree time to practice qigong. By easy time I mean a time period in which one is least affected by worries and thinking. Early morning and bedtime fall into this category. Shortly after waking up in the morning, one's mind is still free from external influences, and therefore it is easier to attain peace of mind if qigong is practiced. Bedtime rings the biological clock of rest, an urge to put all work and thinking behind. So it is also a good time for qigong exercise, as long as one is not too sleepy.

- Wear loose clothes. Loose clothes make one feel relaxed and comfortable, and relaxation leads to concentration and peace of mind.

- Move the bowels if necessary before practicing qigong. Urinate immediately before the qigong exercise.

- Do not practice qigong with an empty or full stomach. An empty or full stomach will divert your attention from qigong, making it hard for you to enter the mental state of tranquillity.

- Look at the tip of your nose while practicing qigong. Since the tip of the nose is more visible and tangible than dantian, some people find this to be a more efficient way of concentrating the mind.

- Look through "the third eye" inward at the route by which the qi moves around your body, imagining that you are literally guiding the flow of qi inside your body;

	Body Position	Respiration	Mental Tranquility	Frequency and Length	Requirements
Stage I	Normal sitting position or lying position for those in delicate health	From natural to partial deep breathing	Mentally count respiration cycles	Three to five times daily, fifteen minutes each	(1) Correct body position (2) Regulated breathing (3) Mind concentrated on qigong exercise
Stage II	Normal sitting or half-lotus position	Deep breathing	Mentally count respiration and try to focus mind on dantian	Two to three times daily, thirty minutes each	(1) Deep breathing down to dantian (2) Initial mental tranquillity
Stage III	Half-lotus or full-lotus position (the latter for those younger and stronger)	Deep breathing with air concentrated on dantian	Mind naturally focused on dantian	Twice a day, longer than forty-five minutes each	(1) Deep, even breathing (2) Complete mental tranquillity (3) Cool or warm sensation around the lower abdomen

Table 7-1
For beginning practitioners of qigong, here is the suggested order of progression.

- Listen to your own breathing while practicing qigong. Normally, it is hard to hear one's own breathing if it is natural. It takes a concentrated mind and quiet environment to accomplish the task. This is exactly what qigong seeks.

- Silently count numbers: 1, 2, 3. . . .

Entering the qigong state of mind can be a long process, especially for people nowadays who have more worries and stress than their predecessors. By persistent effort one will be able to achieve that in due time. Do not feel disappointed if you have trouble expelling distracting thoughts. This is normal. Here, patience is as important as persistence. The more haste, the less speed. The more patient, the easier it is to enter a quiet state of mind.

With regard to the frequency and timing of practice, I recommend that beginners do qigong twice a day, once in the early morning shortly after getting up, and again at bedtime in the evening. The morning session prepares you for a new day's challenges, while the evening session prepares you for a good night's sleep.

Possible Side Effects and Their Solutions

Stiff back or shoulder

This often happens to beginners, and is quite natural because one is not accustomed to standing or sitting in the qigong posture for a long time, or one's posture is not correct. To prevent this from happening, start with the supine position and gradually shift to the sitting position with a single leg crossed. Another way of relieving the situation is to change postures during the practice. Yet another way is to shorten the length of each practice in the light of the individual's physical status.

Numbness in the legs while sitting

This can be prevented by limbering up your legs before sitting in the cross-legged posi-

tions. If numbness persists, massage your legs, and lie down on a bed until it is gone.

Pressure in the chest and difficulty breathing

This situation usually results from artificially prolonging the breathing against the principle of naturalness. To prevent this from happening, breathe completely naturally; do not exert yourself in breathing. To relieve the situation, quit the practice, take a short walk, relax and massage your chest in the fresh air.

Shortness of breath or stitch in the side

This usually happens when you breathe too hard, try to hold your breath for too long, or trap your breath in the chest or throat. The symptoms will disappear once these faults are overcome. To gain relief, stop the exercise, go outdoors, and do some physical exercise such as chest expanding.

Lethargy

This is undesirable in qigong practice, less one will completely fall into sleep and lose control of both breathing and meditation. This phenomenon occurs most often when one practices qigong in a lying posture, or when one is tired and sleepy. To prevent this from happening, do not practice qigong when you are physically tired or feeling sleepy. Ensure that you glance at the tip of the nose during the exercise. Or, if you are really tired and feel like sleep, stop qigong and go to bed. Do not exert yourself.

Qi surging upward

This phenomenon happens because the practitioner cannot hold qi in the dantian area. The reason why one cannot hold qi steadily in dantian is because one's mind is not focused on dantian. Since qi is guided by the mind, if the mind goes wool-gathering, qi will consequently float and ramble in undesired directions. To relieve the situation, stop the exercise, relax, and drink a cup of warm water, or swallow some saliva down to dantian.

Thirsty after practice

This is caused by closing the mouth too tightly during the exercise. To relieve the situation, simply take a cup of water or fruit juice and relax.

Fast heart rate

This happens because one is too nervous about qigong, or one is not relaxed enough either in posture, breathing, or mind. To relieve the situation, relax your posture and forget about the breathing requirements of qigong for a while.

Stomach swelling sensation

This can be caused by either forced long breathing or forced thinking of the lower abdomen. In other words, it results from violating the supreme principle of qigong, i.e., naturalness. To relieve, forget about dantian and breathing for a while or, if necessary, stop the exercise completely and lie down on a bed for a rest.

Appendix 2

Mobile Qigong

This is a series of exercises combining physical movement with qigong. It was designed by a mysterious Taoist immortal named Zhang Shanfeng, who lived about 800 years ago. Zhang is also the inventor of taich'i exercise. Legend goes that one summer afternoon when Zhang was meditating in his mountain hut in central China, he was aroused by a loud noise. Rising and peeping out through the window, he discovered that a snake and a crane were engaged in a bitter life-and-death struggle. The struggle went on for almost an hour, ending in the death of both parties. Zhang closely watched the entire process of the fierce but skillful fighting. For days afterwards, he was lost in serious thought about the fight, and the result was the invention of taich'i, a flexible soft exercise mimicking the sneaky and tactful movements of the snake and the crane, while incorporating into each movement the factor of regulated breathing as a guiding principle.

420 • *Mobile Qigong*

Mobile qigong is another invention of Taoist Zhang. As the name implies, mobile qigong is a breathing exercise in motion. It lies somewhere between static qigong and taich'i exercise. Unlike the static qigong we have already described, it is more mobile and physical. Unlike taich'i, it does not have many physical movements. Its purpose is to strengthen both the internal elixir (the mind and vital energy) and the external elixir (the body and limbs). The idea is to facilitate accumulation and circulation of qi in the body by means of limited body movements together with regulated breathing. It requires greater skills in coordinating body movements and regulated respiration. Therefore, it is recommended that you practice static qigong for a month or two before attempting this variation.

Described below are three forms of mobile qigong that have been shown to have potent therapeutic effects.

Hands Rising and Falling

Starting position
Stand upright with feet shoulder-width apart. Hold your head and neck erect with your chest drawn slightly inward. Put the tip of your tongue against the upper hard palate with your teeth softly clenched. Bend your knees slightly. Hold your shoulders and elbows down with your arms hanging naturally and your thumbs resting against the

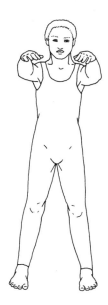

Figure 2-1
As you inhale, raise your arms, and imagine the strength flow to your fingertips.

thighs. Look straight ahead and take three deep breaths.

Performance
1. While you are inhaling, slowly raise both arms in front of the chest to shoulder level, palms facing down, fingers slightly bent and elbows gently dropped. Keep arms shoulder-width apart and imagine that the strength is coming to the fingertips. At the same time, clench your toes and contract your anal muscle. (See Figure 2-1.)

2. As you exhale, guide your qi down to dantian, your lower abdomen. At the same time, let your arms fall down gently

to resume the starting position, thumbs resting against the thighs, while relaxing both the toes and the anal muscle.

3. Repeat the above movements at least a dozen times.

Points to remember

- Make sure that you coordinate your hand movements with your breathing as if in the static breathing exercise.

- Do not use force, but gradually prolong the length of each round of movement as you prolong your breathing.

- Practice this form twice a day, once in the morning and once before going to bed.

Benefits

This mobile form, if practiced regularly and consistently, will promote digestion and circulation of blood and qi energy, help cure stomach ulcers, enhance the function of the heart, lungs, and mind, and relieve the problems of nocturnal emissions and impotence.

Chest Expanding and Contracting

Starting position

Stand with your feet shoulder-width apart. Slightly bend your knees and allow your hands to hang loosely at your sides. Concentrate and take three deep breaths. Your mind should focus on the lower abdomen and your eyes should look straight ahead.

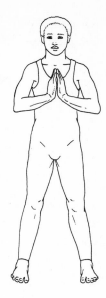

Figure 2-2
As you focus on dantian, bring your palms together in front of your chest.

Performance

1. Slowly raise your hands and place them, palms together, in front of the chest. (See Figure 2-2.)

2. Inhale, and gently separate the palms horizontally across the chest to shoulder width, until you reach the limit of inhalation.

3. Exhale, and gently bring both palms together until they resume the position of step 1 (Figure 2-2) as you reach the end of your exhalation.

4. Repeat steps 2 and 3 for as many times as you want.

5. Once you have finished, let your hands hang loosely to resume the starting position.

Points to remember

· Gradually and naturally increase the depth and length of your breathing as you proceed, but never exert yourself.

· As always, think in general terms of your lower abdomen as you exhale.

· Imagine that you are exerting your strength at your fingertips, which means slightly concentrating your force at the fingertips but never overdoing it.

Benefits

This form of mobile qigong is shown to be able to promote digestion, prevent and relieve heart disease, pneumonia, and hypertension, ease headaches and backache, relieve asthma, and enhance the function of the overall immune system.

Body and Hands Rising and Falling

Starting position

Stand straight with feet together and eyes looking ahead. Take three deep breaths.

Performance

1. Put your hands against each other in front of your abdomen, with the palms facing upward and the fingers closed. (See Figure 2-3.)

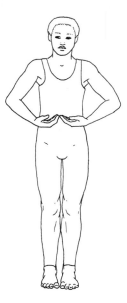

Figure 2-3
Stand straight with your palms curved upward, keeping your fingers together.

2. As you inhale, slowly raise the right hand, with the palm facing upwards until you have reached your limit in terms of both inhaling and hand extension. The left hand remains in the original position. (See Figure 2-4, page 423.)

3. As you exhale, turn the right palm downward and press it down along the chest. At the same time, raise the left hand in exactly the same way as you did for the right hand, palm up and to the position just above your head. At the same time, squat down until you have reached your limit in terms of both exhaling and body movement. (See Figure 2-5, page 423.)

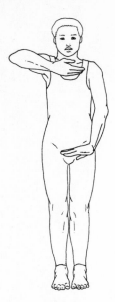

Figure 2-4
Inhale and slowly raise your right hand while turning your left palm downward

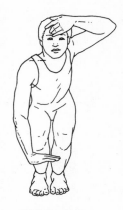

Figure 2-5
As you squat down, lower your right hand while raising your left hand.

4. As you inhale, stand up slowly. At the same time, raise the right hand (palm upwards) and press down the left hand (palm downward) in front of your lower abdomen until you have reached the limit of both your respiration and physical extension.

5. Exhale and squat down again, while pressing the right hand down and raising the left hand up. Repeat the above movements five to seven times.

6. Then cross both hands in front of the abdomen with palms facing upward. (See Figure 2-6.)

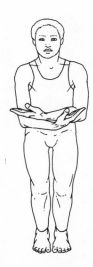

Figure 2-6
Keep your palms facing upward as you cross them in front of your abdomen.

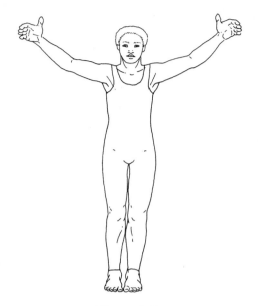

Figure 2-7
Breathe deeply as you raise your arms back in a circle.

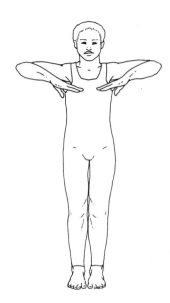

Figure 2-8
Deeply exhale, sending the air down to dantian, and relax.

7. Throw both hands backwards in a circle and raise them to head level while turning the palms to face downward. At the same time, make deep inhalations. (See Figure 2-7.)

8. Press both hands down in front of your body while deeply exhaling and sending the air down to dantian. At the same time, relax completely. (See Figure 2-8.)

9. Round up the whole series of exercises, body straight and looking forwards.

Points to remember
• Practice this exercise outdoors in fresh air.

• Coordinate your breathing with the body and hand movements, i.e., inhale while standing up and exhale while squatting down, with your mind focused on the lower abdomen.

• Try to hold your trunk and head as straight as possible. Always look forward.

Benefits
This form of mobile qigong can strengthen the kidneys, lungs, and heart. It promotes the respiratory as well as circulatory systems, helps relieve lumbago, pneumonia, chest pain, impotence, and back pain.

Appendix 3

Sound Qigong

The use of external sounds for healing purposes has been briefly discussed before. Sound qigong is the use of various sounds made during qigong practice for therapeutic purposes. Again, the ancient Chinese were the first to discover the self-healing effects of the various sounds, and added that tool to the arsenal of their natural health care system. The ancient Chinese believed that the special sounds one makes are associated with special internal organs and meridians. Therefore, by deliberately making specific sounds in qigong practice, one can massage and nourish specific organs in the body, channel the subtle qi energy along the desired routes or meridians, promote blood circulation around the diseased part of the body, dispel the blockage of blood and qi in that area, and eventually effect a cure through self-healing.

We all make different sounds from time to time, consciously or unconsciously. With the exception of laughing, most of these sounds do not lead to healing. Why?

The reason is because sound alone is not enough for healing. Only when it is combined with regulated breathing that sound manifests its therapeutic effects. This ancient Chinese healing theory has been confirmed by modern scientific research which show that making sounds while regulating one's breathing possesses psychological, physiological and therapeutic effects.

Describing sound qigong has become much easier since we have already discussed the art of breathing in great detail. What remains to be told is how to generate different sounds for different healing purposes.

How to Generate Sounds

To generate the sounds needed for healing, you must already be in the process of practicing qigong exercise.

- A sit-bending position is recommended, i.e., you sit on the ground with your belt loosened, and press your bent legs against your chest with both hands.

- In sound qigong, sounds are made while exhaling, not inhaling. This is in symphony with the process of breathing—both exhaling and making sounds are activities that release the qi.

- While inhaling, close your mouth and breathe in through your nose. Do it as slowly, gently, and naturally as your breathing.

- While exhaling, send the qi down to the lower abdomen (dantian) while making specific sounds.

- Make the same sound thirty-six times.

As to the timing and frequency of practice, the ancient Chinese told us to exercise twice a day and that the best time is at bedtime and early in the morning. One important reason why bedtime and the early morning are considered best is because these are times when one is free from external interference and can best concentrate on the exercises, thus enhancing its positive effects.

Healing Sounds

What kinds of sounds should we make? The answer depends on what diseases we want to heal, or which internal organs we want to strengthen. The following are specific sounds with specific medical benefits.

Ge

This sound can reach the liver. Making this sound while exhaling can relieve liver diseases, especially hepatitis and cirrhosis.

Gong

This sound can reach the spleen. Hence, making this sound while exhaling can relieve spleen dysfunction and indigestion, and boost the appetite.

Ha

This sound is related to the kidneys, heart, and blood system. Therefore, making this sound while exhaling can nourish the kidney energy, reduce heart fire and blood pressure, and help cure heart disease and sexual dysfunction.

Hay

This sound is related to the kidneys. Making it while exhaling can promote kidney and stomach function, improve kidney qi energy and therefore relieve diseases such as sexual dysfunction, impotence, incontinence, and excess urination.

He

Making this sound will calm down the heart fire, relieving insomnia, nocturnal emission, ear ringing, and sore throat.

High

This sound is related to the stomach and spleen. Making this sound while exhaling can promote stomach and spleen function, improve digestion, and relieve obesity and high cholesterol.

Huu

This sound is related to the stomach and duodenum. Making this sound while exhaling can nourish and promote the stomach and duodenum, and relieve diarrhea, stomachaches, and ulcers.

Sang

This sound is related to the lungs. Making this sound while exhaling can promote the function of the lungs and relieve related diseases such as asthma, coughing, difficulty in breathing, and lung cancer.

Shi

Making this sound can improve the function of your lungs, and relieve asthma, coughing, and the common cold.

Xu

This sound is related to the liver. Making this sound has the therapeutic effect of brightening the eyes, nourishing the liver, reducing liver fire, relieving dizziness, eye-watering, eyestrain, and especially hypertension and heart disease.

Zhen

This sound can reach the heart so making this sound while exhaling can promote blood circulation, improve heart function, and relieve heart disease.

Appendix 4

Dharma's Morning Exercises

Dharma was a prolific inventor of Chinese fitness exercises as well as a great religious leader. In China, he is widely regarded as the father of Chinese martial arts as well as the patriarch of Chinese Buddhism. The following is a series of exercises he designed for his monks to practice in the morning. As you will see, many of the movements described here smell of martial arts, one of his professions. Regular practice of these exercises will bring you many therapeutic benefits including preventing obesity and keeping you fit and high-spirited. It is also recommended that one practice this set of exercises in the order listed.

This section of movements is aimed at getting rid of the stale air one accumulates during a night's sleep and replacing it with fresh air in the morning. It can cleanse you body and mind, promote your heart and lungs, boost your appetite and improve your digestion. It also greatly enhances one's spirit for a new day's challenge. Therefore, it is best taken as the first set of movements in the morning when one gets up. Remember to move slowly, making sure each step is in sync with your breathing.

Replacing the Stale Air with Fresh Air

Preparation

Stand straight with feet together. Take three deep breaths, sending the air you inhale down to the lower abdomen, or dantian. Look straight ahead with your hands hanging loosely on both sides. Cross your hands in front of your abdomen with palms facing upward.

Performance

1. Slowly raise both hands with palms facing upward until they are right above your head. Keep the elbows pointing out to the sides. At the same time, inhale and raise your head and heels in accordance with the hand movements. (See Figure 4-1.)

2. Once above your head, separate your hands, letting them fall naturally out to the sides in a wide circle until they cross each other in front of the legs. At the same time, exhale and bend your knees and body accordingly. Let your eyes follow your right hand.

3. Repeat steps 1 and 2 six times—three times watching your right hand, three times watching your left hand.

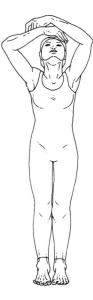

Figure 4-1

As you raise your heels, raise your arms above your head, keeping the palms facing upward.

4. After the last round of letting your hands fall down, deeply inhale and form your hands into fists and place them at your waist. (See Figure 4-2, page 431.) Slowly exhale and think of your lower abdomen (dantian).

5. Finally, lower your hands, palms down, and completely relax.

Points to remember

- Fully coordinate your breathing with your movements. Inhale while you raise your hands and body, exhale when you lower your hands and bend your body.

- Relax and think of dantian.

- Your eyes should follow your right hand three times and your left palm three times to create balance.

Waist Exercise

This section of exercises is aimed at strengthening the waist and kidneys, which are thought to hold the vital primordial qi energy, and are therefore essential for one's sexuality and immunity.

Preparation

Stand straight with your hands hanging naturally on both sides and looking straight ahead. Legs and feet should be together. Take three deep breaths and focus your mind on dantian while exhaling.

Performance

1. Slowly interlock the fingers of both hands in front of your abdomen, palms facing up, fingers straight, and elbows out. As you inhale, slowly raise them above the head as far as you can, turning the palms upward to face the sky. (See Figure 4-3.)

2. Exhale, bend forward at the waist and press both hands down, with fingers remaining interlocked and palms facing down, all the way to the ground in front of you.

3. Press both hands against the ground, first to your left, and then to your right. (See Figure 4-4, page 432.)

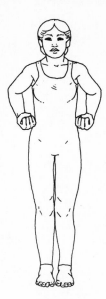

Figure 4-2
Deeply inhale and form your hands into fists.

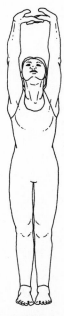

Figure 4-3
Raise your hands above you as you inhale.

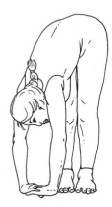

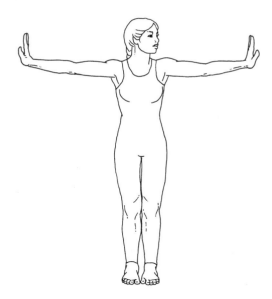

Figure 4-4

Try to press both hands against the ground.

Figure 4-5

Exhale deeply as you slowly let your arms fall down out to the sides.

4. Then firmly wrap both arms around your legs and press your head and upper body against your legs.

5. Slowly straighten and raise your hands, fingers interlocked and palms upwards, as far as you can above your head as in Figure 4-3, page 431.

6. Separate your hands and let them down slowly out to the sides, stopping at shoulder level, with hands bent at the wrist so the fingers are pointing upward. At the same time, exhale deeply and think of your lower abdomen. (See Figure 4-5.)

7. Lower your arms and form your hands into fists as you inhale and place them beside the waist, with the knuckles facing outward, until you reach the limit of inhalation.

8. As you exhale and send the breath down to dantian, relax both hands and let them fall naturally to the sides, fully relaxing.

Leg Exercise

Also known as the Shaolin leg exercise because Dharma once presided over the famous Shaolin Temple in central China, this exercise is aimed at strengthening your legs, preventing arthritis and rheumatism, and enhancing your flexibility, spirit, and work efficiency.

Preparation

Stand straight with both feet together and your hands in fists beside your waist. Your chest is out and you are looking forward. Take three deep breaths.

Performance

1. Advance your right foot and arm simultaneously, bending the right leg. Once you have fully stretched the right arm, turn the right fist into a hook. The left hand remains beside the waist in a fist, and the left leg remains straight while the right leg stays bent. (See Figure 4-6.)

2. Next, advance the left leg and the left arm simultaneously in exactly the same manner as the right arm and leg. At the same time, withdraw the right hand to the side in a fist. This time the right leg should be straight but the left leg bent.

3. Now put both fists at the waist and advance the right leg and kick it as high as you can in an attempt to fold your leg with your upper body. (See Figure 4-7.)

4. Let the right leg fall to the ground and make a 180-degree turn to the left (on

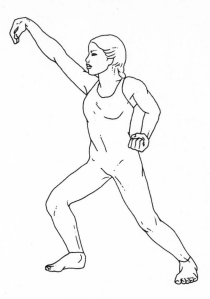

Figure 4-6
This is known as the bow step.

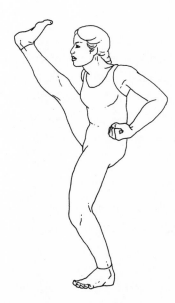

Figure 4-7
With your fists at your waist, kick your right leg as high as you can.

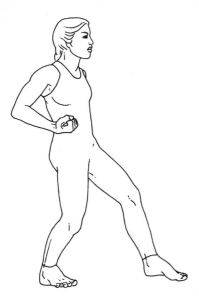

Figure 4-8
Turn 180 degrees to the left so that your right leg is now behind your left leg.

your heels) immediately after the right leg is down. Finish with the left leg half a step ahead of the right, with only the toes touching the ground, and all your weight on the right leg. (See Figure 4-8.) Both legs should be slightly bent.

5. Repeat steps 1 through 4 three times, starting with the left leg.

6. Inhale deeply with your hands in fists beside your waist. Then let them relax as you exhale, sending the breath down to your lower abdomen, relaxing.

Points to remember

- Try to keep your upper body as straight as possible while you kick upward.

- Coordinate your breathing with the movements, i.e., inhale while advancing the leg and kicking, exhale while withdrawing the leg and relaxing.

- Go slowly. It takes some training and practice before you can raise your leg straight and high. So be patient and progress gradually. With persistent practice you will eventually be able to raise your legs above your head, although this is not necessary for the mere sake of health. (It is highly desired, and actually required, in Shaolin martial arts.)

Spinning the Body

This section of exercises strengthens the kidneys, heart, and lungs, and also promotes the qi and blood circulation inside the body. Regular practice of it can help boost your sexual vitality, relieve sexual dysfunction, lumbago, and psoatic strain.

Preparation

Stand with your feet shoulder-width apart and your knees slightly bent. Position your hands in front of the chest, with the right palm facing downward and the left palm facing upward. The right hand should be directly above the left hand. This is called yin-yang hands in Chinese martial arts. Keep your body straight, eyes looking forward.

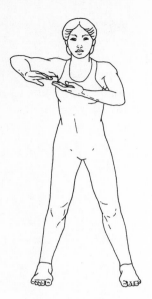

Figure 4-9
Begin rotating your hands counterclockwise, twisting at the waist.

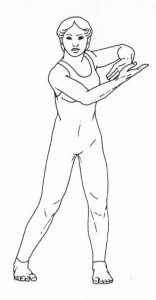

Figure 4-10
Halfway through the rotation, switch the positions of your palms.

Take three deep breaths before you start the movement.

Performance

1. Inhale, and begin rotating both hands counterclockwise, twisting at the waist. (See Figure 4-9.)

2. Half of the way around, switch the positions of your hands so that the right palm now faces upward and the left palm downward. (See Figure 4-10.)

3. Continue the rotation for a full semicircle in this hand position. Then, switch the positions of the hands again and continue whirling until back in the starting position.

4. Repeat these movements for one minute with the left hand facing down and the right hand facing up.

5. Slowly bring your feet together. While squatting down, cross your hands in front of the abdomen with palms facing upward (See Figure 4-11, page 436.)

6. Inhaling deeply, straighten while raising both hands out to the sides and above the head.

7. Push down the hands, palms down and fingers pointing together, while exhaling slowly. (See Figure 2-8, page 424.) Relax.

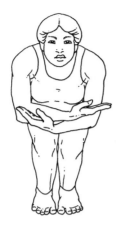

Figure 4-11
Squat down, crossing your hands in front of your abdomen.

Points to remember

- Combine the breathing with the movements. Breathe slowly and deeply, with your mind concentrated on dantian.

- While moving your body, keep your head as still as possible so that it looks as if your head were suspended from a rope during the whole process.

- Your eyes should look forward all the time, and your upper body should be as straight as possible.

Comprehensive Exercise

Preparation

Stand straight with your feet together and eyes looking straight ahead. Put your hands in fists beside the waist with the knuckles facing outward. Take three deep breaths, thinking of dantian while exhaling.

Performance

1. Open your hands and put them in front of your abdomen with the palms facing upward. (See Figure 4-12, page 437.)

2. Slowly raise both hands above the head, uncrossing them. Arms should be straight with the hands bent so the palms face up. Your eyes should follow the hand movement. At the same time, deeply inhale until you reach the end of inhalation. (See Figure 4-13, page 437.)

3. Exhale and lower your hands out to the sides in a semicircle, palms facing outward, and return to the starting position, with your palms in fists beside your waist.

4. Stretch the right arm straight out to the right, with the palm facing downward. (See Figure 4-14, page 437.) Then bring it back to a fist beside your waist.

5. Repeat step 4 with the left arm.

6. Stretch your right arm forward, with the fingers straight and palm up, until the arm is fully stretched and level with your chest. (See Figure 4-15, page 437.)

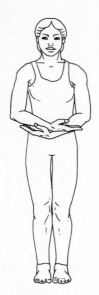

Figure 4-12

Cross your hands in front with the palms facing upward.

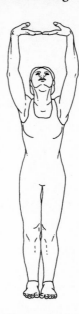

Figure 4-13

Deeply inhale as you raise both hands above your head, keeping the palms facing upward.

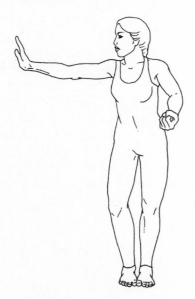

Figure 4-14

Stretch the right arm out to the right side.

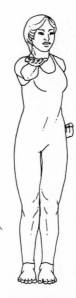

Figure 4-15

Stretch your right arm forward until it is fully extended and level with your chest.

7. Now "draw" a complete circle with the right arm: move downward first, then swinging to the back and up, until your arm falls forward and down to the tip of the right foot, fingertips touching the ground. (See Figure 4-16.) Bend from your waist as far as you can to help the hand reach the ground, exhaling, and keeping the legs straight. Your eyes should follow the movements of your right hand all the time.

8. Inhale and straighten, taking the right arm straight up over your head, and drawing a semicircle out to the right side, ending with both hands in fists beside the waist.

9. Repeat steps 6 through 8 with your left arm.

10. Inhale and interlock the fingers of both hands and raise them upward, with palms facing up until they reach the level of your chin.

11. Then rotate your palms 180 degrees and stretch them over your head, with the fingers still interlocked and your eyes following the movement of the hands. At the same time, deeply inhale and think of dantian.

12. Exhale slowly while pressing your palms against the ground, and bending your upper body as far as you can. Keep your legs straight.

13. Straighten your body and stretch your hands above your head with the fingers

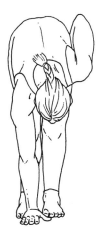

Figure 4-16
Complete the circle by bending forward, your fingertips touching the ground.

interlocked. At the same time, inhale deeply and look up at your palms.

14. Lower the hands gradually out to the sides making a semicircle. At the same time, slowly exhale with your mind concentrated on dantian.

15. Then put your hands in fists and place them beside your waist with the knuckles facing out. At the same time, inhale deeply.

16. Exhale and lower your hands. Relax completely to conclude the exercise.

Points to remember

- Fully coordinate all the movements with your breathing and your mind on dantian. Breathe slowly, naturally, and deeply.

- Keep the legs straight and together.

- Watch the movement of your hands all the time.

Turning the Windlass

Preparation

Stand straight with your feet together and fists at your waists. Look forward. Take three deep breaths, and focus on dantian.

Performance

1. Advance the right leg half a step forward, with the toes gently touching the ground and the left knee bent slightly. (See Figure 4-17.)

2. While inhaling, raise both fists to the sides so they are level with your ears. Elbows should be bent at right angles and your weight on the back leg.

3. As you exhale, advance the right leg in a forward lunge, forming a "horse step," keeping the left leg straight. At the same time, punch out both palms up in the air. (See Figure 4-18.)

4. Swing down to touch the ground, bending forward until your upper body touches your right knee. (See Figure 4-19, page 440.)

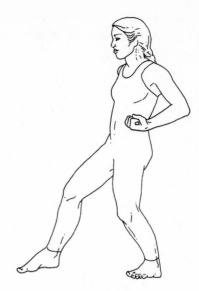

Figure 4-17
Bring your right leg forward, with the toes lightly touching the ground.

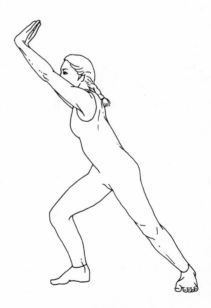

Figure 4-18
Exhale and lunge, creating the "horse step."

5. Inhale, come back up, and place your hands in fists beside your waist, while withdrawing the right leg half a step back to resume the ending position of step 1. (See Figure 4-17, page 439.)

6. Repeat the above movements three times.

7. Now alternate your leg position, advancing the left leg instead of the right leg in step 1. Then repeat steps 1 through 4 three more times.

Overall Recommendations

You do not have to do each and every exercise in the morning, although it is highly recommended that you do so. Actually, you can perform just two or three of your favorites in the morning everyday. The skill requirements and physique needed vary with each exercise, but they all achieve the same effects of improving health and preventing diseases.

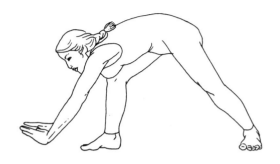

Figure 4-19
Swing down to the ground, bending at the waist.

Appendix 5

Dharma's Internal Exercises

This is a series of self-massage exercises that Dharma developed to promote health, immunity, self-healing, and longevity. It is Dharma's belief that the combined exercise of qigong and self-massage can promote qi and blood circulation in the body. This can enhance immune power, dispel the body of its wastes and toxins, prevent malign tumors from forming, boost sexual vitality, keep the various qi energies in the body well balanced, nurture the body cells and skin, keep one young and fit, and substantially prolong one's life.

Massage is an action that works directly on the skin. Since skin is closely associated with the internal organs and body system, massage indirectly affects the internal organs as well. As a direct and indirect result, the entire central nerve system is promoted, various organs receive nourishment, the immune system becomes strengthened, and diseases (especially chronic, degenerative diseases) are cured. Modern experiments and surveys have provided us with an abundance of clinical evidence pointing to the following physiological benefits of massage:[1]

- It promotes the circulation of the blood, significantly increasing the rate of blood flow and the oxygen capacity of the blood.

- It stimulates the nerve receptors, causing the blood vessels to dilate.

- It promotes the health of internal organs by stimulating the functioning of these organs and providing a greater supply of blood to these organs.

- It keeps the channels of qi energy open throughout the body, improving the nutrition supply to cells and enhancing the immune system.

- It soothes and relaxes contracted, shortened muscles, induces recovery from rigorous exercise and fatigue, and stimulates weak, flaccid muscles.

- It keeps the skin healthy by improving the function of sebaceous and sweat glands, which keep the skin lubricated, warm, smooth, and resilient.

- It expands the pores, and facilitates the excretion of skin fats, sweat, and toxins.

- It increases the body's metabolism rate, as shown by the increase in the excretion of nitrogen, sodium chloride, and inorganic phosphorus.

- It soothes and relaxes the nervous system, reducing stress and inducing sound sleep.

All of these therapeutic effects of massage are doubled when performing Dharma's Internal Exercises. In this series of exercises, massage works side by side with qigong, the Chinese breathing exercise. This is an ideal combination of natural healing. In such a situation, you possess control over both the breathing process and the tempo of the massage. Thus, self-massage is superior to other forms of massage in promoting health and healing disease. It is little wonder that people who start practicing Dharma's internal exercises on a regular basis early in life stay healthy and are never afflicted with illness or degenerative diseases.

Clinical observations in China show that daily practice of these exercises alone have been able to significantly relieve or completely cure severe diseases including cancer, heart diseases, hypertension, diabetes, insomnia, toothaches and tooth decay, tinnitus, myopia, depression, neurasthenia, kidney diseases, stomach ailments, liver problems, constipation, headaches, insomnia, stress and depression. Indeed, it is a drugless, natural therapy in the true sense of the term.

This series of exercises can be performed in a sitting or lying position, and are best performed in conjunction with breathing exercises. Generally speaking, a sitting position is better than a lying position. This is because qi energy flows more freely and smoothly than in a lying position. Its therapeutic effects are significantly enhanced if one can practice it in the nude. This is because when you are naked you act directly on the skin without anything being in your way. Consequently, the vessels and internal organs will receive greater and better therapeutic effects. In addition, the body exposes itself to the air directly in its naked form, which itself is a form of health exercise called "air bath." Believe it or not, clean air is a healer in itself. To achieve the best results of this series of exercises, therefore, you should apply your hand directly to your skin rather than through the clothing. Obviously, you need to ensure that the room is warm enough.

Certainly, there are times when a lying position is a more realistic alternative, such as when one is sick and cannot sit long enough to finish the exercises, or on an early winter morning when the room temperature is low, making one vulnerable to cold. In such situations, it is advised to practice this series of internal exercises in a lying position under the bed covers. However, clothes should be removed to enhance the therapeutic effect.

There is no limitation as to how often you can practice these exercises. In fact, the more frequently you practice them, the greater and faster will you receive the benefits and bring about healing. The therapeutic effects of these series of exercises are most manifest if its practitioner has already mastered the art of qigong.

Throughout the exercises, breathe slowly, deeply, and naturally, focusing your mind on the dantian area. Make sure that there is plenty of fresh air in the room. The rubbing movements should be done gently and rhythmically in time with your respiration.

The amount of force you should use during the exercises is completely up to you, and depends on your physique. If you are overweight and strong, you can exert more force when massaging. On the other hand, if you are weak and lean, less force should be used. The guiding principle is to use appropriate force until you can comfortably feel the effect of the massage penetrating the skin. In no case should you hurt yourself by using too much force. It is important to remember that you should not take a cold bath or shower right after practicing these exercises, indeed, right after practicing any exercise.

While desirable, it is not mandatory that you go through each and every exercise in this series each time you practice it. A more practical approach would be to repeat many times those exercises that bear more directly on your specific medical conditions. Thus, if you are afflicted with hypertension, repeat the exercise of massaging the head, scalp, and soles. If you suffer from sinusitis, you might repeatedly massage the bridge of your nose during each session. If you have an eye problem, you might rotate your eyes many times a day. If you have sexual dysfunction problems, you can just focus on the sections of massaging the neck, abdomen, waist, and soles, or clenching the teeth and shaking the "Heavenly Pillar." In any case, you should feel better after each practice.

To prepare for these exercises, sit on the floor or lie in bed, preferably nude or with your clothes loosened. Take several deep, natural breaths and concentrate on dantian.

Rub the Head and Face

Performance

1. Rub both hands against each other until they are warm.

2. Close your fingers together, and place your hands on your face, with your little fingers against the sides of your nose. (See Figure 5-1.)

3. Rub the entire head and face with both hands, around and around thirty-six times.

Therapeutic effects

This exercise can promote blood and qi circulation to the face, nourish the brain, keep your face smooth and youthful, improve memory and work efficiency, prevent and relieve premature aging, headaches, hair loss, the common cold and flu, stroke, Alzheimer's and Parkinson's diseases, and is especially effective in lowering blood pressure. According to traditional Chinese medicine, the head and face are of vital importance to your health and life because they are the natural meeting place for all kinds of yang energy, which should ascend rather than descend in the body. Massaging the head and face can greatly promote the yang energy to ascend, nourishing and promoting the blood circulation in that portion of the body, and restoring hair to the scalp.

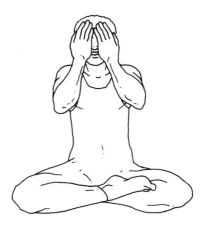

Figure 5-1
Place your warmed hands on your face and rub your entire head and face.

Rub the Bridge of the Nose

Performance

1. Rub the thumbs against each other first until they are warm.

2. Hold both hands in fists, fingers away from the face, with thumbs outstretched. Place your hands on your face and use the thumbs to rub the sides of your nose thirty-six times, in up and down movements. (See Figure 5-2, page 445.)

Therapeutic effects

This exercise can prevent and relieve nasal ailments such as sinusitis and runny nose, as well as prevent the common cold and flu. It can promote local blood circulation, enlarge

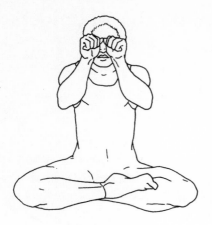

Figure 5-2
Rub the sides of your nose with your warmed thumbs.

the blood capillaries, raise the temperature of the nose tissues, and enhance our adaptability to external cold.

Rub the Neck

Performance

1. Rub both hands until they are warm.

2. Use the hands to rub the neck, rhythmically up and down thirty-six times. Adjust the strength to your comfort level.

Therapeutic effects

This can prevent and relieve the common cold, shoulder and neck pain, hypertension, and sexual dysfunction. The ancient Chinese believed that regularly rubbing the neck can improve your sexual vitality.

Rub the Scalp

Performance

1. Rub both hands until warm.

2. Using your palms, massage the scalp thirty-six times.

Therapeutic effects

This exercise can strengthen your mental power, improve your memory, prevent and relieve Alzheimer's and Parkinson's diseases, hair loss, and gray hair.

Beat the Heavenly Drum

Performance

1. Rub both hands until they are warm.

2. Cover the ears with your palms, with your fingers curled around the back of your head.

3. Press the index fingers on the middle fingers and suddenly slip down the index fingers to flick on the skull, making a drumming sound, hence the name. Do this thirty-six times. Breathe deeply and naturally. (See Figure 5-3, page 446.)

Therapeutic effects

This exercise can prevent and relieve headaches, ear ringing, Alzheimer's disease, Parkinson's disease, hearing loss, ear diseases, and improve memory.

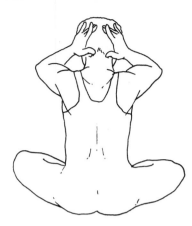

Figure 5-3
Use the index fingers to gently flick the skull, making a drumming sound.

Rub the Chest

Performance

1. Rub both hands until they are warm.

2. Use the right hand to rub the left half of your chest in circles. Repeat this thirty-six times. (One circular motion equals one time.)

3. Then use your left hand to rub the right half of your chest in exactly the same manner for another thirty-six times.

Therapeutic effects

This exercise can help prevent and relieve asthma, chest pain, pneumonia, lung cancer, breast cancer, and heart disease.

Rub the Abdomen

Performance

1. Rub your hands until they are warm.

2. Use your right hand to rub the entire abdomen in clockwise circles twenty times.

3. Alternate and use your left hand to rub the abdomen in exactly the same manner, but counterclockwise this time.

Therapeutic effects

This exercise is particularly beneficial to the stomach and digestive systems. It can prevent and relieve chronic diseases such as hypertension, neurasthenia, constipation, indigestion, gastric ulcer, kidney diseases, sexual dysfunction, stomach ailments and ulcers, stomach and colon cancer, and premenstrual syndrome in women. However, women should avoid practicing this section of exercise during menstruation.

Rub the Waist

Performance

1. Rub your hands until they are warm.

2. Use both hands to massage the back of the waist, up and down, for thirty-six times. Keep your upper body as straight as you can. (See Figure 5-4, page 447.)

Therapeutic effects

Rubbing the waist can greatly nourish the kidney qi energy, improving the overall

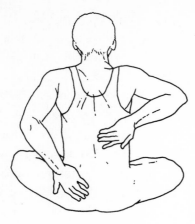

Figure 5-4
Massage the back of the waist in an up and down motion.

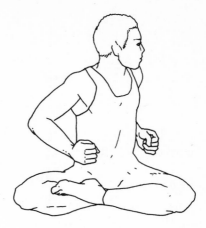

Figure 5-5
Quickly turn your upper body to the left, then right.

functioning of kidneys. It can prevent and relieve kidney ailments and lumbago. It is also very helpful for sexual dysfunction such as premature ejaculation, impotence, and nocturnal emission.

Shake the Heavenly Pillar

Performance

1. Put both hands in fists besides your waist, knuckles facing outward. The body should remain as erect as possible.

2. Turn your upper body and head to the left as fast as possible, eyes looking toward the back. (See Figure 5-5.)

3. Then, reverse the position and turn to the right as fast as possible.

4. Repeat these movements thirty-six times.

Therapeutic effects
This exercise can further enhance the effects of the previous exercise, massaging the waist.

Rub the Arms

Performance

1. Rub your hands until they are warm.

2. With the left hand resting naturally on the left knee, use the right hand to rub the left arm, up and down, from wrist to shoulder, eighteen times.

3. Alternate, using your left hand to rub your right arm in exactly the same manner for another eighteen times.

Therapeutic effects

This exercise can help the circulation of blood and qi energy, and prevent arthritis and rheumatism, as well as pain in the arms and shoulders.

Clench the Teeth

Performance

1. Just like it sounds, simply clench your teeth together as if you were biting or chewing food, keeping your mouth closed. Do this thirty-six times each day.

Therapeutic effects

The Chinese hold that the teeth are closely linked to the stomach, liver, and kidneys. Therefore, clenching the teeth can prevent and delay the decay and loss of teeth, prevent toothaches, and improve digestion and sexual vitality. It costs you nothing, and is considered far more healthier than having your teeth cleaned by a dentist.

Massage the Soles

Performance

1. Rub your hands until they are warm.

2. Turn the left sole upward and rub it with your right hand. Do this thirty-six times.

3. Then repeat on your right sole using your left hand. Do this thirty-six times.

Therapeutic effects

This simple exercise has magical therapeutic effects. It can release the fire in the liver and kidney, greatly improve your sexual vitality, and relieve conditions such as sexual dysfunction and impotence. This is because the ancient Chinese believed that the soles are connected with the kidneys and liver. By massaging the soles, you improve the functioning of the kidneys and liver. As a result, your eyesight strengthens, and your sexuality is enhanced. Also, massaging the sole can induce the blood to flow to that part of the body, relieving health problems such as high blood pressure, palpitation, kidney deficiency, and insomnia.

Rub the Legs

Performance

1. Rub both hands until they are warm.

2. Sit down with both legs fully stretched in front of you.

3. Place your warmed hands on your legs, rubbing all the way from the thigh to the ankle. Do this thirty-six times.

Therapeutic effects

This exercise can promote blood and qi circulation in the legs, strengthen the knees, and prevent and relieve conditions such as rheumatism and osteoporosis.

Rotate the Eyes

This movement serves as the rounding up exercise after you have gone through the previous exercises and are ready to finish. Of particular importance is to practice this shortly after you get up in the morning and right before you go to bed in the evening.

Performance

1. To perform, slowly open your eyes, and pause for a short while.

2. First, rotate your eyes seven times clockwise, and then seven times counterclockwise.

Therapeutic effects

This exercise can prevent and relieve various eye ailments such as cataracts and myopia. It can also improve your eyesight, relieve eye fatigue, and boost your spirits.

Bend the Body and Grasp the Toes

This is an optional exercise depending on which posture you adopt when practicing Dharma's internal exercises. If you adopt the single-lotus or full-lotus posture, then this section is highly recommended as a finishing exercise for a transition to other activities. If you are sitting on a chair while practicing the exercises, you can skip this exercise.

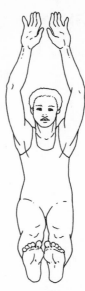

Figure 5-6
With your legs straight out in front and hands above the head, prepare to bend forward.

Performance

1. Sit upright with your legs straight out in front of you, forming a 90-degree angle.

2. Close your legs together and stretch them flat on the ground.

3. Raise both hands above the head with your eyes following the hands in preparation for the grasping of the toes. (See Figure 5-6.)

4. Bend your body forward as far as you can in an attempt to grasp the toes.

5. Once you get hold of the toes of both feet, release and bend your legs, pressing your chest against your legs.

Endnotes

1. Daifeng Gu, *Keep-Fit Massage* (Beijing, China: People's Physical Education Publications, 1962).

Appendix 6

Yijinjing

Yijinjing—limbering-up exercises for the tendons—is yet another invention of the great Dharma that is still widely practiced today in China as a means of keeping fit and curing diseases. Just as the Chinese name implies— yi (limber up or strengthen) plus jin (tendons) plus jing (methods)—this series of exercises is designed to strengthen flaccid and frail muscles and tendons. The movements contained in this series are at once vigorous and gentle, and their performance calls for a unity between mind and body, physical movement, and respiratory control, as is the case with Dharma's internal exercises.

There are altogether eight exercises in this routine. Begin each one by relaxing the body and mind, looking straight ahead, clenching the teeth together, closing the mouth with the tongue gently touching the upper palate to promote the accumulation of saliva in the mouth. Do not exert force; do not throw out the chest or raise the shoulders. Instead, slightly lower your shoulders, bend your knees and bring your chest inward. Breathe naturally, remain relaxed, and focus your mind on dantian exactly as in the qigong exercises.

Regular practice of yijinjing can not only strengthen your hands, but also positively improve your blood circulation and the functioning of internal organs, relieving conditions such as indigestion, lumbago, constipation, chest pain, arthritis, and rheumatism.

Clenching Fists

Starting position

Stand with your feet shoulder-width apart. Clench both fists with the knuckles facing down and the tips of both thumbs pressed lightly against the thighs. (See Figure 6-1.)

Performance

1. Inhale, keeping the fists clenched.

2. Exhale, clenching the fists more tightly than before.

3. Repeat this exercise eighteen times.

Pressing Palms Downward

Starting position

Stand with your feet shoulder-width apart. Press both palms downward with the fingers pointing out to the sides and the fingertips tilted slightly upward. (See Figure 6-2.)

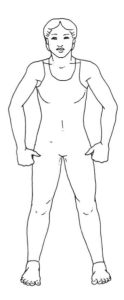

Figure 6-1
Clench your fists with the tips of the thumbs pressed against the thighs.

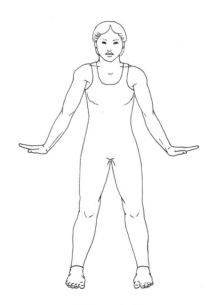

Figure 6-2
Press both palms downward, fingers tilted slightly upward.

Performance

1. Exhale, pressing the palms downward with inner strength, the whole body slightly vibrating and both knees slightly bent.

2. Inhale, keeping the body taut, and then exhale again, pressing the palms further downward with renewed strength and slightly raising the fingertips.

3. Repeat these movements eighteen times.

Holding Weight with Level Arms

Starting position

Stand with your feet shoulder-width apart. Raise both arms to the front, with the palms turned upward.

Performance

1. Inhale to distend the lower abdomen to its fullest.

2. Exhale, concentrating on the palms as if they were holding heavy weights. Each time you exhale, imagine that the weights have become slightly heavier, but maintaining the position of the palms.

3. Repeat these movements eighteen times.

Extending Palms Out

Starting position

Stand with your feet shoulder-width apart. Raise both arms to shoulder level, stretching out to the sides, hands bent with the palms facing outward. Press the fingers towards the head as much as possible.

Performance

1. Exhale, and extend the palms outward with strength as if pushing two enemies away, with the whole body vibrating slightly.

2. Inhale, holding on to this position.

3. Exert a bit more strength with each exhale as if the palms were extending further and further outward.

4. Repeat these movements eighteen rounds of breathing.

Propping Up the Sky

Starting position

Move the left foot a step to the left side and bend the left leg at the knee, keeping the right leg straight. The body remains erect. Raise the left hand with the palm facing upward, while the right hand hangs naturally on the side with the palm facing downward and the fingers touching the thigh. (See Figure 6-3, page 454.)

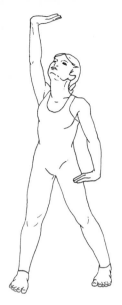

Figure 6-3
*Raise the left hand with the palm facing up-
ward, while the right faces downward.*

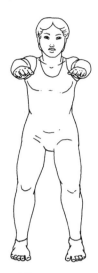

Figure 6-4
Turn the palms downward as you squat down.

Performance

1. Exhale, and extend both arms further
   apart as much as possible by using inner
   strength.

2. Inhale, holding on to the position.
   Thus, the upper arm keeps going higher
   and higher, and the lower arm lower
   and lower. You may feel a vibration in
   the body at this time. This is quite
   natural.

3. Repeat these movements eighteen times.
   Then reverse the starting position and
   repeat for another eighteen times.

Up and Down
With Arms

Starting position
Stand with feet shoulder-width apart.

Performance

1. Inhale and stretch the arms forward,
   raising them to shoulder level, with the
   arms bent slightly and palms facing
   upward.

2. Exhale and turn the palms downward
   while at the same time squatting down
   slowly, keeping the upper body straight.
   (See Figure 6-4.)

3. Straighten slowly, turning the palms up again to return to the position of step 1.

4. Repeat these movements eighteen times.

Bending and Straightening

Starting position

Stand with feet shoulder-width apart. Take three deep breaths.

Performance

1. Exhale and bend over slowly to an angle of 90 degrees, at the same time letting your hands hang down naturally. The palms should be facing inward and the fingertips pointing downward, touching the ground. Do not exert any force with the hands. (See Figure 6-5.)

2. Inhale when standing up to resume the starting position.

3. Repeat these movements eighteen times.

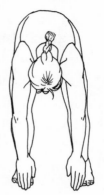

Figure 6-5
Let your hands hang down naturally.

Twisting the Body

Starting position

Stand erect, but feeling relaxed, with your feet shoulder-width apart.

Performance

1. Move the left foot a step to the left.

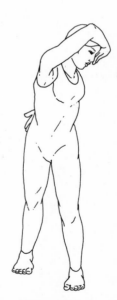

Figure 6-6
Twist to the left; your left hand on your back and your right arm arched over your head.

2. Twist the body to the left, placing the left hand on the lower back with the palm facing outward.

3. Bend the right arm to form an arch and place it over the forehead, with the palm facing outward, about a fist's distance away from the forehead. Look at your right heel which remains on the ground. (See Figure 6-6, page 455.)

4. Stretch the waist as the body twists to the left; when breathing out, imagine that the center of gravity is shifting to the right heel. Gradually twist the waist further with each round of breathing.

5. Repeat these movements for seven rounds of breathing.

6. Then turn to the right and repeat the above movements another seven times.

Appendix 7

Acupressure

Acupressure has been in use in China for thousands of years. It is one member of the family of Chinese massage, which contains five variations characterized by different styles of hand manipulation—pressing, pushing, rubbing, holding, and punching. Acupressure is by far the most commonly used variation of massage, because it is so convenient and effective. The unique nature of acupressure makes it accessible and affordable to virtually everybody. Its greatest beauty lies in its complete naturalness and simplicity. Moreover, it has no side effects, and is very effective in both preventing and healing diseases.

Even if one is healthy, one can regularly apply acupressure on certain points of the body to promote health and work efficiency. For instance, acupressure is now widely used in the field of sports to boost the competitiveness and performance of athletes. It can also prevent and relieve bodily damage caused during sports, and relieve fatigue after rigorous competition.

It is universally acknowledged that this natural health care method was first developed in China thousands of years ago. It is well documented that Qi Bo, the private doctor and medical advisor to the Yellow Emperor, had written ten volumes of books on massage and acupressure. More than two thousand years ago, a famous doctor in the early Han Dynasty (206 B.C.–220 A.D.), named Pian Que, successfully cured Prince Zhao of his night-blindness by means of acupressure. In the Tang dynasty (618–907 A.D.), the position of Doctor of Massage was formally created for the palace hospital. According to historical documents published at that time, there were fifty-six massage doctors and fifteen massage interns in the imperial hospital. It is around this time that a Japanese doctor came to China to learn massage and acupressure. Since that time, acupressure has been very popular in Japan.

Also known as "contact healing" or "digital massage," acupressure applies finger pressure on vital points of the body known as "acupoints." It accomplishes the same healing effects as acupuncture, which uses needles instead to effect a cure. Acupressure is based on exactly the same principles underlying the practice of acupuncture; indeed, they are like brothers and sisters of the same family. Both are widely used for circulating and replenishing qi energy and restoring the delicate balance between yin and yang forces inside the body. Acupressure's healing effects include promoting the preservation and circulation of vital qi energies, nourishing the cells and internal organs, restoring the dualistic balance between yin and yang, relaxing muscles, relieving body pains, boosting immunity, and balancing the hormonal functions in the body.

According to traditional Chinese theory, qi energy is the commander of blood, and blood is the basis of qi energy. Together, they nourish the body and mind, and fight against disease. As long as qi and blood are moving and flowing uninterrupted inside the body, one will enjoy normal biological functions and good health. However, once qi or blood is interrupted in their circulation, even if only locally, disease will occur.

The channels along which qi and blood move inside the body are called meridians and collaterals, which spread out through the entire body as a complex fabric, balancing yin and yang, linking the inner, outer, upper, and lower parts of the body, and constituting the body's great wall of natural defense. Qi energy moves to and fro, nourishing the body and fighting disease. The two main channels are the Functioning channel (Ren) and the Governing channel (Du). (See Figures 7-1 and 7-2 on page 459) Connected, they form a circular line around the body, which is referred to as the middle line, or midline.

There are literally hundreds of such vital points scattered throughout the body, between the bones and tendons. The acupoints along the Governing and Functioning channels as well as twelve regular meridians are called the classical points of the fourteen

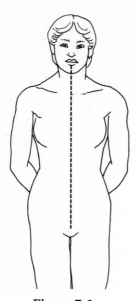

Figure 7-1
Functioning channel or Ren channel.

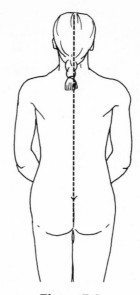

Figure 7-2
Governing channel or Du channel.

meridians. Each point has a designated name and location. The twelve meridians are the Heart Meridian, Lung Meridian, Kidney Meridian, Liver Meridian, Stomach Meridian, Spleen Meridian, Large Intestine Meridian, Small Intestine Meridian, Pericardium Meridian, Triple Energizer Meridian, Bladder Meridian, and Gallbladder Meridian.

Although invisible from a botanic perspective, meridians and collaterals certainly exist in every human body. They connect with the visceral organs internally and extend to the skin on the body surface, forming a crisscross network through which qi energy flows and circulates around the body,

to nourish the body and treat diseases. The ancient Chinese found that there are fourteen meridians or channels spreading out in the body, each with its own route and functions. Along the meridians and collaterals are located hundreds of acupoints, at which needles are inserted (acupuncture) or finger pressure (acupressure) is applied.

As the Chinese ancients see it, when disease attacks the body, it first comes in touch with the skin and the exposed parts of the body. From there it enters the body, reaches the meridians and collaterals, and finally invades the internal organs. If these channels of qi are open and the qi can move through them freely, a strong reinforcement of qi will rush to the point of attack and engage in battle with the disease. If our qi energy is strong enough, as is the case when we are healthy, the virus will be killed on the spot and the battle of health versus disease won without our knowing it. However, if some of these qi channels are blocked, the reinforcement for the body's defense against disease will be delayed when it is most needed, giving the disease a free hand and sufficient time to do its dirty job. In this sense, we can say that all diseases are the result of a blockage of qi in the meridians and collaterals.

Of course, disease can do its job the other way round, i.e., from the inside out. We have already discussed the relation between mind and body, emotional change, and physical health. The fact is that not only can external viruses attack the meridians and collaterals; our own emotions can also cause these qi channels to become blocked. For instance, when we are furious, we often find ourselves short of breath, or short of qi. Apparently, fury has blocked the smooth flow of qi energy inside our body. Also, if we are depressed or worried, our yang qi will become excessive and we will have yin disease as a consequence of this imbalance. Such yin diseases can be insomnia, premature aging, and hair loss.

Also, since the meridians and collaterals are connected and related to specific organs, blockage of certain channels will trigger diseases related to these organs. Thus, if qi energy in the Large Intestine Meridian is blocked, ailments such as toothaches, eyestrain, nasal bleeding, and neck pain will follow. Through the meridians and collaterals, dysfunction and pathological changes of internal organs are reflected at the body's surface. Therefore, disorders of the meridians and collaterals, either due to the impact of emotional factors (excessive joy, anger, melancholy, worry, sorrow, fear, and fright) or exogenous pathogenic factors (wind, cold, summer heat, damp, dryness, and fire), will lead to a blockage of the qi channels, interrupting the qi flow in the body, and eventually causing diseases.

It is essential that we keep these meridians and collaterals open to qi flow all the time. Otherwise, the balance between yin and yang will be disturbed, blood circulation interrupted, and various diseases can occur. In case the qi flow is blocked or hindered, as is reflected in various diseases, we can apply pressure to specific acupoints along the meridians and collaterals to remove the blockage, promoting the qi energy flow, and eventually bringing about a healing, a self-healing, of the disease. This is how acupressure works.

By accurately and delicately triggering or pressing on these acupoints with a finger, we can promote and facilitate the flow of qi energy, nourish the internal organs, remove the blockage in qi channels, enhance the body's immunity, reinforce what is deficient and reduce what is in excess, maintain and restore the yin-yang balance, and cure diseases. In particular, the following diseases lend themselves well to the treatment of acupressure: arthritis, asthma, bronchitis, polio, arthritis and rheumatism, chronic fatigue, trauma, common cold, constipation, diarrhea, headache, hemorrhage, indigestion, insomnia, impotence, hypertension, myopia, nausea, sinusitis, toothache, morning sickness during pregnancy, stroke, and various physical pains. Like the meridians and collaterals, acupoints are also related to internal organs. When an organ is ill, the corresponding acupoints become painful if touched.

So far, the meridians and collaterals along with the acupoints cannot be seen with the naked eye. The reason why they cannot be seen is because they are related to the living body only. Once the body is dead, the meridians and channels disappear, too. But for living people, their existence is undeniable. The fact that a tiny needle inserted at the right location can generate a sense of an electricity current itself is a powerful proof of their existence. They are not nerve distributions in the body, but the carriers and travel routes of qi energy.

As part of the basic training in acupressure treatment, you have to familiarize yourself with the acupoints. Acupoints are those points along the meridians and collaterals where qi energy concentrates. They are the sites where the qi energy and blood of the visceral organs reach the body surface.

Accurately locating the right acupoint is the first prerequisite for a successful application of acupressure. Anyone who wants to use this natural, economical tool of self-healing should, therefore, try to familiarize himself with the correct location of acupoints. This involves accurately locating each acupoint—exactly the same acupoints used in acupuncture—and knowing what their respective therapeutic effects and functions are.

Knowing and understanding these acupoints is no small task, but it is an effort worth taking. The good thing is that you do not need to learn them all. In fact, only about 100 of these points are commonly used for self-healing. Another good thing about acupressure is this: unlike acupuncture which requires accurate allocation of acupoints before a needle can be inserted into the body, acupressure does not have the same requirement of accuracy for it to be effective. Since the area affected by a touch of the finger is wider than that affected by a needle, accuracy in locating the acupoint is not as big an issue in acupressure as it is in acupuncture. In acupuncture, if a needle is not accurately inserted at an acupoint, bleeding usually ensues. By contrast, acupressure is totally devoid of bleeding—another blessing of this technique.

For your convenience, I have listed the name, location, and therapeutic effects of 120 acupoints in the following pages in alphabetic order. But first, you need to learn the three methods of how to locate the acupoints.

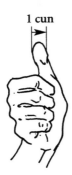

1 cun

Figure 7-3
One cun is equal to the width of your thumb.

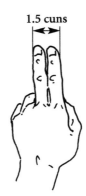

1.5 cuns

Figure 7-4
The width of your two middle fingers equals 1.5 cuns.

Locating Acupoints

By proportional unit of the body

Since the length and breadth of your fingers are in proportion to other parts of your body, the fingers can be used as units of measurement. If applying acupressure to another person, that person's fingers should be used instead. Typically, the width of the interphalangeal joint of the receiver's thumb is taken as one measurement unit, known as a "cun" in Chinese acupuncture. (See Figure 7-3.) The breadth of the middle segments of the index and middle fingers together is measured as 1.5 cuns (see Figure 7-4), and the breadth of the middle segments of the index, middle, ring, and little fingers together is measured as 3 cuns. (See Figure 7-5.)

By bone length

The location of an acupoint can be measured by the length of evenly divided portions of

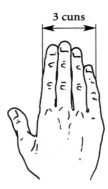

3 cuns

Figure 7-5
The width of all four fingers equals 3 cuns.

the body, no matter whether the patient is male or female, tall or short, obese or lean. Figure 7-6, page 463, shows several bone measurements. The distance from the anterior fold of the armpit to the transverse fold of the elbow is considered to be 9 cuns. The

By landmarks of the body surface

Acupoints can also be located with the aid of the natural landmarks, or features, of the body's surface. Thus, the acupoint Quchi is found in the elbow crease. The acupoint Danchong is at the midpoint between the two nipples. The acupoint Yintang is located at the midpoint between the inner ends of the two eyebrows, in the open space right above the nose bridge.

Once the acupoint is accurately located, you need to apply finger pressure to it. Thus, the second requirement of a successful acupressure session lies in the proper manipulation of the fingers. The correct manipulation of the fingers should be lasting, energetic, but at the same time even and gentle, so that the effect will penetrate to the meridians. "Lasting" means that the finger pressure should be continuous and uninterrupted for a period of time. "Energetic" means that the pressure should carry sufficient strength with it. "Even and gentle" means that the pressure should be rhythmic, caring, and free from violent and brutal force.

Theoretically, all ten fingers can be used for acupressure. In practice, it is the thumbs, index fingers, and middle fingers that are most often employed, possibly because for most people these are the stronger fingers. To be able to use your fingers in an effective way, you have to strengthen them through conscious training so that you can project inner force—delicate but penetrating force—via the fingertips. Fortunately for practitioners of natural healing methods, all the soft exercises

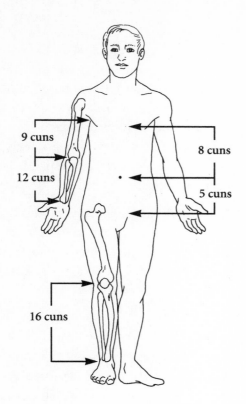

Figure 7-6
Using bone length to locate acupoints.

distance from the center of the sternum to the center of the navel is considered to be 8 cuns. The distance from the center of the umbilicus to the upper margin of the pubic bone is 5 cuns. The distance from the inferior border of the kneecap to the tip of the ankle bone is 16 cuns. The distance from the transverse fold of the elbow to the transverse fold of the wrist is 12 cuns.

introduced in this book have the additional benefit of strengthening the fingers. This is true of Dharma's morning exercises, mobile qigong, yijinjing, as well as taich'i. All these exercises require that the practitioner guide his or her force to the fingertips. It must be said that fingers so strengthened are best fitted for acupressure, because their force is gentle rather than violent, enduring rather than tempestuous, penetrating rather than superficial. Another way to train the fingers is to press them against hard objects, such as a table or wall, for ten to thirty minutes.

How To Perform Acupressure

Once you have learned how to locate the acupoints and have sufficient strength in your fingers, you are now ready to perform acupressure itself. You can use one of the following four methods to perform acupressure:

1. Carefully and accurately locate the relevant acupoints you want to press (two at the most). Press lightly with one finger at each acupoint. Gradually and firmly increase the pressure until you can feel the strength penetrating into the acupoint. Maneuver a bit around the acupoint with the finger as if kneading dough, never losing contact with the skin. Vary the force and speed up a little to fit the patient's individual conditions. Press steadily for three to five minutes until

you begin to feel a very faint sense, even pulse at the acupoint.

2. Exert pressure against the skin at a certain acupoint with a finger, and push the finger forward steadily, slowly and evenly with rhythmic movements. You can also pinch the acupoints by placing the thumb and index finger on it, gripping, twisting, and lifting the skin and muscles with the fingers.

3. You can rub the acupoints with your fingers or palms. To do that, place your finger on the acupoint and move it forward and backward in a series of movements until you can feel a sense of warmth or light electricity in it.

4. You can also tap the acupoints. Press your index finger against the thumb, and give quick, light blows on the acupoints. Exert strength from the wrist. The movement of the fingers should be steady, nimble, and flexible. Tap with both hands alternately, as if playing a drum.

List of Acupoints

The following is a list of the most commonly used acupoints and their locations and medical assessments, arranged in alphabetic order, according to their pronunciation in Mandarin Chinese. Refer to Figures 7-7 through 7-16 on pages 477–481 for illustrations showing their location.

1. Baihui
Located 1.5 cuns from the very top of the head to the back along the middle line. This acupoint is useful for treating headaches, dizziness, amnesia, common cold, cataract, dizziness, heat stroke, insomnia, hypertension, stroke, ear ringing, deafness, psychosis, hemorrhoids, neurasthenia, and declining memory.

2. Baixie (Yemen)
Located on the back of the hand between the small heads of the fourth and fifth palm bones, i.e., the bones connecting the fingers to the wrist. This is used to relieve headaches, toothaches, eyestrain, and throat pain.

3. Burong
Located on the abdomen, 6 cuns above the navel, 2 cuns beside the anterior median line, this acupoint is used to relieve stomachaches, vomiting, abdominal distention, and gastroptosia.

4. Changgu
Located on the abdomen about 2.5 cuns lateral to the center of the navel, this acupoint is used for treating acute and chronic enteritis, indigestion, and chronic fatigue syndrome.

5. Changqiang
Located below the tip of the coccyx, at the midpoint of the line connecting the tip of the coccyx and anus. This acupoint is used to treat hemorrhoids, prolapse of the rectum, bloody stools, dysentery, enuresis (bed wetting), mental disorder, and lumbar and spinal pains.

6. Chenfu
Located on the back of the thigh, in the center of the inferior gluteal crease, this acupoint is useful for treating insomnia, sexual dysfunction, and arthritis.

7. Chengjiang
Located in the depression of the chin right below the lower lip, this acupoint is used to prevent and relieve hemiplegia, diabetes, toothaches, headaches, stroke, indigestion, and facial swelling.

8. Chengshan
Located in the depression between the two heads of the stomach muscle. This acupoint is used to relieve piles, prolapse of the anus, constipation, hemorrhoids, lumbago, back pain, stiff neck, and sciatica.

9. Chuanzhu
There are two of these acupoints. One is located at the end of each eyebrow. They are useful for treating myopia and eyestrain.

10. Daheng
Located 4 cuns lateral to the navel. This acupoint is used to relieve abdominal pain, diarrhea, and constipation.

11. Daling
Located in the middle of the crosswise line of the wrist, between the tendons of the major and minor muscles which bend the wrist. This acupoint is used to relieve chest pain, eyestrain, headaches, shortness of breath, stroke, heat stroke, laryngitis, stomachache, vomiting, and heartburn.

12. Danzhong

Located in the middle of the chest between the two nipples. This point is used to relieve asthma, severe chest pain, heart disease, and heartburn.

13. Dazhui

Located 1 cun directly below the neck along the middle line of the back. This acupoint is used to relieve asthma, coughing, and chronic fatigue syndrome.

14. Diji

Located on the posterior border of the tibia and 3 cuns below the middle of the tibia. This acupoint is used to relieve leukopenia, menstrual pain and dysfunction, abdominal distention, and edema.

15. Earlobe

Pressing the earlobe can relieve impaired hearing and toothaches, boost sexual vitality, and improve sexual performance.

16. Erbai

Located 4 cuns above the transverse crease of the wrist, on the anterior aspect of the forearm. This acupoint is used to relieve hemorrhoids and proctitis (rectum inflammation).

17. Fengchi

Located at the base of the skull, in the depression below the skull and behind the ear. This acupoint is used to prevent and relieve the common cold, headaches, stiff neck, impaired hearing, asthma, sinusitis, hypertension, toothaches, eyestrain, night blindness, dizziness, and even Alzheimer's and Parkinson's diseases.

18. Fengfu

Located on the middle line of the back of the neck, in the depression just below the occipital protuberance and 1 cun above the hairline. This acupoint is used for relieving the common cold, stiff neck, shoulder pain, headaches, dizziness, nasal blockage, deaf-mutism, stroke, and hemiplegia.

19. Fenglong

Located at the middle of the outer side of the lower leg. This acupoint is used for relieving asthma, common cold, stroke, dizziness, insomnia, and phlegm.

20. Fengmen

Located 1.5 cuns lateral to the midpoint between the second and third thoracic vertebrae. This acupoint is useful for improving sexual performance, treating sexual dysfunction, impotence, stroke, common cold, asthma, and bronchitis.

21. Fengshi

Located on the outside of the thigh, 7 cuns above the inferior border of the patella. It is used for treating muscle pain, arthritis, hypertension, and stroke.

22. Ganshu

Located 1.5 cuns lateral to the midpoint between the ninth and tenth chest bones. It is used in the treatment of hepatitis, leukopenia, amenorrhea, and myopia.

23. Geshu

Located 1.5 cuns lateral to the midpoint between the spinous process of the seventh and eighth thoracic vertebrae. It is used for treating leukopenia, amenorrhea, and myopia.

24. Gongsun

Located on the bottom of the foot, 6 cuns above the end of the big toe, on the interior border of the foot. This acupoint is used for treating diabetes, incontinence, jaundice, and prostate ailments.

25. Guanyuan

Located 3 cuns below the umbilicus. This acupoint is used to relieve gastroptosis, prostatitis, impotence, nocturnal emission, premature ejaculation, incontinence, frequent urination due to deficiency in kidney qi energy, difficulty in urination, diarrhea, stroke, neurasthenia, hypertension, abdominal pain after delivery, uterus bleeding, morbid leucorrhea, and menstrual pain and dysfunction.

26. Guanzhong

This is one of the most obvious acupoints, commonly known as the naval. It is used in treating impotence and incontinence.

27. Guilai

Located on the lower abdomen, 4 cuns below the navel and 2 cuns from the midline. This acupoint is used to relieve hernia, abdominal pain, impotence, amenorrhea, leucorrhea, and irregular menstrual cycle.

28. Hegu

Located between the thumb and forefinger on the back of the palm. This acupoint is used to relieve asthma, bronchitis, common cold, cough, dispel phlegm, headaches, loss of hearing, heat stroke, hypertension, stroke, diarrhea, diabetes, eyestrain, hysteria, sore throat, rheumatism, difficulty in urination, painful menstruation, amenorrhea, sinusitis, nasal bleeding, jaundice, toothaches, and lactation problems.

29. Houding

Located 1.5 cuns behind Baihui along the midline of the head. This acupoint is used to relieve headaches, migraines, and dizziness.

30. Huiyin

Located in the middle of the perineum at the midpoint joining the anus and the genitals in females. This acupoint relieves menstrual syndrome, nocturnal emission, constipation, difficulty in urination, piles, anal fistula, metroptosis, and feminine itching.

31. Huagai

Located in the middle chest line at the interval between the first and second ribs. This acupoint is used to treat asthma, heartburn, and throat pain.

32. Hukou

This acupoint is located in the depression on the back of the hand between the thumb and the forefinger. It is useful for treating headaches, dizziness, insomnia, hypertension, bladder ailments, night sweating, toothaches, and heartburn.

33. Jiache
Located 1 cun lateral to the front of the jawbone. It is used in relieving toothaches.

34. Jianjing
Located at the highest point of the shoulder muscle midway between the outer tip of the shoulder and the spine, joining the spinous process of the seventh thoracic vertebra and the acromion. This point is used for treating myopia, relieving stress and painful shoulders, and is highly recommended for AIDS patients.

35. Jianyu
Located in the depression anterior to the end of the shoulder when the arm is straightened. It is used in treating all kinds of shoulder pains.

36. Jingming
Located in the depression on the inner end of the eye. It is useful for preventing and treating myopia, dizziness, eyestrain, and night blindness.

37. Jiuwei
Located in the upper abdomen, 1 cun below the junction of the chest and xiphoid. This acupoint is used for relieving asthma, vomiting, coughing blood, pain in the throat, heartburn, stomachaches, and palpitation.

38. Jujiao
Located outside the "groove" between the nose and upper lip, below the wings of the nose and directly in line with the pupils. This acupoint is used to relieve facial spasms, sinusitis, myopia, nose bleeds, common cold and ailments related to the common cold.

39. Juque
Located along the middle line of the chest, 8 cuns directly above the navel. This acupoint is used for treating heartburn, heart disease, vomiting, jaundice, abdominal distention, diarrhea, gastroenteritis, and sexual dysfunction such as impotence and premature ejaculation.

40. Kunlun
Located 3 cuns above the protruding angle of the anklebone. It is used for ankle sprains, heel pain, and arthritis.

41. Kongzui
Located 7 cuns above the wrist on the anterior aspect of the forearm, at the depression between the two radius bones of the forearm. This acupoint is useful in the treatment of asthma, coughing, expectorating blood, and arm pain.

42. Laogong
Located in the center of the palm at its depression. This acupoint is used in treating diabetes, stroke, jaundice, and toothaches.

43. Lianquan
Located on the neck above the Adam's apple, in the depression at the edge of the thyroid. This acupoint is used to relieve asthma, diabetes, deaf-mutism, cough, and a swollen tongue.

44. Lieque

Located 1.5 cuns above the transverse crease of the wrist, on the anterior aspect of the forearm. This acupoint is used for relieving headaches, migraines, asthma, toothaches, throat pain, cough, sinusitis, stroke, hiccups, fatigue syndrome, and hemiplegia.

45. Longmen

Located at the external orifice of the vagina. This acupoint is used for treating menstrual syndrome, female infertility, and incontinence. (Not shown.)

46. Meichong

Located on the head, 0.5 cun above the hairline, and 0.5 cun lateral to the midline. This acupoint is used to relieve headaches, nasal congestion, epilepsy, sinusitis, dizziness, and eyestrain.

47. Mingmen

Located along the middle line on the back at the midpoint between the kidneys. This acupoint is used for improving sexual performance, treating nocturnal emission, incontinence, impotence, ear ringing, piles, menstrual dysfunction, morbid leucorrhoea, and neurasthenia.

48. Muchuang

Located 1.5 cuns lateral to the midline, on the top of the head. This acupoint is used to relieve headaches, dizziness, edema of the head and face, red eyes, eyestrain, and epilepsy.

49. Neiguan

Located on the forearm, 2 cuns directly above the midpoint of the wrist crease. This acupoint is used to relieve headaches, cough, severe chest pain, diabetes, heart disease, heartburn, vomiting, hiccups, neurasthenia, bronchitis, hysteria, dizziness, stomachaches, abdominal distension, hemorrhoids, indigestion, jaundice, gastrointestinal ailments, diabetes, stroke, nocturnal emission, diarrhea, and menopausal syndrome.

50. Nose-tip

The location of this acupoint is self-explanatory. It is used for treating hypertension and toothaches.

51. Nuxi

Located at the boundary of the foot on the middle line of the heel, right above the heel. This acupoint is used to relieve vomiting, diarrhea, psychosis, toothaches, and gum disease.

52. Pishu

This acupoint is located 1.5 cuns lateral to the midpoint between the spinous processes of the eleventh and twelfth thoracic vertebrae. It is used for treating leukopenia (abnormally low white cell count).

53. Qianding

Located at the very peak of the head along the middle line of the Governing channel. This acupoint is useful for treating headaches, insomnia, and dizziness.

54. Qichong

Located 5 cuns below the navel and 2 cuns outside the anterior median line near the groin. The acupoint is used to relieve and cure vaginal discharge, menstrual syndrome, urine leakage.

55. Qihai

This acupoint is located 1.5 cuns below the navel. Pressing it can relieve gastroptosis, gastrointestinal neurosis, difficulty in urination, constipation, nocturnal emission, impotence, stroke, chronic fatigue, incontinence, hypertension, insomnia, hearing loss, sexual dysfunction, abdominal pain after delivery, indigestion, and menstrual dysfunction.

56. Qimen

Located 3 cuns below the navel, and 3 cuns sideways from the middle line of the upper body. This acupoint is used for treating postpartum abdominal pain, uterus bleeding, excessive bleeding, irregular periods, female infertility, and urinary troubles.

57. Qixue

Located 3 cuns below the navel, and 0.5 cun beside the middle line of the upper body. This acupoint is used for relieving premenstrual syndrome, vaginal discharge, female infertility, and diarrhea.

58. Quchi

Located in the depression at the lateral end of the elbow crease as the elbow is flexed. This acupoint is often used for the prevention and treatment of asthma, rheumatism, common cold, diabetes, vomiting, hypertension, irregular menstruation, impaired hearing, stroke, dizziness, diarrhea, breast cancer, and lack of milk during nursing.

59. Quanmen

Located in the female's lower margin of the pubic bone and the superior border of the front of the labia. This acupoint is used to treat female infertility, menstrual ailments, and abnormal vaginal discharge.

60. Quepen

Located at the center of the depression of the clavicle, 4 cuns lateral to the anterior middle line. This acupoint is used for treating hiccups and heartburn.

61. Renzhong

Located midway between the nose-tip and the upper lip. It is used in treating diabetes, stroke, heat stroke, uterus bleeding, shock and dizziness, hysteria, toothaches, fainting after delivery, and chronic fatigue syndrome.

62. Ruzhong

Located at the midpoint between the two nipples. It is considered the Gate of Life for women, equivalent to the midpoint between the kidneys for men. Pressing this acupoint can nourish female qi energy, promote female sexual drive, and relieve menstrual dysfunction and menopausal syndrome, as well as rheumatism.

63. Sanyinjiao

Located 3 cuns above the tip of the ankle bone, just posterior to the tibia. This acupoint is used to nourish the kidney energy and help relieve diabetes, leukopenia, kidney diseases, chronic fatigue syndrome, neurasthenia, headaches, insomnia, dizziness, prostatitis, difficulty in urination, incontinence, impotence, seminal emission, premature ejaculation, amenorrhea, menstrual disorders and pain, excessive leucorrhea, indigestion, menopausal syndrome, lactation problems, and neurasthenia.

64. Saoshang

Located on the ulnar side of the thumbnail, right below the thumbnail corner. This acupoint is used to relieve influenza, acute tonsillitis, and high fever.

65. Shangjuxu

Located 6 cuns below the lateral aspect of the knee. It is used for treating constipation, and indigestion.

66. Shangwan

Located on the Functioning channel, 5 cuns above the navel. This acupoint is used for relieving vomiting, indigestion, stomachache, hiccups, diarrhea, and jaundice.

67. Shangxing

Located on the midline of the head about 1 cun into the hairline on the forehead. This is used to prevent and relieve headaches, eyestrain, myopia, nasal bleeding, sinusitis, and Alzheimer's and Parkinson's diseases.

68. Shaohai

Located on the inner bone of the forearm at the end of the elbow lines as the elbow is flexed. This acupoint is used in treating stress, depression, toothaches, dizziness, nasal congestion, and neurosis.

69. Shenmen

Located just above the end of the wrist crease on the side of the inner bone of the forearm. This is used to relieve hypertension, heart disease, indigestion, lack of appetite, chronic fatigue syndrome, asthma, spitting blood, insomnia, and neurasthenia syndrome.

70. Shenshu

Located 1.5 cuns lateral to the midpoint between the second and third lumbar vertebrae. This acupoint is used for improving eyesight, treating night blindness, difficulty in urination, impotence, seminal emission, premature ejaculation, rheumatism, amenorrhea, indigestion, and impaired hearing.

71. Shimen

Located 2 cuns below the navel. This acupoint is used to relieve acute pain in the abdomen, abdominal distention, difficulty in urination, indigestion, and gonorrhea.

72. Shousanli

Located 2 cuns below the depression at the side of the elbow crease as the elbow is flexed. This acupoint is used for relieving painful arms and elbows, muscle pain, lumbar and abdominal pain, stroke, loss of voice, and toothaches.

73. Shouwuli

Located 3 cuns above the acupoint of Quchi on the lateral side of the upper arm. This acupoint is used for relieving paralysis in the upper arm, arthritis, rheumatism, scrofula (form of tuberculosis), and pain in the arm and elbow.

74. Shuidao

Located on the lower abdomen, 3 cuns inferior to the navel and 2 cuns lateral to the anterior midline. This acupoint is used for treating difficulty in urination, irregular periods, urinary tract infection, menstrual pain, infertility, and abdominal pain.

75. Shuitu

Located at the front side of the neck on the border of the thyroid and the margin of the bone at the opening for the ear. This acupoint is used to relieve sore throat, asthma, goiter, bronchitis, hoarseness, and loss of voice.

76. Sibai

Located on the face immediately below the pupil at the depression under the eye. This acupoint is used to treat red or painful eyes, headaches, dizziness, facial nerve paralysis, and myopia.

77. Taichong

Located on the dorsum of the foot in the depression 2 cuns proximal to the articulation of the first and second toes. This acupoint is used for treating headaches, colds, fatigue, hiccups, insomnia, neurasthenia, menstrual syndrome, hepatitis, menopause, hypertension, gastrointestinal neurosis, and hysteria.

78. Taixi

Located at the midpoint between the central ankle bone and Achilles tendon. It is used to relieve toothaches, asthma, coughing, diarrhea, diabetes, kidney diseases, and menstrual dysfunction.

79. Taiyang

Located in the depression 1 cun superio-lateral to the outer corner of the eye. This acupoint is used to prevent and relieve the common cold, headaches, hypertension, eyestrain, insomnia, sinusitis, neurasthenia, and Alzheimer's and Parkinson's diseases. Regularly pressing it can prevent disease and is conducive to longevity.

80. Taiyi

Located 2 cuns above the navel. This acupoint is useful for relieving stomachaches, abdominal flatulence, indigestion, acute and chronic gastritis, depression, and mania.

81. Taiyuan

Located at the arterial pulse close to the line of the wrist. This acupoint is used for relieving the common cold, asthma, coughing, heartburn, deaf-mutism, amenorrhea, hemoptysis, and sore throat.

82. Tianshu

Located 2 cuns lateral to the navel. This acupoint is used in treating gastrointestinal neurosis, constipation, neurasthenia, diarrhea, vomiting, menstrual dysfunction, indigestion, and stomachaches.

83. Tiantu

Located at the central depression at the bottom of the throat, bordering on the uppermost chest bone. This is used for relieving asthma, cough, coughing blood, esophagitis, cancer of the esophagus, vomiting, jaundice, acute gastroenteritis, and deaf-mutism.

84. Tianyou

Located at the depression 3 cuns below each ear. This acupoint can relieve toothaches and improving sexual performance.

85. Tianzhong

Located on the back of the shoulder, 1.5 cuns lateral to the spine, and 4 cuns below the top of the shoulder. This is used in treating hiccups, stiff neck, and shoulder pain.

86. Tinggong

Located in the depression anterior to the tragus and posterior to the condylar process of the mandible. This acupoint is used for treating ear ringing and impaired hearing.

87. Tonggu

Located 2 cuns below the breast. This acupoint is used to treat cardiac pain, heartburn, mastitis, and intercostal neuralgia.

88. Tongli

Located 1 cun above the transverse crease of the wrist, on the anterior aspect of the forearm, on the interior side. This is used to relieve all kinds of heart disease, heartburn, headaches, dizziness, palpitation, aphasia, incontinence, insomnia, and menorrhagia.

89. Waiguan

Located on the lateral side of the forearm, 2 cuns above the transverse crease of the wrist, and between the ulnar and radius. This acupoint is used for relieving asthma, common cold, headaches, toothaches, sore throat, cough, heat stroke, tinnitus, deaf-mutism, flu, pneumonia, and arthritis.

90. Wailaogong

Located at the center of the dorsum of the hand. This acupoint is used for treating the inability of fingers to stretch, numbness in the fingers or palms, indigestion, abdominal pain, diarrhea, and neck rigidity.

91. Weizhong

Located on the posterior aspect of the knee, at the center of the popliteal skin crease. It is used for the treatment of incontinence, prostate ailments, lumbago, stomachaches, and headaches.

92. Xiaguan

Located in the depression between the mandibular notch and the inferior border of the zygotic arch. It is used for relieving toothaches and rheumatism.

93. Xialian

Located on the radial aspect of the forearm, 4 cuns under the cross striation of the elbow. This acupoint is used to relieve headaches, abdominal pain, indigestion, and stool bleeding.

94. Xiawan

Located at a point 3 cuns beneath the navel. This acupoint is used to treat indigestion, stomachaches, abdomen pain and distention, and vomiting.

95. Ximen

Located on the anterior aspect of the forearm, 5 cuns superior to the wrist crease and between the two soft bones. This acupoint is used to relieve chest pain, spitting up blood, nosebleeds, heart disease, and neurasthenia.

96. Xinjian

Located at the soft spot between the first and second toes. This acupoint is useful for relieving toothaches, especially the upper rank toothache, dizziness, eyestrain, insomnia, stroke, and menstrual dysfunction.

97. Xinshu

Located 1.5 cuns lateral to the midpoint between the spinous processes of the fifth and sixth thoracic vertebrae. Pressing it can relieve severe chest pain and treat myopia.

98. Xuanji

Located on the central line of the sternum, paralleling the first joint of chest and elbow, 1 cun beneath the acupoint of Tiantu. This acupoint is used to relieve heartburn, asthma, cough, sore throat, and indigestion.

99. Xuehai

Located at the central side of the thigh, 2 cuns above the upper border of the knee cap. This acupoint is used for treating leukopenia, menstrual disorder, uterus bleeding, amenorrhea, distention, and urticaria.

100. Yangchi

Located on the radial depression on the wrist crease. It is used for relieving asthma, coughing, gastralgia, and abdominal pain.

101. Yaoyangguan

Located along the middle line of the upper back, at 2 cuns below the acupoint of Mingmen. This acupoint is used for boosting sexual performance, treating nocturnal emission, impotence, leucorrhea, lumbago, and rheumatism.

102. Yifeng

Located in the depression right behind the earlobe. This acupoint is used for relieving dizziness, sore throat, ear ringing, and impaired hearing.

103. Yingxiang

Located at the depression right next to the nose wing. It is used for treating sinusitis, nasal bleeding, the common cold, and strokes, and has the effect of prolonging one's life and prevent disease.

104. Yinjiao

Located 1 cun below the navel. This acupoint is used to treat menstrual disorders, uterine bleeding, morbid leucorrhoea, and abdominal distention.

105. Yinlingquan

Located in the depression on the medial aspect of the knee, below the medial condyle of the tibia. This acupoint is useful in relieving prostatitis, difficulty in urination, impotence, menstrual dysfunction, stomachaches, rheumatism, and excessive leucorrhea.

106. Yintang

Located at the midpoint between the inner ends of the eyebrows, in the open space right above the nose. This acupoint is used to relieve headaches, common colds, flu, sinusitis, hypertension, dizziness, faintness after delivery of a baby, and neurasthenia.

107. Yongquan

Located at the center of the sole in the depression. This acupoint is used to nourish the kidney qi energy, enhance sexual vitality, prolong life, and help relieve hypertension, hysteria, stroke, stress, and difficulty in urination.

108. Youmen

Located on the upper abdomen, 6 cuns above the navel, and 0.5 cun off the midline. This acupoint is used to treat vomiting, stomachaches, diarrhea, and dysentery.

109. Yuji

Located on the border of the front palm and 1.5 cuns above the thumb toward the wrist. This acupoint is used for treating fever, cough, breast cancer, and pain in the throat due to swelling.

110. Yutang

Located on the chest at the midline depression between the third and fourth ribs of the chest. This acupoint is used for relieving asthma, vomiting with cold phlegm, chest pain, lung and heart diseases.

111. Yuwei

Located at the end of the transverse crease of the eye. This acupoint is used to relieve headaches, dizziness, eye diseases, migraine, and gum disease.

112. Zhigou

Located on the dorsal aspect of the forearm, 3 cuns above the wrist crease between the radius and ulna. It is used for treating constipation and indigestion.

113. Zhishi

Located 3 cuns lateral to the midpoint between the spinous processes of the second and the third lumbar vertebrae. This acupoint is used for treating nephritis, nocturnal emission, indigestion, prostate disease, impotence, pain in the penis, and diarrhea.

114. Zhongdu

Located in the center of the inner side of the tibia (larger of the two bones of the leg, below the knee), 7 cuns above the center of the ankle bone. This acupoint is used to relieve menstrual disorders, excessive menstruation, abdominal pain, and loss of sensation in the lower part of the foot.

115. Zhongfu

Located on the outer side of the thorax, 6 cuns from the anterior median line. This acupoint is used to relieve asthma, cough, heartburn, pneumonia, and tuberculosis.

116. Zhongji

Located about 4 cuns below the navel on the midline. This acupoint is used for treating prostatitis, urinary retention, nuresis, urinary infection, nocturnal emission, menstrual dysfunction and pain, frequent urination, uterus bleeding, morbid leucorrhoea, incontinence, and impotence.

117. Zhongwan

Located 4 cuns superior to the umbilicus. This acupoint is useful for relieving headaches, gastroptosis, stomachaches, indigestion, gastrointestinal neurosis, diarrhea, vomiting, hypertension, premenstrual syndrome, insomnia, jaundice, constipation, and asthma.

118. Zhongzhu

Located on the lower abdomen, 0.5 cun lateral to the anterior median line and 1 cun below the navel. This acupoint is useful for relieving menstrual disorder, diarrhea, constipation, and abdominal pain.

119. Zigong

Located on the Functioning channel on the chest, at the space between the second and third ribs. This acupoint is used for relieving heartburn, asthma, breast pain, indigestion, and vomiting.

120. Zusanli

Located 3 cuns below the lateral aspect of the knee and one finger's breadth lateral to the tibia crest. Pressing or massaging this point can nourish the vital kidney energy and help relieve headaches, asthma, hypertension, hepatitis, gastroptosis, gastrointestinal neurosis, stomachaches, vomiting, diabetes, jaundice, leukopenia, indigestion, chronic fatigue syndrome, rheumatism, neurasthenia, impaired hearing, deaf-mutism, stroke, dizziness, seminal emission, incontinence, diarrhea, constipation, amenorrhea, premenstrual syndrome, abdominal pain after delivery, and lactation problems. Regular acupressure of this point can also strengthen the immune system, prevent the common cold, and prolong life.

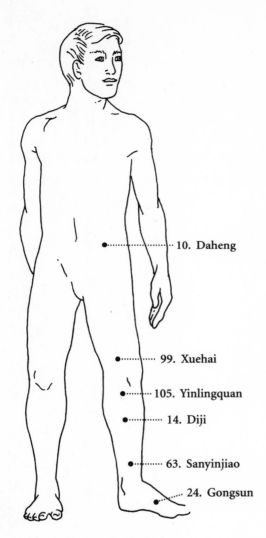

Figure 7-7
Acupoints along the Spleen Meridian.

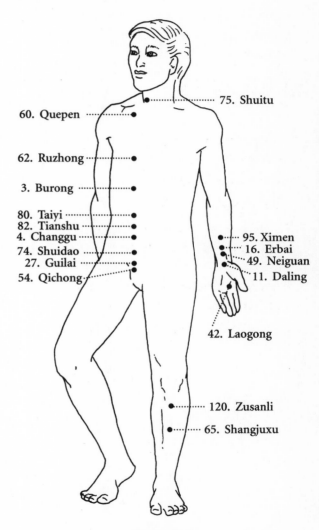

Figure 7-8
*Acupoints along the Pericardium Meridian
and the Stomach Meridian.*

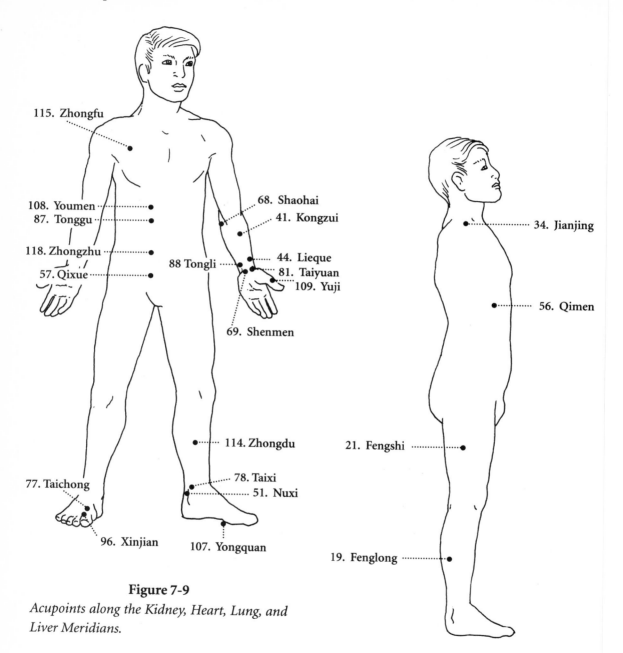

115. Zhongfu

108. Youmen
87. Tonggu

118. Zhongzhu
57. Qixue

68. Shaohai
41. Kongzui

88 Tongli

44. Lieque
81. Taiyuan
109. Yuji

69. Shenmen

114. Zhongdu

78. Taixi
51. Nuxi

77. Taichong

96. Xinjian
107. Yongquan

Figure 7-9

Acupoints along the Kidney, Heart, Lung, and Liver Meridians.

34. Jianjing

56. Qimen

21. Fengshi

19. Fenglong

Figure 7-10

Acupoints on the side of the body.

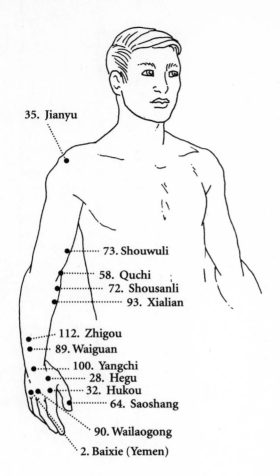

Figure 7-11
Acupoints located on the Liver Meridian and the Lung Meridian.

35. Jianyu

73. Shouwuli
58. Quchi
72. Shousanli
93. Xialian
112. Zhigou
89. Waiguan
100. Yangchi
28. Hegu
32. Hukou
64. Saoshang
90. Wailaogong
2. Baixie (Yemen)

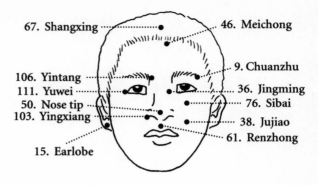

67. Shangxing
46. Meichong
106. Yintang
111. Yuwei
50. Nose tip
103. Yingxiang
9. Chuanzhu
36. Jingming
76. Sibai
38. Jujiao
61. Renzhong
15. Earlobe

Figure 7-12
Closeup of the acupoints located on the face and head.

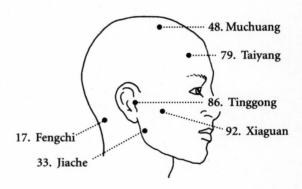

48. Muchuang
79. Taiyang
86. Tinggong
92. Xiaguan
17. Fengchi
33. Jiache

Figure 7-13
Closeup of the acupoints located on the side of the face and head.

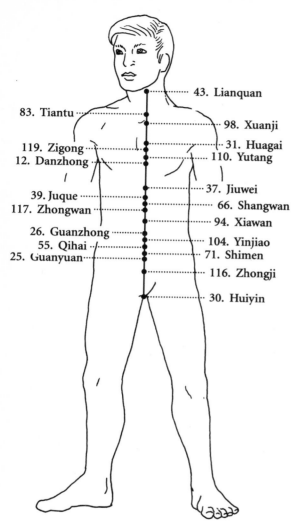

43. Lianquan
83. Tiantu
98. Xuanji
119. Zigong
12. Danzhong
31. Huagai
110. Yutang
39. Juque
117. Zhongwan
37. Jiuwei
66. Shangwan
94. Xiawan
26. Guanzhong
55. Qihai
25. Guanyuan
104. Yinjiao
71. Shimen
116. Zhongji
30. Huiyin

Figure 7-14
Acupoints along the Functioning channel.

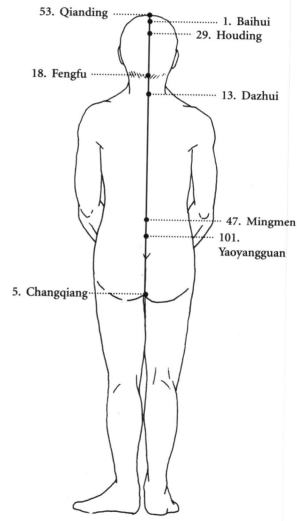

53. Qianding
1. Baihui
29. Houding
18. Fengfu
13. Dazhui
47. Mingmen
101. Yaoyangguan
5. Changqiang

Figure 7-15
Acupoints along the Governing channel.

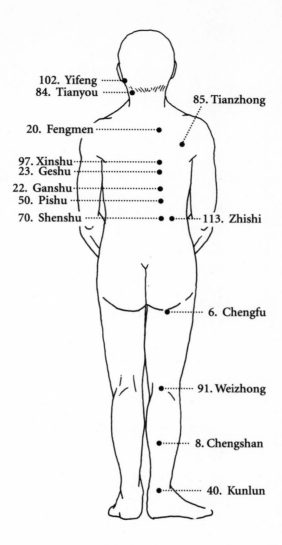

102. Yifeng
84. Tianyou
85. Tianzhong
20. Fengmen
97. Xinshu
23. Geshu
22. Ganshu
50. Pishu
70. Shenshu
113. Zhishi
6. Chengfu
91. Weizhong
8. Chengshan
40. Kunlun

Figure 7-16
*Acupoints along the Bladder Meridian and
Triple Energizer Meridian.*

Glossary

Acupoints: These are points used in acupressure and acupuncture that are located along fourteen meridians, or channels, in the body. These meridians, channels, collaterals and acupoints are closely connected with the functioning of the internal organs and central nervous system. They are believed to be closely associated with the flow of qi energy inside the body, and therefore with our health. By exerting pressure on them (acupressure) or inserting a needle at these points (acupuncture) qi circulation and health is promoted, immunity is enhanced, and diseases healed. Each acupoint delivers different therapeutic effects.

Acupressure: This is considered a variation of massage, and a brother of acupuncture. It involves pressing acupoints on the body with the fingers, knuckles, or palm. Therapeutically, acupressure can promote blood and qi circulation, relieve pain and stress, soothe the muscles, dissipate qi blockage and blood stasis, activate collaterals, and enhance the immune system and the central nervous system. Therefore, it can relieve a number of ailments, including muscle pain, stress, diarrhea, nausea, stroke, hypertension, and even cancers.

Acupuncture: Like acupressure, acupuncture is based on the traditional Chinese medical theory of qi energy, meridians, channels, and collaterals that spread throughout the body, with hundreds of acupoints located along these invisible routes. Acupuncturists insert needles into these to bring about healing effects in exactly the same manner as acupressure.

Amino acids: These are organic acids in which one or more of the hydrogen atoms are replaced by the amino group NH_2. They are the end product of protein hydrolysis and from them the body resynthesizes its own protein.

Biological clock: This is the clock that comes with life and resides in our body. We all have a biological clock that keeps us attuned to a twenty-four-hour cycle. Pathologically, we are all more susceptible to disease symptoms at certain times of the day, and therefore more responsive to medication at such times. For instance, the morning is a high-risk time for those afflicted with heart disease (risk peaks around 9 A.M.); pain in the knees and joints typically worsens toward the end of the day for arthritis patients; the stomach produces 20 percent more acid after dinner and during the night; hay fever tends to be most bothersome in the early morning when the upper airways and nasal cavities are most inflamed; asthma tends to worsen at night, and so on. Physiologically, the biological clock gets the feedback and messages as to what time to do what. Once set at a definite time and kept unchanged, it will facilitate the biological activities and enhance our health. It is highly desirable, therefore, that we stick to a regular schedule of daily activities such as the timing for sleep, meal, and bowel movement. If changed frequently, our biological clock will become confused as to what to do. As a result, our bodily functions will be degraded and our health affected.

Bodhidharma Dharma: Born into the family of an Indian king named Sughanda, Dharma belonged to an Indian warrior caste and grew up in a Buddhist province in southern India, where he received his Buddhist training and was later revered as the 278th reincarnation of Gautama Buddha, the founder of Buddhism. At the invitation of Emperor Liang Wu, Dharma came to China in the fourth century A.D. in the Five Dynasty Period. Legends abound about his supernatural power, as well as his superb mental and physical skills. One of these legends tells how he crossed the turbulent Yellow River into the domain of the Liang realm by standing on a mere reed leaf instead of a boat. He served for a while as a philosophical and medical advisor to the emperor, lecturing the latter on the philosophy of life and Buddhism, and the ways to promote health and longevity. He later settled in the Shong San Mountains in Honan province in central China to set up the now famous Shaolin Temple, the home of Chinese martial arts, and to teach Buddhism philosophy. He spent nine years in the mountains and imprinted the shadow of his entire body on the wall of his cave dwelling upon his leaving. During the course of his stay, he founded a unique school of Buddhism known as Zen Buddhism, which combines meditation with teaching and reading of Buddhist classics. He was concerned that his disciples would get sick by sitting all day long with little exercise, and created a number of exercises for them, both internal and external. He further explored the art of qigong and meditation, and invented Dharma's internal exercises, and the ways to purify the marrow and brain for the sake of attaining immortality. Dharma created a number of physical exercises including yijinjing (methods of strengthening the tendons), Dharma's morning exercises, and martial arts skills to defend oneself against the attack of either humans or animals. Consequently, he is widely recognized as the father of Chinese martial arts.

Chinese medicine: Traditional Chinese medicine is based on the Taoist philosophy of yin-yang correlation and the five element system, plus the vital concept of qi. It recognizes the inseparable link between the mind and body, mental and physical activities, internal emotions and external environment. In diagnosis, it applies a number of techniques such as pulse feeling, sound listening, face reading, looking at the tongue and urine, and so on. In treatment, it uses herbs, foods, acupressure, acupuncture, and other more natural methods. It is generally believed that traditional Chinese medicine is more effective than Western medicine in treating degenerative diseases, but the two can be combined to enhance the therapeutic effects.

Classic of the Plain Girl: This book is the first Chinese classic on bedroom arts and sexual yoga, based on years of detailed and profound discussions between the Yellow Emperor and his sexual advisor and girlfriend, the Plain Girl. The idea is to enhance mutual health and pleasure through regulated sex, in which the harmonious interflow between the female yin and the male yang energy serves to promote mutual health and longevity.

Collaterals: Collaterals are invisible branches of the channels that run to various parts of the body which the regular channels cannot reach. Collaterals include fifteen main channels and many superficial and minute channels, which are connected with the regular channels.

Confucius (551–479 B.C.): The founder of Confucianism, the Chinese ethical and moral system in traditional China, and one of the greatest thinkers and educators in the world. Born into a poor family in Shandong province, he took up the task to educate himself, and became a teacher at the age of twenty. Except for serving three months as premier of the feudal Lu State in his home province, he devoted all the rest of his life to education and writing. As a great educator in feudal society, he boldly declared that education should know no social class. As a philosophical thinker, he advocated a set of ethical codes of behavior. For thousands of years, he has been revered as the greatest sage in China, and his teachings have been essential reading for students and scholars for more than 2,000 years. Chinese veneration and worship for him can be seen from the following praise offered to him by generations of scholars: "If Confucius had not been born, we would still be living in the Dark Age." He is said to have died shortly after he saw a unicorn in the countryside of Shangdong province.

Cun: The unit of measurement used in acupressure and acupuncture. It is roughly equal to the breadth of the thumb.

Dantian: This is a small area located 3 cuns below the navel and between the kidneys. It is the area where a man's seminal chamber and a woman's uterus are located. It is considered the "sea of qi" by Chinese fathers, and is the area of mental concentration during qigong practice.

Daoyin: This is a series of soft exercises designed in ancient China to be used in the palace. It was the first of its kind in human history to deliberately and purposefully exercise the body in order to prevent disease and promote health. Significantly, this series of exercises combines regulated breathing with proper movement of the body to derive the maximum health and therapeutic results. The movements in this method are rather simple, but the system paved the way for more complex and elaborate systems of exercise therapy in China.

Dietary therapy: The branch of Chinese natural health care that employs natural foods and drinks, prepared in special ways with the addition of special seasonings, to relieve and cure medical conditions. The Chinese have a long history of using common foods to promote health and cure diseases, but it was systematically studied and developed into a science of its own by famous doctors such as Sun Simiao, Hu Sicong, and Zhang Zhongjing.

Essence: This is a fundamental substance constituting the body and maintaining the life's activities. It is considered one of the three elements making up the microcosmic trinity of life. The other two elements are qi and spirit.

External elixir: Also known as waidan, external elixir is an important concept in the Chinese natural health care system. There are different definitions regarding this term. According to Dr. Wan Laisheng, it refers to the body, the limbs, and the eyes.

External evils: Alternatively known as "external excesses" in traditional Chinese medicine,

external evils refer to extreme weather types or dramatic changes in weather that often cause diseases. These evils are considered to be external causes of disease.

Feng shui: Technically known as geomancy, feng shui is a unique product of Chinese culture that has a history of three thousand years. Literally meaning the "wind" and the "water," feng shui seeks to design residential, commercial buildings, and tombs in such a way to maximize the harmony among the macrocosm; that is, among heaven, earth, and humans, so that the residents of the building or those working in it will benefit by the natural force of the environment, rather than be punished by the environment. The Chinese understanding is that the environment in which we live has a great impact on our well-being and fortune. Feng shui is an involved, complex subject which draws heavily upon the Taoist theories of yin-yang, the five element system, and eight characters of the birthday.

Five elements: The five elements in Chinese philosophy refer to water, fire, wood, metal, and earth, which are regarded as the most basic materials by which everything in the universe, including human fate, is made. Each element stands for a host of objects, tangible and intangible, in the world. For instance, kidneys correspond to water, heart to fire, liver to wood, lungs to metal, and spleen to earth. There are two basic kinds of relations between the elements: mutual production and mutual destruction. The relationship of mutual creation works as follows: water creates wood, wood creates fire, fire creates earth, earth creates metal, and metal creates water, thus completing the cycle of mutual creation. On the other hand, there is the cycle of mutual destruction among the five elements, which works as follows: water quenches fire, fire melts metal, metal cuts wood, wood looses earth, and earth stops water flow, thus completing the cycle of mutual destruction. The relationships among these five elements embody and signify the growth and development of life and disease, and the five element system is widely used in diagnosis and fortune telling.

Five sound families: Corresponding to the five elements of earth, wood, fire, metal, and water, the ancient Chinese classified different sounds in nature into five major families, i.e., Gong, Shang, Jiao, Zhi, and Yu. Significantly, the Chinese ancients found that these five sounds can not only make beautiful melodies, they also possess the magic power of healing because they are associated with our internal organs in a subtle way.

Five-animal Play: This is a series of exercises in imitation of the movements of five animals: tiger, bird, bear, monkey, and deer. It was invented in the second century by a great Chinese doctor and the father of Chinese anathema named Hua Tuo. Hua's idea was to teach his students and fellow countrymen to regularly exercise their bodies so as to prevent disease and promote health. In introducing this creative series of exercises to the world, Hua Tuo made the following ageless declaration: "Running water never gets stagnant, and the door-hinge never gets worm-eaten. For the same reason, by regularly exercising our body, we can maintain health and keep the disease at bay."

Flowery pond: This is a metaphorical term in Taoist regimen referring to the sublingual part in the mouth. Hence, water of the flowery pond means "saliva," which is considered a precious substance and of great value to health and healing. It is alternatively referred to as jade juice, and the golden liquid. Therefore, Chinese fathers urge us to save this precious liquid as much as possible by two means: first, speak as little as possible and second, accumulate saliva as much and frequently as possible. Once the mouth is full of saliva, one should slowly swallow it down to the lower abdomen in three small mouthfuls, with the aid of the mind.

Functioning channel: Also known as the Ren channel. One of the Eight Extra Channels defined in Chinese acupuncture. Its route starts inside the lower abdomen and ascends from the perineum along the midline of the abdomen, passes the throat and lower jaw, and ends under the eyes.

Gate of Life: In the literature of Taoist regimen, there are two locations in the body called the Gate of Life. One is the right kidney, and the other is dantian, which is found 3 cuns below the navel. These are vital places which serve as the pivot and reservoir of essence and qi energy. Therefore, it is highly recommended that these places be kept warm all the time so as to nourish the essence and qi energy.

Governing channel: One of the Eight Extra Channels defined in Chinese acupuncture, also known as the Du channel. Its main route begins from the perineum going first backward along the inner part of the spinal column, then upward, all the way to the brain. It keeps on ascending, passing the top of head and forehead, then starts to descend along the bridge of the nose to the teeth.

Hu Sicong (1260–1355): A native of Mongolia, Hu was an expert in medical nutrition during the Yuan Dynasty (1279–1638). He held the position of Royal Diet Physician during the reigns of Ghengis Khan and his son, and was responsible for the dietary affairs of the royal family. Based on his thirty years of experience and incorporated material medica, effective prescriptions used by famous physicians, as well as his understanding of the tonifying property of various food, he compiled three volumes of *Principles of Correct Diet* in 1330, making significant contributions to the subject of dietary therapy and natural health care.

Hua Tuo (124–208 A.D.): An outstanding physician and surgeon in Eastern Han Dynasty. Hua Tuo came from Anhui province in central China. He was the most famous doctor and medico-athlete of his day, being proficient in internal medicine, pediatrics, gynecology, acupuncture, surgery, and exercises. According to historical records, he performed abdominal tumor excision and gastroenterectomy under general anesthesia invented by himself and attained good results. He also made significant contributions to the art of acupuncture. For good reasons, he is considered the father of acupuncture and anesthesia. He emphasized the supreme importance of preventing disease in the first place, and for this purpose he invented Five-animal Play. He also wrote many books on medicine.

Huang-jing-bu-nao: A technique used in qigong practice, especially in regulated sex, that refines essence into spirit through a set procedure. It is believed that if one can transform essence into spirit, one will greatly enhance his health and feel invigorated and full of spirit.

I-Ching: One of the oldest and most significant classics in China. It is regarded as the source of traditional Chinese culture. It explains in detail the theory and implications of yin and yang, the trigrams, as well as the origin of the universe and how man is related to the universe. Its original purpose was to be a tool in divination, but the theories contained in it are so profound and universal that Chinese in later generations have used the book for a number of applications including medicine, geomancy, military strategy, politics, science, astronomy, and business administration.

Immortality: This refers to the life after physical death. The ancient Chinese hold that immortality can be cultivated, and the process of cultivating immortality is known as *xiutao*, which is achieved through the long, persistent practice of qigong, so that human essence, qi energy, and spirit can be refined to an immortal state or nirvana. Once attained, immortality allows one to live up to several hundred years, assuming various life forms.

Internal elixir: Known as *neidan* in Taoist literature, internal elixir refers to the trinity of life, i.e., essence, qi, and spirit, as contrasted with the more tangible and visible external elixir of body, limbs, and eyes.

Lao Tze: Founder of Taoism and the author of *Tao Te Ching* who lived in the sixth century B.C. His real name is Li Er. Since he was born a white-haired, old-looking child, people called him Lao Tze, which literally means "the Old Boy." He was the teacher of Confucius, and advocated simplicity, naturalness, and spontaneity in all the essentials of life.

Macrocosmic trinity: In traditional Chinese philosophy, this refers to the trinity of heaven, man, and earth. The Chinese ancients do not regard humans as an isolated entity, but think of human beings as closely related to their environment. Therefore, for human beings to be healthy, we should act in accordance with the laws of nature and cooperate with, rather than exploit, the environment in which we live.

Magpie bridge: This is a metaphorical term for the tongue. In qigong practice, it is advisable to put the tongue slightly against the upper hard palate in order to complete the Minor Heavenly Cycle. This serves as a link that bridges the Functioning channel and Governing channel that would otherwise be disconnected. Hence the name of the bridge. Magpie bridge is a literary allusion in China. It comes from a fairy tale which says that a loving couple in heaven are forced by the Heavenly Mother to separate as a punishment for their violation of rules. They are thus allowed to meet only once a year, which happens on the night of the seventh day of the seventh month in the lunar calendar. Even then, they are not able to embrace each other since there is the Milky Way separating them. On such occasions, a huge group of magpies—the harbingers of love—always come to the couple's aid by laying themselves down across the Milky Way so that the couple can walk over these magpies to eventually embrace each other.

Major Heavenly Cycle: This is an invisible route through which qi energy travels in the body. Basically, the route runs the whole distance of the Minor Heavenly Cycle, plus two legs. The Major Heavenly Cycle starts from both soles and ascends upwards along the legs

as one inhales. As one inhales, it continues to ascend to the acupoint of Huiyin located near the anus, and then climbs up along the Governing channel all the way to the acupoint of Baihui located at the very top of the head until it finally reaches the nose bridge. This movement coincides with the action of inhalation. Then as one exhales, the major heavenly cycle starts to descend from the nose bridge along the Functioning channel down to dantian and Huiyin. From there it separates into two branches and continues its downward travel along the two legs until it finally returns to the soles, thus completing a full cycle as one completes a round of respiration. Opening the Major Heavenly Cycle is considered a must for the cultivation of immortality. From the standpoint of health, it is believed that if one can guide the qi energy to flow around such a cycle, one's health will be significantly improved, and many kinds of disease will be cured.

Meditation: It is a technique for attaining a state of physical relaxation and mental peace by regular practice of a relaxation procedure. Although there are different forms of meditation, all share the basic requirements of sitting or resting quietly, with eyes closed or semi-closed, and performing mental exercises designed to focus concentration. In traditional Chinese culture, meditation is a vital part of qigong, the Chinese breathing exercise. The ancient Chinese saw meditation as the way to purify the mind, keep the spirit in the body, promote qi buildup and conservation, guard the essence from loss, combat diseases, and create a bond between man and nature. Meditation often results in peace, if not void of mind, minimization of desires, and an optimal balance between yin and yang of life. Such a mental and physical state contributes greatly to the enhancement of the immune system.

Mencius: The second greatest Confucian scholar and philosopher, who lived in the time period known as Warring States in China's history. Mencius was a great thinker with a strong democratic orientation. He unambiguously declared to the world: "People are more important than emperors." He also drew an interesting and significant conclusion regarding human nature: "Food and sex are just human nature, wherein lie the greatest desires of mankind."

Meridians: These are invisible biological channels spreading out like a complex network of nerves in the body, carrying qi energy to various parts of the body. The ancient Chinese believed that there are fourteen bodily meridians in each person. Twelve of these are symmetrical or bilateral; that is, they have identical versions on both sides of the body. Only two of them are unilateral or asymmetrical, running along the midline of the body. These two unilateral meridians are named Functioning (or Ren) and Governing (or Du) meridians, or channels. The twelve bilateral meridians are bladder, gallbladder, heart, kidneys, large intestine, small intestine, spleen, stomach, lungs, liver, pericardium, and triple warmer. Hundreds of acupoints are aligned along these meridians, and the bodily functions of an organ are affected when acupoints along a specific meridian are stimulated, either by a needle, or by means of naked fingers.

Microcosmic trinity: A term referring to the unity of body, mind, and soul; the three treasures of life.

Minor Heavenly Cycle: This is a qi flowing route located in the upper part of the human body. Starting from the acupoint of Huiyin located near the anus between the two legs, the Minor Heavenly Cycle ascends along the Governing channel in the midline of the back all the way to the acupoint of Baihui at the very top of the head. From there it descends to the bridge of the nose as one reaches the limit of inhalation. Then it begins its downward trip as one starts to exhale descending from the nose to the lower jaw and throat, all the way down along the Functioning channel in front of the body, through dantian until it eventually returns to the acupoint of Huiyin where the route started, completing a full cycle in the upper part of the body in coincidence with a full round of respiration. The Minor Heavenly Cycle is a preparation and prerequisite for the Major Heavenly Cycle.

Physiognomy: This is the ancient Chinese art of face reading. Invented by a Taoist immortal named Gui Gu Tze, physiognomy is a highly involved subject that classifies facial organs and bodily features into dozens of classes, each of which possess some specific features and properties. By means of such understanding, an experienced face reader can tell the personality and fortune of people by just looking at them.

Principle of the mean: This is an important principle in Confucian philosophy. It states that excess is as bad as deficiency in almost everything, as too much can be as bad as too little. This is true for all kinds of human affairs and endeavor. Therefore, we should follow, in everything we do, the mean which lies somewhere between the extremes of too much and too little.

Qi: Qi is an encompassing concept in Chinese medicine, philosophy and indeed, the entire traditional Chinese culture. The operation of the human body as well as the universe depends on this vital qi. Disturbance, disharmony, and deficiency of qi will cause disease and natural calamities. Broadly, qi can be defined as the life energy on which depends life itself and the universe. In Chinese medicine, qi in the human body can be classified into various kinds, such as prenatal, postnatal, primordial, organic, or defensive. The stronger the qi one possesses, the stronger will be one's immunity, and the healthier one will be. As such, the conservation, promotion, and circulation of qi became one of the central themes in traditional Chinese natural health care and medicine, as well in Chinese philosophy. In terms of the universe, qi very much determines the brightness of the celestial objects such as the sun and stars, and the weather type. Therefore, it is the link between man and nature.

Qi Bo: A famous doctor and high ranking magistrate of the Yellow Emperor in charge of the national and royal affairs on astrology, astronomy, and medicine. He was the tutor to the Yellow Emperor, and was revered as the "Emperor's teacher." He was profoundly studied in herbology, acupuncture, regimen, astrology, and astronomy. His name repeatedly appears in *The Yellow Emperor's Classic of Internal Medicine*. He is regarded as the father of Chinese medicine. The combined name of Qi Bo and the Yellow Emperor has been a synonym of traditional Chinese medicine.

Qigong: This is a unique breathing exercise invented by the Chinese ancients and widely practiced in China for centuries. It emphasizes regulating physical posture, mental state, and respiration while exercising. In terms of posture, there are sitting, lying, and standing postures. The mental state during qigong exercise should be one of meditation. The mind should be completely focused on the exercise itself, with no distractions allowed, and the breathing should be deep, slow, and smooth, letting the mind guide the qi energy to flow along set routes in the body, clearing the meridian passages.

Qu-yin-bu-yang: An important belief in regulated sex that if the male partner can avoid ejaculation during intercourse, he will benefit greatly from the essence and qi of the female partner, thus promoting health, preventing disease, and delaying the aging process.

Regulated sex: The guiding principle of ancient Chinese bedroom arts. It is an integral component of Chinese natural health. Regulated sex advocates frequent intercourse but very infrequent ejaculation. The Chinese ancients believed that this can promote health and bring about rejuvenation.

Reincarnation: A central belief of Buddhism and Taoism that on death our soul is separated from our body, and is afterwards implanted into a new body of the same or different species. This process goes over and over again, mainly to serve nature's purpose of punishment or reward for one's behavior in the prior life. To jump out of this cycle of reincarnation, one has to cultivate Tao, or perform many good deeds for several generations.

Ruo-cun-ruo-wang: An ideal state of breathing in qigong practice. Literally, it means that a practitioner of qigong enters into a state in which his or her breathing seems to be somewhere between existence and nonexistence. This is known as "tortoise breathing" in Chinese natural health care.

Seven emotions: According to the ancient Chinese, there are both internal and external factors of diseases. The external causes include change in the weather, air and water pollution, contamination of disease elements (the equivalent of bacteria), as well as friction and hurt. The internal factors of disease are mainly the excess of the seven emotions: joy, anger, worry, pensiveness, grief, fear, and fright. Joy affects the heart, which is considered to be the home of the spirit. Excessive joy causes over-excitement and damages the heart. This may result in insomnia, irritability, shortness of breath, and hypertension. Likewise, excess anger damages the liver, the factory of blood. Consequently, blood circulation will become blocked, and qi energy dampened. In a worst case scenario, the person can collapse and die at the outburst of anger. Excess worry will hurt the spleen, which regulates the process of digestion, absorption, and distribution of postnatal qi. Excessive pensiveness affects the stomach, resulting in indigestion, jaded appetite, constipation, diarrhea, ulcers, and other stomach ailments. Excess grief affects the lungs, and may cause lung disease, coughing, shortness of breath, blocking of qi, and therefore the pathological changes in cells. Excessive fear damages the kidneys, leading to kidney qi deficiency and resulting in incontinence, bed-wetting, nocturnal emission, and other diseases. Excessive fright will affect the heart and bladder, causing qi flow to stop in an extreme case.

Spirit: Spirit is one member of the microcosmic trinity of life, the other two being essence and qi. Spirit is materially based on the congenital healthy energy of viscera, and is the ultimate determinant of life and death, man and superman.

Sui-huo-ji-ji: This is an important concept in the art of qigong and xiutao, the search for immortality. Literally water and fire working in harmony, it is used to refer to the communion between the kidneys and heart. This is because the heart stands for fire and the kidneys stand for water. The kidney is the house of essence, while the heart is the house of spirit. So the whole idea is to refine essence into spirit so as to achieve optimal health and possibly immortality.

Sun Simiao (581–682): As the greatest doctor of the Tang Dynasty in China, Sun Simiao was profoundly studied in Chinese medical theories, Taoism, and Buddhism. His early affliction with rheumatism caused him to devote himself to the study of medicine. He refused to work as an official even at the repeated invitation of emperor Taizhong of Tang, and lived with the common people to study medicine, treat patients, and write books. He made no distinction between the rich and poor among his patients, but treated them all to the best of his ability. He systematically summarized the rich experience of medical development passed down by his predecessors. In particular, he crystallized methods of dietary therapy popular among the people, such as dietary methods to prevent and treat goiter with animal thyroid glands, to treat nyctalopia with animal livers, and to perform urethral catheterization with leaves of green onion for patients with diuresis. He paid special attention to the science of regimen and prevention of disease, elaborating it into a well-founded subject. Included in this subject are regular exercise, proper diet, and the practice of regulated sex. Based on his eighty years of rich clinical experience, he wrote two great medical classics: *Priceless Prescriptions* and *Supplement to Priceless Prescriptions,* each containing thirty volumes. In addition, he wrote *The True Records of Regimen, Secrets of Bedroom Arts,* and *Essentials of Longevity.* He made great contributions to the theory and practice of Chinese medicine and natural health care, and is justifiably referred to by the Chinese people as the "King of Medicine" and "Sun the Superman."

Taich'i: A form of Chinese martial arts combining meditation and slow, delicate, flowing physical movements. For this reason, taich'i is sometimes called "meditation in motion." It was originally designed for the dual purposes of self-defense and health promotion. As mankind entered the age of hot weaponry, taich'i gradually lost its luster as a means of self-defense. However, its value in promoting health and curing diseases has become greatly enhanced as many more people die of degenerative diseases each year than in the battlefield. This is because taich'i exercise can positively affect the flow of qi energy and bring about physical self-awareness. Clinical experiments in China and many other countries have shown that taich'i is effective in relieving a wide array of medical conditions, chronic and degenerative diseases in particular. There are three major schools of taich'i in existence.

They are: Zhang style, Yang style, and Chen style. As well, there are many minor variations of taich'i based on these three major styles.

Tao Te Ching: This is the bible of Taoism written by Lao Tze, the founder of Taoism, in the sixth century B.C. The book contains about 5,000 Chinese characters, and is full of profound, philosophical insights about the origin of the universe and the rules of human society. The major themes of the book is that Tao is the source and ultimate principle of everything in the universe, including human beings; that nature is our teacher, and we should live peacefully in accordance with the laws of nature, if we want peace in the world and good health for ourselves. According to Lao Tze, tragedies in life and human society are largely resulted from man's attempt to outsmart nature.

Tao: The essence of Taoism. According to the teaching of Lao Tze and Chuang Tze, Tao, or the Way of Nature, is the source and supreme, ultimate principle of the whole universe of which humankind is a part.

Taoism: A school of thought and a philosophy created by Lao Tze, which advocates simplicity of life and obedience to the laws of nature.

Three treasures of life: Refers to essence, energy, and spirit.

Waidan: See "External Elixir."

Waiqi: The qi energy that flows out of the body deliberately for the sake of diagnosis, detection, healing, and self-defense. The commonly used points of outflow of qi energy are acupoint Laogongxue in the middle of the palms, and the midpoint between the eyebrows, eyes, and fingers.

Wo-gu-bu-xie: A guiding principle of Chinese regulated sex. Literally, it means holding on to one's semen and not ejaculating during sexual intercourse. The ancient Chinese believed that this was the way to a healthy, long life.

Wu-chu-wu-wang: A guiding principle of qigong which requires that one do not use force to push qi to flow inside the body, nor should one forget about the circulation of qi during qigong exercise. Only thus can one promote the qi energy without incurring negative side effects.

Xiutao: The process of cultivating immortality. Xiutao is a determined attempt on the part of the Chinese to transcend reincarnation forever and become immortal. The process involves four interrelated steps: refining diet into essence; refining essence into qi energy; refining qi into primordial spirit; and merging primordial spirit into nature. When one's primordial spirit becomes strong enough and is merged into nature, one is said to have attained immortality. One's soul can be separated from one's physical body, assume various life forms, and live anywhere from 500 years to eternity, depending on one's level of achievement.

Yellow Emperor's Classics of Internal Medicine: This Chinese classic is the first synthesis of medical treatments. It is based on the Taoist principles and methods jointly discovered by the Yellow Emperor and his medical advisors. The theme of this classic is preventing and treating disease, promoting health and longevity, and searching for immortality.

Yellow Emperor: The Yellow Emperor was the first recorded ruler in ancient China. He reigned a loosely combined empire in the now northern part of China along the Yellow River valley around 2600 B.C. He is considered the father of Chinese civilization and a highly wise sage who ruled China according to the laws of nature. For this reason, he is also regarded as the father of Taoism in China. His name is often associated with Lao Tze to stand for the philosophy of Taoism. Besides he made great contributions to the art of natural health care, Chinese medicine, and Chinese civilization. His name, together with that of his medical advisor, Qi Bo, has long been the synonym of Chinese medicine. He is said to have lived to an agile age of 111 and attained immortality upon his death.

Yin and yang: Yin-yang dichotomy is one of the philosophical bases of traditional Chinese culture. This pair of polarities stands for almost everything and every phenomenon in the universe. Broadly speaking, yin is the principle realized on earth, while yang is the principle realized in heaven. Individually, both polarities command a bizarre constellation of objects, properties, and phenomena. Thus, yin stands for the earth, the female, the moon, the night, benevolence, darkness, softness, water, etc. On the contrary, yang represents the heaven, the male, the sun, the day, righteousness, brightness, hardness, fire, etc. It is in the combination, interrelation, and interdependence that everything in the universe has, and will, come into being.

Zhang Shanfeng: A Taoist immortal living in the late Yuan Dynasty and early Ming Dynasty. Zhang was a native of Manchuria. He traveled widely around China, treating patients and visiting famous mountains. He could stay alive without any food for several months, and came back to life himself after death in the Jintai Mountains. Several emperors in the early Ming Dynasty sent many people out to find him, but all to no avail. Nonetheless, the Ming emperors granted him the title of "Superman Who knows the Future" and "Genuine Immortal With Lofty Ideas Who Hides His Capacities." Zhang is also acclaimed as the father of taich'i, or shadow boxing. He wrote *Superman Zhang Shangfeng's Magic Prescriptions*.

Zhang Zhongjing: The greatest doctor of the Eastern Han Dynasty in China, Zhang is considered a "Sage of Medicine," and his classical *Synopsis of Prescriptions in Golden Chamber* is reputed to be the "origins of all medical prescriptions." He was the father of enema, and an expert in acupuncture and acupressure. His influence by way of his classics *On Febrile Dis-* *eases* and *Synopsis of Prescriptions in Golden Chamber*. His influence on Chinese medicine is far reaching and enduring.

Zhuang Tze: Living in the fourth century B.C., Zhuang Tze is the greatest of Taoist writers, and the greatest inheritor of the thoughts of Lao Tze. Actually, another name for Taoism in China is "the study of Lao (Tze) and Zhuang (Tze)." His writings as collected in *Zhuang Tze* are full of humor, philosophical insight, and literary genius. His influence on all Chinese schools of thought is profound. His subtle, mystical reasoning has left a permanent mark on Chinese culture as a whole. In his book, there is a great deal of teaching about simplicity, humility, and childish naiveté. For Zhuang Tze, to lose one's life is to save it, and to seek to save it for one's petty, selfish sake is to lose it.

Bibliography

Aldred, Heather E. *Women's Health Concern Sourcebook*. Detroit, MI: Omnigraphics, Inc., 1997.

Alman, W. "Preventing or at Least Postponing Brain Drain. How to Decrease the Effects of Aging on Mental Ability." *Forbes*, 1995.

Beers, M. *Aging in Good Health*. New York, NY: Simon & Schuster, 1992.

Berger, S. *Forever Young*. New York, NY: William Morrow, 1989.

Blate, Michael. *The Natural Healer's Acupressure Handbook*. Pembroke Pines, FL: Falkynor Books, 1976.

Blofeld, John. *Gateway to Wisdom*. Boulder: Shambhala, 1980.

———. *Taoism: The Road to Immortality*. Boulder, CO: Shambhala, 1978.

———. *Taoist Mystery and Magic*. Boulder, CO: Shambhala, 1982.

Bragg, Paul. *The Miracle of Fasting*. Santa Barbara, CA: Health Science, 1985.

Braverman, E. R. *The Healing Nutrients Within: Facts, Findings and New Research on Amino Acids.* New Canaan, CT: Keats Publishing, 1987.

Brosche, T. "Garlic as Phytogenic Antilipemic Agent. Recent Studies with a Standardized Dry Garlic Powder Substance." *Fortschritte Der Medizin* 108, no. 36 (Dec. 20, 1990): 703–6.

Chang, Jolan. *The Tao of Love and Sex.* New York, NY: Dutton, 1983.

Cook, Allen R. *Men's Health Concerns Sourcebook.* Detroit, MI: Omnigraphics, Inc., 1998.

———. *Environmentally Induced Disorders Sourcebook.* Detroit, MI: Omnigraphics, Inc., 1997.

———. *The New Cancer Sourcebook.* Detroit, MI: Omnigraphics, Inc., 1996.

Edstrom, Krs. *Healthy, Wealthy and Wise: A Step-by-Step Plan for Success Through Healthful Living.* Englewood, NJ: Prentice Hall, 1988.

Frahm, David and Anne Frahm. *Reclaim Your Health.* Colorado Springs, CO: Pinon Press, 1995.

Fujiki, H. "Anticarcinogenic Activity of Green Tea Polyphenols." *Preventive Medicine* (1992).

Green, E. and Green A. *Beyond Biofeedback.* New York: Delacorte, 1977.

Gulik, R. H. *Sexual Life in Ancient China.* Leiden: E. J. Brill, 1974.

Harris, Dan R. *Fitness and Exercise Sourcebook.* Detroit, MI: Omnigraphics, Inc., 1996.

Heart and Stroke Facts: 1996 Statistical Supplement. American Heart Association, 1996.

Holmes, T. H. and M. Masuda. "Life Change and Illness Susceptibility." Paper presented as part of Symposium on Separation and Depression: Clinical and Research Aspects, Chicago, December 1970.

Hu, Shichong. *Essentials of Healthy Diets.* Shanghai, China: The Commercial Press, 1948.

Hu, Haitian et al. *Dietary Therapy.* Canton, China: Science and Technology Press, 1985.

Ishihara, Akira and Howard Levy. *The Tao of Sex.* Japan: Shibundo, 1968.

Jiang, Linzhu. *Common Menus of Dietary Therapy.* Hong Kong: Honye Book Company, 1968.

Kinoshita, Haruto. *Illustration of Acupuncture Point.* Tokyo, Japan: Ido No Nippon Sha, 1995.

Klein, Donald F. *Understanding Depression: A Complete Guide to its Diagnosis and Treatment.* New York, NY: Oxford University Press, 1993.

Lao Tze. *Tao Te Ching.* Guiyang: Classical Chinese Publisher, 1965.

Leiblum, S. R. "High Incidence of Coexisting Sexual Dysfunction and Psychopathology." *Primary Psychiatry* (1996).

Lin, Yutang. *The Wisdom of China.* New York, NY: Modern Library, 1963.

Liu, Da. *The Tao of Health and Longevity.* London: Routledge and Kegan Paul, 1979.

Lopez, D. A. *Enzymes: The Fountain of Life.* Charleston, SC: Neville Press, 1994.

Lu, Henry C. *Chinese System of Food Cures.* Selangor Darul Ehsan, Malaysia: Pelanduk Publications, 1989.

Mary Kane et al. *Sound Decisions.* Boston, MA: Mosby Consumer Health, 1995.

McLaughlin, J. H. et al. "Study Finds Green Tea May Protect Against Esophageal Cancer." *Cancer Facts.* Washington, D.C.: National Institutes of Cancer, 1994.

Moyers, Bill. *Healing and the Mind.* New York, NY: Doubleday Books, 1993.

Mukhtar, H. "Cancer Chemoprevention by Green Tea Compounds." *Diet and Cancer.* London, England: Plemum Press, 1994.

Murray, M. T. "PCO sources: Grape Seed vs. Pine Bark." *American Journal of Natural Medicine* (1995).

National Center for Health Statistics. *Advance Report of Final Natality Statistics,* 1991.

Ohno, Y. "Tea Consumption and Lung Cancer Risk: A Case-control Study in Okinawa, Japan." *Japanese Journal of Cancer Research* (1995).

Pace-Asciak, C. R. et al. "The Red Wine Phenolics Trans-resveratrol and Quercetin Block Human Platelet Aggregation and Eicosanoid Synthesis: Implications for Protection Against Coronary Heart Disease." *Clinica Chimica Acta* (1995).

Palos, Stephan. *The Chinese Art of Healing.* New York, NY: MaGraw Hill, 1971.

Pendergrass, E. "Host Resistance and Other Intangibles in the Treatment of Cancer." *American Journal of Roentgenology* (1961).

Rake, Susan. *The Hormone of Desire.* New York, NY: Harmony Books, 1996.

Roman, Mark. "The Good Sex Workout." *Men's Health,* September 1994.

Rosenthal, Saul. *Sex Over 40.* Los Angeles, CA: Jermy P. Tarcher, Inc., 1987.

Shen, Lirong. *A Collection of Foods and Herbs.* Wuhan, China: Jinchan Book Publisher, 1902.

Shimkin, Michael B. *Science and Cancer.* National Institute of Health, 1980.

Soo, Chee. *The Taoist Ways of Healing.* Wellingborough, Northants: The Aquarian Press, 1986.

Stensvold, I. "Tea Consumption. Relationship to Cholesterol, Blood Pressure, and Coronary and Total Mortality." *Preventive Medicine* (1992).

Tilden, J. H. *Food: Its Influences as a Factor in Disease and Health.* New Canaan: Keats Publishing, 1976.

U.S. Department of Health and Human Services. *The Health Benefits of Smoking Cessation: A Report of the Surgeon General.* DHHS/CDC, Washington, D.C., 1990.

U.S. Department of Health, Education, and Welfare. *The Health Consequence of Smoking.* DHEW/HSM, Washington, D.C., 1973.

Veith, Ilza. *The Yellow Emperor's Classic of Internal Medicine.* Berkeley, CA: University of California Press, 1966.

Wan, Laisheng. *A Summary of Chinese Martial Arts.* Shanghai, China: The Commercial Press, 1928.

Wang, Yin. *Special Diagnosis with Qigong.* Beijing, China: China Medical Science and Technology Press, 1993.

Wilcox, Wendy. *Public Health Sourcebook*. Detroit, MI: Omnigraphics, Inc., 1998.

Wilhelm, Richard (translator). *The Secret of the Golden Flower: A Chinese Book of Life.* New York: Harvest Books, 1970.

Wilhelm, Richard and Cary Baynes. *The I Ching, or Book of Changes*. Princeton, NJ: Princeton University Press, 1966.

Williams, David. *Secrets of Life Extension: 10 Simple All-Natural Steps to Achieving Your Maximum Lifespan*. Ingram, Texas: Mountain Home Publishing.

Williams, Redford. *Anger Kills: Seventeen Strategies for Controlling the Hostility that Can Harm Your Health*. New York, NY: Times Books, 1993.

Yu, C.P. et al. "Green Tea Consumption and Risk of Stomach Cancer. A Population-based Case Control Study in Shanghai, China." *Cancer Causes and Control* (1995).

Yu, Yunrui. *Massage Therapy*. Hong Kong: The Commercial Press, 1963.

Zhao, K. S. et al. "Enhancement of the Immune Response in Mice by *Astragalus membranaceus* Extracts." *Immunopharmacology* (1990).

Zheng, Dakun. *Highly Nourishing Foods Lightly Taken*. Jilin, China: Science and Technology Press, 1989.

Index

Acne, 94, 204–205

Acupoint (*see also individual acupoint names*), 2, 171, 181, 190–192, 208, 213, 216–217, 221, 226, 231, 236, 240, 243, 246, 249, 253, 257, 259, 261–262, 264–265, 274–276, 283, 286–287, 289, 293, 300, 302, 305–306, 310–312, 318, 321, 324–325, 327–328, 331, 333, 337, 339, 341, 346, 354, 356, 358, 363, 366, 368, 371, 373, 375, 394–395, 397, 409, 412, 458–481

Acupressure, 4, 262, 368, 385, 395, 457–481

Acupuncture, 4, 318, 322, 385, 394, 458–459, 461–462

AIDS, 4, 11, 29, 38, 140, 143, 148, 150, 205–208, 231, 255, 267, 295, 337, 389, 395, 468

Alcohol, 9–10, 55–58, 64, 72, 120, 149–150, 158, 204, 208–209, 211–212, 214, 216, 223, 226, 232, 234, 250–251, 254–255, 258, 265, 267, 271, 273, 275–276, 280, 283–284, 290–291, 295–296, 307, 313, 315–316, 319, 322, 327, 329, 332–333, 335, 337, 339, 342–345, 347, 352, 357, 361, 369–370, 372, 404

Alcoholism, 58, 94, 208

Allergies, x, 4, 83, 116, 134, 204, 209–210, 218, 258, 260, 288, 332, 357, 375–376

☾ REACH FOR THE MOON

Llewellyn publishes hundreds of books on your favorite subjects! To get these exciting books, including the ones on the following pages, check your local bookstore or order them directly from Llewellyn.

ORDER BY PHONE

- Call toll-free within the U.S. and Canada, 1-800-THE MOON
- In Minnesota, call (651) 291-1970
- We accept VISA, MasterCard, and American Express

ORDER BY MAIL

- Send the full price of your order (MN residents add 7% sales tax) in U.S. funds, plus postage & handling to:

    Llewellyn Worldwide
    P.O. Box 64383, Dept. K434-0
    St. Paul, MN 55164–0383, U.S.A.

POSTAGE & HANDLING

(For the U.S., Canada, and Mexico)

- $4.00 for orders $15.00 and under
- $5.00 for orders over $15.00
- No charge for orders over $100.00

We ship UPS in the continental United States. We ship standard mail to P.O. boxes. Orders shipped to Alaska, Hawaii, The Virgin Islands, and Puerto Rico are sent first-class mail. Orders shipped to Canada and Mexico are sent surface mail.

International orders: Airmail—add freight equal to price of each book to the total price of order, plus $5.00 for each non-book item (audio tapes, etc.).

Surface mail—Add $1.00 per item.

Allow 2 weeks for delivery on all orders.
Postage and handling rates subject to change.

DISCOUNTS

We offer a 20% discount to group leaders or agents. You must order a minimum of 5 copies of the same book to get our special quantity price.

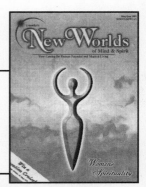

FREE CATALOG

Get a free copy of our color catalog, *New Worlds of Mind and Spirit*. Subscribe for just $10.00 in the United States and Canada ($30.00 overseas, airmail). Many bookstores carry *New Worlds*—ask for it!

Visit our web site at www.llewellyn.com for more information.

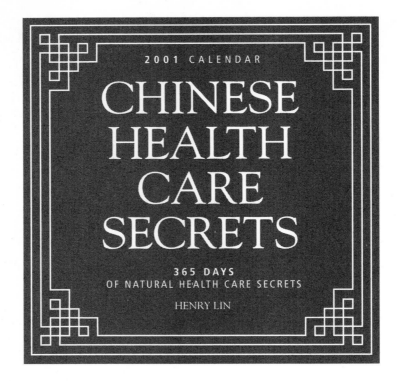

2001 CALENDAR

CHINESE HEALTH CARE SECRETS

365 DAYS
OF NATURAL HEALTH CARE SECRETS

HENRY LIN

CHINESE HEALTH CARE SECRETS

2001 DAY-TO-DAY CALENDAR

Chinese natural health care methods, which focus on the causes of diseases, rather than suppressing the symptoms, have been used for centuries. To help you learn these secret methods of natural health, this calendar brings daily advice from Chinese natural health care expert Henry Lin. You will find simple, natural treatments for a range of problems, and there is also sensible advice on all aspects of daily life to help you take good care of your own health for year-round wellbeing.

The Ink Group USA
PO Box 5517
Novato CA 94948-5517, USA
Telephone: +1 415 883 6797
Facsimile: +1 415 883 6798

blackink@inkgroup.com
Offices in Australia, New Zealand, USA and UK

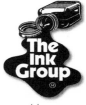

www.inkgroup.com